Gastrointestinal Bleeding

Editor

PATRICK PFAU

GASTROINTESTINAL ENDOSCOPY
CLINICS OF NORTH AMERICA

www.giendo.theclinics.com

Consulting Editor
ASHLEY L. FAULX

April 2024 • Volume 34 • Number 2

ELSEVIER

1600 John F. Kennedy Boulevard ● Suite 1800 ● Philadelphia, Pennsylvania, 19103-2899

http://www.theclinics.com

GASTROINTESTINAL ENDOSCOPY CLINICS OF NORTH AMERICA Volume 34, Number 2
April 2024 ISSN 1052-5157, ISBN-13: 978-0-443-13047-2

Editor: Kerry Holland
Developmental Editor: Malvika Shah

Gastrointestinal Endoscopy Clinics of North America (ISSN 1052-5157) is published quarterly by Elsevier Inc., 360 Park Avenue South, New York, NY 10010-1710. Months of issue are January, April, July, and October. Business and Editorial Offices: 1600 John F. Kennedy Blvd., Suite 1800, Philadelphia, PA, 19103-2899. Periodicals postage paid at New York, NY and additional mailing offices. Subscription prices are $392.00 per year for US individuals, $100.00 per year for US and Canadian students/residents, $432.00 per year for Canadian individuals, $516.00 per year for international individuals, and $245.00 per year for international students/residents. For institutional access pricing please contact Customer Service via the contact information below. To receive student/resident rate, orders must be accompanied by name of affiliated institution, date of term, and the *signature* of program/residency coordinator on institution letterhead. Orders will be billed at individual rate until proof of status is received. Foreign air speed delivery is included in all *Clinics* subscription prices. All prices are subject to change without notice. **POSTMASTER:** Send address change to *Gastrointestinal Endoscopy Clinics of North America*, Elsevier Health Sciences Division, Subscription Customer Service, 3251 Riverport Lane, Maryland Heights, MO 63043. **Customer Service: 1-800-654-2452 (US). From outside the United States, call 1-314-447-8871. Fax: 1-314-447-8029. E-mail: JournalsCustomerService-usa@elsevier.com (for print support) or JournalsOnlineSupport-usa@elsevier.com (for online support).**

Reprints. For copies of 100 or more, of articles in this publication, please contact the Commercial Reprints Department, Elsevier Inc., 360 Park Avenue South, New York, NY 10010-1710. Tel. 212-633-3874; Fax: 212-633-3820; E-mail: reprints@elsevier.com.

Gastrointestinal Endoscopy Clinics of North America is covered in *Excerpta Medica, MEDLINE/PubMed (Index Medicus), and MEDLINE/MEDLARS.*

Contributors

CONSULTING EDITOR

ASHLEY L. FAULX, MD, MASGE, FACG
Professor of Medicine, Case Western Reserve University School of Medicine, University Hospitals Cleveland Medical Center, Louis Stokes Veterans Affairs Medical Center, Cleveland, Ohio

EDITOR

PATRICK PFAU, MD
Chief of Clinical Gastroenterology, Head of Pancreato-biliary Endoscopy, Advanced Endoscopy Fellowship Director, Section of Gastroenterology and Hepatology, Department of Medicine, University of Wisconsin School of Medicine and Public Health, Madison, Wisconsin

AUTHORS

NEENA S. ABRAHAM, MD, MSCE, MACG, FASGE, AGAF
Professor of Medicine, Division of Gastroenterology and Hepatology, Mayo Clinic, Scottsdale, Arizona

ALI A. ALALI, MB, BCh, BAO, MSc (Clinical Epidemiology)
Assistant Professor, Division of Gastroenterology, Department of Medicine, Kuwait University, Jabriyah, Kuwait

KATHERINE BAKKE, MD, MPH
Assistant Professor, Acute Care and Regional General Surgery, University of Wisconsin School of Medicine and Public Health, Clinical Science Center, Madison, Wisconsin

ALAN N. BARKUN, MD, CM, MSc (Clinical Epidemiology)
Professor, Department of Medicine, Division of Gastroenterology and Hepatology, Associate Department of Clinical Epidemiology and Biostatistics, Director of Endoscopy, Division of Gastroenterology, McGill University Montréal, Quebec, Canada

SOFI DAMJANOVSKA, MD
Fellow, Department of Medicine, University Hospitals Cleveland Medical Center, Case Western Reserve University, Cleveland, Ohio

AMANY ELSHAER, MBBS
Internal Medicine Resident, Department of Internal Medicine, Mayo Clinic, Scottsdale, Arizona

MARK A. GROMSKI, MD
Assistant Professor, Department of Medicine, Division of Gastroenterology and Hepatology, Indiana University School of Medicine, Indianapolis, Indiana

ADITYA GUTTA, MD
Director of Advanced Endoscopy, Department of Medicine, Division of Gastroenterology and Hepatology, Indiana University School of Medicine, Indianapolis, Indiana

ZACHARY HENRY, MD, MSc
Associate Professor, Division of Gastroenterology and Hepatology, University of Virginia School of Medicine, Charlottesville, Virginia

GERARD ISENBERG, MD, MBA
Chief Medical Quality Officer, University Hospitals Digestive Health Institute, Associate Chief and Director of Clinical Operations, Division of Gastroenterology and Liver Disease, University Hospitals Cleveland Medical Center, UH Master Clinician, Professor of Medicine, Case Western Reserve University, Cleveland, Ohio

DENNIS M. JENSEN, MD
Professor of Medicine, David Geffen School of Medicine at UCLA, Staff Physician, UCLA Medical Center, VA Greater Los Angeles Healthcare System, Los Angeles, California

KENDRA JOBE, MD
Resident, Department of Medicine, University of Virginia School of Medicine, Charlottesville, Virginia

ALI KHALIFA, MD
Internist, Digestive Disease Research Center, Medical University of South Carolina, Charleston, South Carolina

MARK KLEEDEHN, MD
Associate Professor, Department of Radiology, University of Wisconsin School of Medicine and Public Health, University of Wisconsin Hospitals and Clinics, Madison, Wisconsin

ANDREW S. MA, MD
Fellow, Internal Medicine, Institute for Digestive Health and Liver Disease Mercy Medical Center, Baltimore, Maryland

ECE MERAM, MD
PGY5 Radiology Resident, Department of Radiology, University of Wisconsin School of Medicine and Public Health, University of Wisconsin Hospitals and Clinics, Madison, Wisconsin

ORHAN OZKAN, MD
Professor, Department of Radiology, University of Wisconsin School of Medicine and Public Health, University of Wisconsin Hospitals and Clinics, Madison, Wisconsin

DON C. ROCKEY, MD
Professor, College of Medicine, Department of Medicine, Digestive Disease Research Center, Medical University of South Carolina, Charleston, South Carolina

ELLIOTT RUSSELL, MD
PGY4 Integrated Interventional Radiology Resident, University of Wisconsin School of Medicine and Public Health, University of Wisconsin Hospitals and Clinics, Madison, Wisconsin

JOHN R. SALTZMAN, MD
Professor of Medicine, Harvard Medical School, Division of Gastroenterology, Hepatology and Endoscopy, Brigham and Women's Hospital, Boston, Massachusetts

STEPHANIE SAVAGE, MD, MS
Professor, Acute Care and Regional General Surgery, University of Wisconsin School of Medicine and Public Health, Clinical Science Center, Madison, Wisconsin

TERESA SOLDNER, MD
Surgical Critical Care Fellow, Acute Care and Regional General Surgery, University of Wisconsin School of Medicine and Public Health, Clinical Science Center, Madison, Wisconsin

DANIEL JOSEPH STEIN, MD, MPH
Instructor, Harvard Medical School, Division of Gastroenterology, Hepatology and Endoscopy, Brigham and Women's Hospital, Boston, Massachusetts

DURGA THAKRAL, MD, PhD
Clinical Fellow, Harvard Medical School, Division of Gastroenterology, Hepatology and Endoscopy, Brigham and Women's Hospital, Boston, Massachusetts

PAUL J. THULUVATH, MD, FRCP
Director, The Institute for Digestive Health and Liver Disease, Mercy Medical Center, Clinical Professor, Department of Medicine, University of Maryland School of Medicine, Baltimore, Maryland

NIMISH VAKIL, MD, FASGE, AGAF, FACG
Clinical Adjunct Professor of Medicine, University of Wisconsin School of Medicine and Public Health, Madison, Wisconsin

HISHAM WEHBE, MD
Chief Resident, Department of Internal Medicine, Indiana University School of Medicine, Indianapolis, Indiana

Contents

Upper gastrointestinal bleeding (UGIB) continues to be an important cause for emergency room visits and carries significant morbidity and mortality. Early resuscitative measures form the basis of the management of patients presenting with UGIB and can improve the outcomes of such patients including lowering mortality. In this review, using an evidence-based approach, we discuss the initial assessment and resuscitation of patients presenting with UGIB including identifying clues from history and physical examination to confirm UGIB, preendoscopic risk assessment tools, the role of early fluid resuscitation, utilization of blood products, use of pharmacologic interventions, and the optimal timing of endoscopy.

Managing gastrointestinal bleeding in patients using antithrombotic agents remains challenging in clinical practice. This review article provides a comprehensive and evidence-based approach to managing acute antithrombotic-related gastrointestinal bleeding, focusing on the triage of patients, appropriate resuscitation, and timely endoscopy. The latest clinical practice guidelines are highlighted to guide decisions concerning the use of reversal agents, temporary interruption, and resumption of antithrombotic drugs. Additionally, preventive measures are discussed to lower the risk of future bleeding and minimize complications among patients prescribed antithrombotic drugs.

Peptic ulcer bleeding is a major cause for hospital admissions and has a significant mortality. Endoscopic interventions reduce the risk of rebleeding in high-risk patients and several options are available including injection therapies, thermal therapies, mechanical clips, hemostatic sprays, and endoscopic suturing. Proton-pump inhibitors and *Helicobacter pylori* treatment are important adjuncts to endoscopic therapy. Endoscopic therapy is indicated in Forrest 1a, 1b, and 2a lesions. Patients with Forrest 2b lesions may do well with proton-pump inhibitor therapy alone but can also be managed by removal of the clot and targeting endoscopic therapy to the underlying lesion.

Cirrhosis is associated with a high morbidity and mortality. One of the most serious and unpredictable complication of cirrhosis, with a high mortality rate, is bleeding from esophagogastric varices. Endoscopic screening of varices followed by primary prophylactic treatment with beta blockers or band ligation in the presence of large esophageal varices will reduce the variceal bleeding rates and thereby reduce mortality risks in those with advanced cirrhosis. There is a paucity of data on primary prophylaxis of gastric varices but secondary prophylaxis includes glue injection, balloon-occluded retrograde transvenous obliteration, or transjugular intrahepatic portosystemic shunting with coil embolization.

Acute variceal bleeding is a serious complication of portal hypertension. This most often manifests as bleeding from esophageal varices. Although less likely to occur, bleeding from gastric varices is usually more severe. The best endoscopic management for acute esophageal variceal bleeding is band ligation and this often proves to be definitive therapy for these patients. For gastric variceal bleeding, the best endoscopic therapy is endoscopic cyanoacrylate injection but this can be cumbersome to perform and is not a readily available resource at most centers in the United States.

Portal hypertensive gastropathy (PHG) and gastric antral vascular ectasia (GAVE) are 2 distinct gastric vascular abnormalities that may present with acute or chronic blood loss. PHG requires the presence of portal hypertension and is typically associated with chronic liver disease, whereas there is controversy about the association of GAVE with chronic liver disease and/or portal hypertension. Distinguishing between GAVE and PHG is crucial because their treatment strategies differ. This review highlights characteristic endoscopic appearances and the clinical features of PHG and GAVE, which, in turn, aid in their appropriate management.

For over 60 years, diagnostic and interventional radiology have been heavily involved in the evaluation and treatment of patients presenting with gastrointestinal bleeding. For patients who present with upper GI bleeding and have a contraindication to endoscopy or have an unsuccessful attempt at endoscopy for identifying or controlling the bleeding, interventional radiology is often consulted for evaluation and consideration of catheter-based intervention.

The use of surgery in managing upper gastrointestinal (GI) bleeding has rapidly diminished secondary to advances in our understanding of the pathologies that underlie upper GI bleeding, pharmaceutical treatments for peptic ulcer disease, and endoscopic procedures used to gain hemostasis. A surgeon must work collaboratively with gastroenterologist and interventional radiologist to determine when, and what kind of, surgery is appropriate for the patient with upper GI bleeding.

Occult and obscure bleeding are challenging conditions to manage; however, recent advances in gastroenterology and endoscopy have improved our diagnostic and therapeutic capabilities. Obscure gastrointestinal (GI) bleeding is an umbrella category of bleeding of unknown origin that persists or recurs after endoscopic evaluation of the entire bowel fails to reveal a bleeding source. This review details the evaluation of patients with occult and obscure GI bleeding and offers diagnostic algorithms. The treatment of GI bleeding depends on the type and location of the bleeding lesion and an overview of how to manage these conditions is presented.

Approximately 5% of all gastrointestinal (GI) bleeding originates from the small bowel. Endoscopic therapy of small bowel bleeding should only be undertaken after consideration of the different options, and the risks, benefits, and alternatives of each option. Endoscopic therapy options for small bowel bleeding are like those treatments used for other forms of bleeding in the upper and lower GI tract. Available endoscopic treatment options include thermal therapy (eg, argon plasma coagulation and bipolar cautery), mechanical therapy (eg, hemoclips), and medical therapy (eg, diluted epinephrine injection). Patients with complicated comorbidities would benefit from evaluation and planning of available treatment options, including conservative and/or medical treatments, beyond endoscopic therapy.

This is a description and critical analysis of current diagnosis and treatment of diverticular hemorrhage. The focus is on colonoscopy for identification and treatment of stigmata of recent hemorrhage (SRH) in diverticula. A classification of definitive, presumptive, and incidental diverticular hemorrhage is reviewed and recommended. The approach to definitive diagnosis with urgent colonoscopy is put into perspective of other management strategies including angiography (of different types), nuclear medicine scans, surgery, and medical treatment. Advancements in diagnosis, risk stratification, and colonoscopic hemostasis are described including those that obliterate arterial blood flow underneath SRH and prevent diverticular rebleeding. Recent innovations are discussed.

Hisham Wehbe, Aditya Gutta, and Mark A. Gromski

Post-polypectomy bleeding (PPB) remains a significant procedure-related complication, with multiple risk factors determining the risk including patient demographics, polyp characteristics, endoscopist expertise, and techniques of polypectomy. Immediate PPB is usually treated promptly, but management of delayed PPB can be challenging. Cold snare polypectomy is the optimal technique for small sessile polyps with hot snare polypectomy for pedunculated and large sessile polyps. Topical hemostatic powders and gels are being investigated for the prevention and management of PPB. Further studies are needed to compare these topical agents with conventional therapy.

GASTROINTESTINAL ENDOSCOPY CLINICS OF NORTH AMERICA

SERIES OF RELATED INTEREST

Gastroenterology Clinics
(www.gastro.theclinics.com)
Clinics in Liver Disease
(www.liver.theclinics.com)

THE CLINICS ARE AVAILABLE ONLINE!
Access your subscription at:
www.theclinics.com

GASTROINTESTINAL ENDOSCOPY CLINICS
OF NORTH AMERICA

FORTHCOMING ISSUES

July 2024
Interventional Pancreatobiliary Endoscopy
Tarek H. Baron, Editor

October 2024
Advances in Bariatric and Metabolic Endoscopy
Violeta Popov and Shelby Sullivan, Editors

January 2025
Updates on Endoscopic Diagnosis in IBD:
From White Light to Molecular Imaging
D. Nageshwar Reddy and Partha Pal, Editors

RECENT ISSUES

January 2024
The Endoscopic Oncologist
Kenneth J. Chang and Jason B. Samarasena, Editors

October 2023
Updates in Pancreatic Endotherapy
D. Nageshwar Reddy and Rupjyoti Talukdar, Editors

July 2023
Advances in Diagnosis and Therapy of Pancreatic Cystic Neoplasms
James A. Gonda, Editor

SERIES OF RELATED INTEREST

Gastroenterology Clinics
(www.gastro.theclinics.com)
Clinics in Liver Disease
(www.liver.theclinics.com)

Foreword

State-of the-Art in Gastrointestinal Bleeding Diagnosis and Management

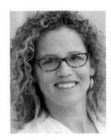

Ashley L. Faulx, MD, MASGE, FACG
Consulting Editor

Endoscopy continues to be the mainstay in the diagnosis and management of gastrointestinal bleeding, as we continue to develop new and evolving endoscopic techniques. Gastroenterologists are further challenged by the increasing numbers of patients on antiplatelet medications and anticoagulants, complicating management in these patients. In this issue, Dr Patrick Pfau has selected a broad range of topics related to gastrointestinal bleeding, from the management of overt variceal and nonvariceal bleeding to diagnosis and management of occult bleeding as well as postpolypectomy bleeding. He has brought in experts from surgery and interventional radiology to better understand the multidisciplinary approach often needed in patients with bleeding refractory to endoscopic intervention. This issue will be an excellent guide for the endoscopist in the management of gastrointestinal bleeding, and the data supporting these interventions.

Ashley L. Faulx, MD, MASGE, FACG
Case Western Reserve University School of Medicine
UH Cleveland Medical Center
Louis Stokes VAMC
11100 Euclid Avenue, Wearn 2nd Floor
Cleveland, OH 44106, USA

E-mail address:
Ashley.faulx@uhhospitals.org

Gastrointest Endoscopy Clin N Am 34 (2024) xiii
https://doi.org/10.1016/j.giec.2023.11.001
1052-5157/24/© 2023 Published by Elsevier Inc.

Preface

Gastrointestinal Bleeding and the Endoscopist

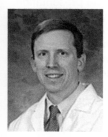

Patrick Pfau, MD
Editor

Gastrointestinal bleeding and gastrointestinal endoscopy are intricately involved with an extensive range of diseases in the field of gastroenterology. Endoscopy is the diagnostic mainstay, from the exsanguinating variceal bleeder to the occult small bowel arteriovenous malformation. The primary therapy of gastrointestinal bleeding is endoscopy, again ranging from treatment of the actively spurting visible vessel to the slowly oozing gastric antral vascular ectasia. Endoscopy and gastrointestinal bleeding come together at 2 AM in the ICU with the intubated cirrhotic patient and in clinic for the fourth opinion on a case of anemia and hemoccult-positive stools.

This broad range of patient types and gastrointestinal diseases demonstrates the need to understand the scope and latest data and research on the diagnosis and treatment of gastrointestinal bleeding with gastrointestinal endoscopy. With this goal, we have brought together experts in the field of gastrointestinal bleeding to present state-of-the-art articles discussing and examining gastrointestinal bleeding and endoscopy and just as importantly how this is applied to benefit patient care. The topics in this issue of *Gastrointestinal Endoscopy Clinics* cover the complete range of disease in which endoscopy and gastrointestinal bleeding interact.

Before any endoscopic intervention, diagnostic or therapeutic, is performed, it is crucial that the patient is prepared for the endoscopy to help ensure the planned endoscopy can be carried out in a safe and effective manner. This includes a thorough assessment of the patient and administration of the correct medical therapies before the scope is even put down. With the increasing number of blood thinners, anticoagulants, and antiplatelet agents, it must be clear how to use and adjust these medications to prevent bleeding initially and in the patient who is actively bleeding.

After a patient is safely prepared and stabilized, endoscopy plays an essential role in the diagnosis and treatment of upper gastrointestinal bleeding. We review the

Gastrointest Endoscopy Clin N Am 34 (2024) xv–xvi
https://doi.org/10.1016/j.giec.2023.10.001
1052-5157/24/© 2023 Published by Elsevier Inc.

diagnostic role and latest treatment in patients with peptic ulcer disease, esophageal and gastric varices, as well as portal gastropathy and gastric vascular ectasia.

While endoscopy is the primary tool in the evaluation and therapy of gastrointestinal bleeding, it should be understood that endoscopy can fail and, in some cases, may not be the first or most successful line of management. Thus, it is important to understand the indications for and complementary role to endoscopy of interventional radiology and surgery for patients with gastrointestinal bleeding.

Gastrointestinal bleeding does not always have a dramatic or acute presentation. Endoscopy also plays a role in finding the diagnosis for bleeding when the cause is not obvious and other diagnostic/imaging modalities are unsuccessful. Often the occult and obscure bleeding source is found in the small bowel, and thus, we cover the latest endoscopic technology and data used to treat small bowel bleeding.

Finally, this issue explains in detail two of the most common large bowel gastrointestinal bleeding disorders treated by the endoscopist, diverticular bleeding and post-polypectomy bleeding. The latest research and guidelines on the diagnosis, outcomes, and therapy of these frequently encountered colonic bleeding sources are covered in-depth.

With this range of subjects on gastrointestinal bleeding, we believe this issue of *Gastrointestinal Endoscopy Clinics* will be a readily and frequently used reference for the endoscopist. We hope bringing the expertise of true leaders in the field of gastrointestinal bleeding will expand the readers' knowledge and improve how patients, bleeding in many ways from many different areas of the gastrointestinal tract, are cared for.

DISCLOSURE

The guest editor has no disclosures nor conflicts of interest to declare.

Patrick Pfau, MD
University of Wisconsin School of
Medicine and Public Health
MFCB Building 4th Floor
1685 Highland Avenue
Madison, WI 53705, USA

E-mail address:
prp@medicine.wisc.edu

Assessment, Resuscitation and Medical Management of Variceal and Nonvariceal Gastrointestinal Bleeding

Ali A. Alali, MB, BCh, BAO, MSc (Clinical Epidemiology)[a],
Alan N. Barkun, MD, CM, MSc (Clinical Epidemiology)[b],*

KEYWORDS

• UGIB • Peptic ulcer • Varices • Resuscitation • Risk assessment

KEY POINTS

- Acute upper gastrointestinal bleeding (UGIB) remains a common emergency that carries significant morbidity and mortality.
- The initial assessment of patients with acute UGIB should focus toward ensuring patient's airway protection, hemodynamic stabilization, and evaluation of risk factors and comorbidities that can exacerbate the bleeding.
- Preendoscopic risk assessment scores, particularly the Glasgow-Blatchford score, are useful clinical tools that allow early patient triage and safe discharge of low-risk patients.
- Early resuscitative measures including appropriate fluid resuscitation and blood transfusion strategies, selective use of vasoactive drugs and prophylactic antibiotics coupled to timely endoscopy can improve the outcomes of patients with UGIB from both nonvariceal and variceal causes.
- Endoscopy remains the gold standard test for confirming and the cornerstone of treating patients with UGIB but should only be performed once the patient is adequately resuscitated and stabilized.

INTRODUCTION

Upper gastrointestinal bleeding (UGIB) is a common emergency that carries significant morbidity and mortality and accounts for more than 250,000 hospitalizations in

This article has not been published previously in print or electronic format and is not under consideration by another publication or electronic medium.
Source of funding: None.
[a] Division of Gastroenterology, Department of Medicine, Faculty of Medicine, Kuwait University, Jabriyah, Kuwait; [b] Division of Gastroenterology, McGill University Health Center, McGill University, 1650 Cedar Avenue, D7.346, Montréal, Quebec H3G1A4, Canada
* Corresponding author. McGill University and the McGill University Health Centre, 1650 Cedar Avenue, D7.346, Montréal, QC H3G1A4, Canada.
E-mail address: alan.barkun@muhc.mcgill.ca

the United States.[1] As a result of recent advances in general supportive care and the endoscopic management of UGIB, the all-cause case fatality of UGIB has decreased in the last few years to approximately 2%.[2] The initial resuscitative measures provided in the emergency department (ED) remain among the most important interventions to improve outcomes for patients presenting with UGIB, including a decrease in mortality. Such interventions have traditionally included hemodynamic stabilization, adopting an appropriate blood transfusion strategy, correcting coagulopathies in select circumstances, and the use of certain pharmacologic therapies.[3] Furthermore, the use of preendoscopic risk stratification is important to ensure proper triaging of patients with UGIB, including identifying patients at low-risk of a negative outcome who can potentially be managed safely in an outpatient setting. In this article, we review the evidence relating to initial resuscitative strategies for patients presenting with UGIB. We exclude the management of the rare patients with UGIB presenting with massive hemorrhage whose approach is described elsewhere.[4]

DEFINITION AND CAUSES

UGIB is defined as bleeding proximal to the ligament of Treitz and the pathologies can be broadly divided into nonvariceal (NVUGIB) and variceal etiologies. Even though the initial management of UGIB is similar regardless of the cause, subsequent stratification into NVUGIB and variceal UGIB is useful since variceal bleeding carries a higher mortality and requires more targeted pharmacologic and endoscopic therapies adapted to the presence of liver disease with portal hypertension.[5] The most common cause of UGIB remains peptic ulcer disease (PUD) despite a decreasing prevalence worldwide (20%–40%).[6] Variceal bleeding is the second most common cause of UGIB (4%–16%) but its prevalence varies geographically and according to local patient mix, being typically higher in tertiary referral centers.[7] Even though tumor bleeding accounts for a minority of severe UGIB (3%–4%), hospitalization due to UGIB from malignancy has increased by 50% during the last decade.[2] Management is especially challenging due to the lower efficacy of available pharmacologic and endoscopic therapies and the overall poor patient prognosis.[2] Other important causes of UGIB include esophagitis, gastritis/duodenitis, angiodysplasia, Mallory-Weiss tear, and Dieulafoy lesion (**Table 1**).

HISTORY AND PHYSICAL EXAMINATION

The initial history should focus on identifying symptoms that are suggestive of UGIB, patient comorbidities that may increase the risk of developing UGIB (eg, chronic liver disease) or its complications (eg, underlying cardiovascular disease), medications use (eg, aspirin or anticoagulants), and general risk factors for worsened outcomes (eg, alcohol abuse or smoking). Melena (ie, black tarry stool) is a classic symptom of UGIB but is nonspecific because some patients with slow gastrointestinal bleeding of the lower GI tract (usually right-sided origin) may occasionally present with melena. Furthermore, certain medications (eg, iron) can produce black stools that can be mistaken for melena. Hematemesis is more specific for an upper gastrointestinal source of bleeding, whereas hematochezia can be seen in lower GIB but also in massive UGIB–more specifically up to 15% of patients presenting with hematochezia and initial or persistent hemodynamic instability.[8] Symptoms such as lightheadedness and syncope imply intravascular volume depletion and can be seen in more severe episodes. Historical factors that increase the probability of upper gastrointestinal source of bleeding include an earlier history of UGIB (Likelihood ratio [LR] = 6.2 [2.8–14.0]), age less than 50 years (LR = 3.5 [2.0–6.1]), melena (LR range = 5.1–5.9), and

Table 1
Causes of upper gastrointestinal bleeding

Cause	Approximate Prevalence (%)
Inflammatory/ulcerative	
PUD	40–63
Esophagitis	8–20
Gastritis/duodenitis	18–22
Mallory-Weiss tear	5.0–7.4
Cameron lesion	<1
Variceal	
Esophageal/gastric varices	4–16
Vascular	
Angiodysplasia	4–6
Gastric antral vascular ectasia	2.3–4.0
Dieulafoy lesion	1.5–2.3
Neoplasm	
Esophageal/gastric/duodenal	2.6–4
Others	
Hemosuccus pancreaticus	<1
Hemobilia	<1
Aortoenteric fistula	<1
No lesions identified	10–15

Reference Alali and Barkun with modification.[7]

epigastric pain (LR = 2.3 [1.2–4.4]).[9] Identifying melena on examination increases the probability of an upper source of GIB significantly (LR = 25.0 [4.0–174.0]), whereas the presence of clots in the stools makes it less likely (LR = 0.05 [0.01–0.38]). Furthermore, resting tachycardia and hypotension are suggestive of a more hemodynamically significant bleeding event. These historic and physical clues are important to seek out in order to ensure that appropriate patient triage and management are implemented while awaiting further confirmatory testing. Clinical clues to prediction of a variceal source of UGIB include a history of liver disease (OR = 6.36 [3.59–11.3]), excessive alcohol use (OR = 2.28 [1.37–3.77]), hematemesis (OR = 2.65 [1.61–4.36]), hematochezia (OR = 3.02 [1.46–6.22]) and stigmata of chronic liver disease (OR = 2.49 [1.46–4.25]). Patients treated with antithrombotic therapy were more likely to experience nonvariceal causes of hemorrhage (OR = 0.44 [0.35–0.78]).[10]

LABORATORY EVALUATION

Complete blood count, liver enzymes, renal function (blood urea nitrogen [BUN] and creatinine), type and screen, and a coagulation profile are some of the routine blood tests that should be performed at presentation, with the hemoglobin level checked serially to ensure stability. It should be noted that the initial hemoglobin and hematocrit values can be misleading in the acute setting because they can be normal despite significant blood loss. Once the patient has undergone fluid resuscitation, the true degree of blood loss becomes clearer. In addition, a low platelet count can be an indirect sign of the presence of portal hypertension and underlying cirrhosis. An important clue to an upper gastrointestinal source of bleeding is a raised BUN-to-creatinine ratio. A

BUN-to-creatinine ratio more than 30 displays a good positive LR for diagnosing an upper source of GIB (LR = 7.5 [2.8–12.0]) rendering it a useful clinical parameter.[9] The role of correcting an identified coagulopathy is discussed further below.

RISK ASSESSMENT

Appropriate early patient risk stratification is important to ensure optimal patient disposition from the ED or initial point of presentation. Predicting patients who are likely to require a hospital-based intervention (blood transfusion, therapeutic endoscopy, interventional radiology, or surgery) during the initial encounter is useful for patient triaging and prognostication. Several preendoscopic risk assessment scores have been described but only a few have been widely implemented in clinical practice, mostly due to a paucity of supportive data and their modest discriminatory capacity.

The best-validated preendoscopic risk assessment scores include the Glasgow-Blatchford (GBS), clinical Rockall (CRS), and AIMS65 scores. More recently, the Age, Blood tests and Comorbidities (ABC) score has been described but has been the subject of less validation studies.[11,12] These scores are based on preendoscopic clinical data that are easily obtainable during the initial patient encounter in the ED, making them useful for an early risk stratification (**Table 2**). The GBS is a validated scoring system that is quite simple to calculate using readily accessible clinical and biochemical parameters determined during the initial patient assessment in the ED. A low GBS (score 0–1) has demonstrated high sensitivity (98.6%) in identifying low-risk patients, who are unlikely to require a hospital-based intervention and hence can be safely discharged and managed as an outpatient (including a deferred endoscopy).[13] A high GBS (score ≥ 7) has been associated with an increased risk of a patient requiring blood transfusions and an endoscopic intervention.[7] The CRS is less accurate at predicting low-risk patients but a high score (≥4) can be useful in prognosticating an increased mortality.[13] Similarly, the AIMS65 and ABC scores do not adequately discriminate low-risk patients (who can be safely managed in an outpatient setting) but are accurate at predicting mortality.[7] Based on the available evidence, clinical practice guidelines recommend using a GBS cutoff of 1 or lesser to identify low-risk patients with resulting outpatient endoscopy and further management.[14–16] More recently, an updated meta-analysis concluded that a low GBS (cutoff ≤1) was accurate at predicting patients who are unlikely to require a hospital-based intervention, experience rebleeding, or die.[17] Furthermore, the authors also suggested that extending the GBS cutoff to 2 or lesser maintains prognostic accuracy while allowing more patients to be managed safely as outpatients (30% for GBS ≤2 compared with 19% with GBS ≤1).[17] No risk assessment score is currently recommended by guidelines for use in predicting patients at a high risk of worse outcomes. Several other risk assessment scores have been described recently but are limited by the requirement of endoscopic assessment for full calculation (eg, Progetto Nazionale Emorragia Digestiva score) or limited validation studies (eg, Canada-United Kingdom-Adelaide score).[12] Of note, the risk assessment scores described previously have been validated on cohorts presenting mostly with an NVUGIB etiology. Their prognostic abilities may thus not be as accurate in patients with a variceal source of bleeding. In patients with underlying liver cirrhosis who present with a suspected upper variceal bleed, the use of the Child-Pugh classification and the Model for End-Stage Liver Disease (MELD) score may provide more useful prognostic information.[18] In general, patients with a Child-Pugh class B (with active bleeding on endoscopy) or C, and/or a MELD score of 19 or greater are considered at high risk for poor outcomes.[18] Additional scores have also been proposed for more specific prognostication of patients

Table 2
Components of preendoscopic risk assessment scores for upper gastrointestinal bleeding

Glasgow-Blatchford Score		Clinical Rockall Score		AIMS65 Score		ABC Score	
Variable	Point	Variable	Point	Variable	Point	Variable	Point
BUN (mg/dL)		Systolic BP, mm Hg		Albumin		Age	
>18.2 to <22.4	2	<100	2	<3.0 g/dL	1	60–74 y	1
>22.4 to <28.0	3					≥75 y	1
>28.0 to <70.0	4						
≥70	6						
Hemoglobin men (g/dL)		Age		International Normalized Ratio (INR)		Blood tests	
≥12.0 to < 13.0	1	<60 y	0	>1.5	1	Urea >10 mmol/L	1
≥10.0 to < 12.0	3	60–79 y	1			Albumin <3.0 g/dL	2
<10.0	6	>80 y	2			Creatinine	
						100–150 μmol/L	1
						>150 μmol/L	2
Hemoglobin women (g/dL)		Comorbidities		Altered mental status		Comorbidities	
≥10.0 to < 12.0	1	None	0		1	Altered mental status	2
<10.0	6	Any	2			Cirrhosis	2
		Renal or liver failure or advanced malignancy	3			Disseminated malignancy	4
						ASA score	
						3	1
						≥4	2
Systolic BP, mm Hg				Systolic BP, mm Hg			
100–109	1			<90 mm Hg	1		
90–00	2						
<90	3						
Others				Age			
Heart rate >100/min	1			>65 y	1		
Melena	1						
Syncope	2						
Liver disease	2						
Heart failure	2						

Modified from Simon et al.[3]

with liver disease presenting with UGIB including the cirrhosis acute gastrointestinal bleeding, which showed promising results at predicting mortality but further validation studies are required.[19]

INITIAL MANAGEMENT

The initial management of patients presenting with UGIB follows the principles of any medical emergency with specific focus on airway, breathing, and circulation. This protocol is appropriate regardless of the cause of bleeding and aims to protect the patient's airway and breathing while ensuring hemodynamic stability before performing endoscopy. The management of the rare UGIB patient presenting with massive hemorrhage is discussed elsewhere.[4] An overall approach to the initial management of suspected UGIB is shown in **Fig. 1**.

- *Airway and Breathing:* Supplemental oxygen is usually administered to ensure adequate tissue oxygenation, with special care when oxygen is administered via face mask given the risk of aspiration.[20] Patients presenting with UGIB may be at increased risk of aspiration especially if they have a reduced level of consciousness, for example, in patients with hepatic encephalopathy. However, prophylactic intubation does not reduce the incidence of pneumonia, length of hospital stay, or mortality and it may, in fact, increase the risk of such adverse

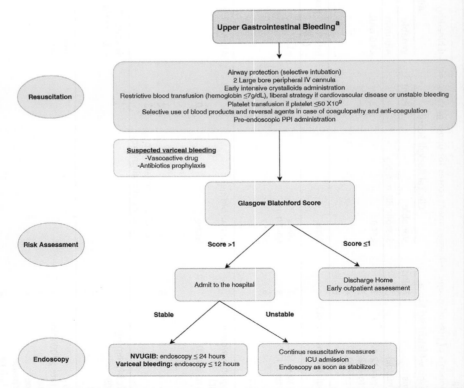

Fig. 1. Approach to the initial resuscitation and management of patients presenting with suspected UGIB. [a]Patients with massive hemorrhage are excluded from this management algorithm.

outcomes.[21,22] Therefore, a routine intubation before urgent endoscopy is not recommended. Prophylactic intubation for airway protection is suggested for patients presenting with ongoing active hematemesis, agitation, or encephalopathy who are unable to protect their airway with early extubation postendoscopy.[18]

- *Circulation:* The goal of early resuscitative measures is to preserve tissue perfusion and prevent organ damage while steps are taken to stop bleeding. This is achieved by volume restitution, typically with crystalloids given intravenously, to maintain hemodynamic stability. Patients with a resting tachycardia and/or hypotension at presentation are more intravascularly volume depleted and require early aggressive fluid resuscitation to restore intravascular volume. The most efficient method of delivering intravenous fluid to the patient is via 2 large-bore peripheral intravenous cannulas (typically 18 gauge or larger). Low-quality evidence suggests lower mortality and myocardial infarction among patients with UGIB treated with intensive early fluid resuscitation.[23] Current evidence does not support the superiority of colloid; hence, crystalloids are currently recommended as the fluid of choice for initial resuscitation.[16] If the patient fails to respond to the initial fluid resuscitative measures, more aggressive fluid resuscitation, and intensive care unit management are appropriate.[4]

Blood Transfusion

To maintain adequate tissue oxygenation and avoid ischemia, an appropriate hemoglobin level must be maintained among patients with UGIB. High-quality evidence supports a restrictive blood transfusion strategy (blood transfusion at hemoglobin threshold 7 g/dL aiming for 9 g/dL) in patients presenting with a stable UGIB and without underlying cardiovascular disease. A meta-analysis of 5 randomized controlled trials (RCTs) concluded that a restrictive blood transfusion strategy was associated with lower mortality (relative risk (RR) = 0.65 [0.44–0.97]) and reduced rebleeding (RR = 0.58 [0.40–0.84]) compared with a liberal transfusion strategy.[24] This restrictive transfusion strategy is particularly important among patients with a variceal source of bleeding because overtransfusion may result in an increased portal pressure, further exacerbating the bleed. This was shown in a subgroup analysis of an RCT of restrictive versus liberal blood transfusion strategies in which overall benefit, including improved mortality, was shown among patients with cirrhosis and variceal bleeding who were managed with the restrictive transfusional approach.[25] It should be noted that patients with underlying cardiovascular disease may be at higher risk of developing ischemic complications with lower hemoglobin levels, hence a more liberal strategy should be considered. Furthermore, patients with exsanguinating bleeding who are hemodynamically unstable may require blood transfusion at a higher hemoglobin level. Current guidelines recommend a restrictive transfusional approach in patients with a stable UGIB and without underlying cardiovascular disease (transfuse at hemoglobin level 7 g/dL with a target level of 7–9 g/dL), using a more liberal strategy in patients with underlying cardiovascular disease (transfuse at hemoglobin level 8 g/dL with a target level of 10 g/dL or greater).[14,15]

Management of Patients with Thrombocytopenia

Limited evidence exists to guide platelet transfusional strategy in patients with UGIB. Among patients with NVUGIB, platelet transfusion for a threshold of 50 × 10^9 platelets/L or lesser has been suggested by experts.[26] The role of thrombocytopenia is even more confusing among patients with cirrhosis and portal hypertension who are typically thrombocytopenic. Among this group of patients, there is a lack of evidence to suggest that platelet count correlates with an increased risk of failure to control bleeding or rebleeding. The Baveno VII consensus suggests considering platelet transfusion among patients with variceal bleeding and thrombocytopenia on a case-by-case basis only.[27] Platelet transfusion should not be used in patients presenting with a UGIB who are on antiplatelets agents (see later discussion).[28,29]

Correction of a Coagulopathy for Patients Not on Anticoagulants

No threshold INR should be used to determine whether to proceed with an early gastroscopy.[14,15] Abnormalities in clotting factors are common among patients with cirrhosis. However, abnormalities in coagulation parameters are not an accurate measure of bleeding tendency in patients with cirrhosis, and hence an elevated prothrombin time may not be prognostic in this group. In fact, the use of fresh frozen plasma (FFP) transfusions to correct a coagulopathy has been associated with worse outcomes among patients with cirrhosis and variceal bleeding, including increased mortality, failure to control bleeding, and longer hospital stay.[30] Similarly, the use of prothrombin complex concentrate (PCC) and recombinant factors VIIa have failed to show any benefits in patients with variceal bleeding.[31] Based on the available literature, correcting a coagulopathy in patients with cirrhosis is not recommended.[18,27] Correction of a coagulopathy for patients on vitamin K antagonists (VKA) or direct oral anticoagulants (DOAC) is not routinely recommended except in cases of life threatening bleeding (see later discussion).[28,29]

Patients on Anticoagulants

In patients on VKA, vitamin K administration and FFP should not be used, whereas PCC could be used in cases of life-threatening bleeds (or if the INR is well beyond the supratherapeutic range).[28,29] Among patients having taken their last DOAC dose within 24 hours of presentation, PCC or DOAC drug-specific reversal agents could be considered if bleeding is considered life threatening.[28,29] Aspirin should not be stopped (unless given for primary cardiovascular prevention, in which case it should never be restarted), and P2Y12 inhibitors should be stopped for 5 to 7 days. Platelet transfusion is not recommended in the absence of thrombocytopenia.[28,29]

Tranexamic Acid

The antifibrinolytic agent tranexamic acid is not recommended because it has failed to show any benefit in improving outcomes in patients with UGIB. In the HALT-IT study, tranexamic acid did not improve mortality among patients with UGIB, and in fact was associated with an increased risk of thromboembolic events.[32]

Preendoscopy Proton Pump Inhibitors

Proton pump inhibitors (PPIs) act by reducing gastric acid secretion by the parietal cells, hence reducing gastric acidity. The increase in gastric pH facilitates clot formation and stabilization, platelet plug aggregation, and aid in ulcer healing.[7] These physiologic properties form the basis for the administration of PPIs during the initial resuscitation of patients presenting with suspected UGIB, before performing an endoscopy. However, evidence for improved patient outcomes attributable to the use of preendoscopy PPI is lacking. A Cochrane review of 6 RCTs (n = 2223 patients) concluded that preendoscopy PPI therapy did not reduce mortality, risk of rebleeding, or need for surgery.[33] However, preendoscopy PPI administration causes a downgrading of high-risk endoscopic stigmata in patients with NVUGIB, resulting in a 32% reduction in the need for endoscopic hemostatic treatment at the index endoscopy.[33] Furthermore, preendoscopy PPI administration has been found to be a cost-effective measure among patients presenting with suspected UGIB when modeling for potential downstream benefits.[34] Recent societal guidelines have either suggested against,[35] suggested the routine use of preendoscopy PPI,[15] or could not make a recommendation for or against the routine use of preendoscopy PPI.[14] PPIs are not indicated in the acute management of variceal bleeding. However, because many patients with cirrhosis who present with UGIB may be hemorrhaging from a nonvariceal cause, intravenous PPIs are commonly started preendoscopy but should be reassessed and discontinued postendoscopy once a variceal cause is identified.[18,27]

Vasoactive Drugs

Vasoactive drugs cause splanchnic vasoconstriction resulting in reduction in pressure in the portal vein and the varices. Hence, these drugs have traditionally been used to manage patients presenting with acute variceal hemorrhage. Several vasoactive drugs are available (somatostatin, terlipressin, and octreotide); high-quality data have demonstrated varying significant decreases in overall mortality and transfusion requirements resulting from the use of these medications in patients with cirrhosis presenting with acute variceal bleeding.[36] The choice of the drug used depends on local availability.[37] These drugs should be started as intravenous infusions at presentation and continued for up to 5 days following endoscopic therapy.[18,27,38] Such vasoactive drugs are not recommended in the routine management of patients with NVUGIB.[16]

Antibiotics

Patients with cirrhosis presenting with acute UGIB are at high risk of developing bacterial infections (up to 50%) with associated increased risks of rebleeding and overall mortality.[39] This observation forms the basis of initiating prophylactic antibiotics in patients with cirrhosis who present with UGIB. Data from 2 meta-analyses have demonstrated significant reductions in the rates of bacterial infections, rebleeding, length of hospital stays, and overall mortality among patient with advance chronic liver disease and UGIB.[40,41] Third-generation cephalosporins are preferred to fluoroquinolones as an empiric choice, given increasing regional prevalences of fluoroquinolone resistance, and this choice is also supported by RCT data.[42] However, local antibiotic resistance must be considered when deciding on the choice of prophylactic antibiotics, which should be continued intravenously for up to 7 days.[18,27,38] Furthermore, it is unclear from the available literature if antibiotics administration improves the outcomes among cirrhotic patients with variceal bleeding only or any gastrointestinal bleeding (eg, PUD). In the absence of underlying advanced chronic liver disease, prophylactic antibiotics are not typically recommended.

Prokinetic Agents

The rational for using prokinetic agents in the setting of UGIB is to clear the stomach from gastric contents, including blood, hence improving endoscopic visualization. This may help in identifying the bleeding lesion, thus optimizing endoscopic therapy, if indicated. The most studied prokinetic agent is erythromycin, a macrolide antibiotic, which has motilin-like properties. It is typically given at a dose of 250 mg intravenously 30 to 120 minutes before the endoscopy.[15] A meta-analysis of 8 RCTs concluded that erythromycin administration was associated with significantly improved gastric mucosal visualization, reduced need for second-look endoscopy, and shorter hospital stays for patients with variceal and nonvariceal UGIB.[43] Furthermore, this practice has been shown to be cost-effective, mostly by reducing the need for a repeat endoscopy to subsequently locate the bleeding lesion.[44] Current practice guidelines recommend using erythromycin before endoscopy in acute UGIB, especially among patients with clinically severe or ongoing active bleeding.[14,15] Metoclopramide does not seem to be useful for this indication.[45]

Nasogastric Tube

The use of a nasogastric (NG) tube in the setting of acute UGIB theoretically serves 2 purposes, namely the detection of blood, confirming an UGIB source, and the ability to carry out lavage to clear the stomach from blood and clots, improving subsequent endoscopic visualization. However, the NG aspirate displays a low sensitivity in confirming an upper gastrointestinal source of bleeding and has a poor negative predictive value (<1%) based on a negative aspirate.[46] However, a positive NG aspirate for blood can confirm an UGIB (LR = 9.6 [4.0–23.0]) and may suggest an increased severity of bleeding (LR = 3.1 [1.2–14.0]).[9] Unfortunately, given the relatively small caliber of regular-size NG tubes, they are not useful to remove large blood clots from the stomach and are unlikely to improve endoscopic visualization. In the absence of strong evidence to support the use of NG tube to improve outcomes in patients with UGIB, this practice is not recommended on a routine basis.[15]

TIMING OF ENDOSCOPY

Endoscopy is the gold standard test for evaluating and treating UGIB. A timely endoscopy allows for prompt identification of the cause of the UGIB and the delivery of appropriate endoscopic hemostatic therapy, if indicated, which in turn may improve patient outcomes and lower hospital costs.[47] Conversely, performing endoscopy in the acute setting before adequate resuscitative measures are implemented, coupled with less available endoscopy resources during off-hours can potentially worsen patients outcomes.[48] Hence, the optimal timing of endoscopy in UGIB has been the subject of several studies adopting heterogenous methodologies.[7] Different definitions have been proposed for the timing of endoscopy but, in general, urgent endoscopy is defined as endoscopy within 12 hours while early endoscopy is defined as endoscopy within 24 hours from presentation.[15] Despite the limited data, the recommended timing of performing endoscopy in the setting of acute UGIB depends on the suspected cause, namely NVUGIB or variceal bleeding. Therefore, each scenario will be discussed separately but adequate resuscitation before endoscopy remains critical, regardless of the cause.

- *NVUGIB*: The optimal timing of endoscopy in patients presenting with suspected NVUGIB has been the subject of several observational and randomized studies with variable conclusions. Several observational studies have yielded conflicting conclusions with some showing improved outcomes with urgent endoscopy,[49] whereas others showed no or even worse outcomes, including increased mortality with urgent endoscopy.[16,50] A meta-analysis of 5 RCTs and 10 observational studies failed to show any improvement in patient outcomes with urgent endoscopy compared with early endoscopy, including similar rates of rebleeding, surgery, blood transfusion, and mortality.[51] Furthermore, the mortality was significantly higher in patients receiving urgent endoscopy (within 12 hours) compared with early endoscopy (OR = 1.66 [1.27–2.18]).[51] Patients who underwent urgent endoscopy were more likely to have high-risk lesions identified requiring endoscopic therapy (RR = 1.24 [1.06–1.46]) but did not translate into better patient outcomes.[52] Hence, based on the current available evidence, early endoscopy (within 24 hours from presentation) is appropriate for patients presenting with stable UGIB. It should be noted that many of the published studies excluded patients who presented with hemodynamically unstable UGIB; therefore, more urgent intervention may be required in such patients. However, adequate resuscitation of these patients takes priority over urgent endoscopy as highlighted by a large Danish prospective cohort study of patients with PUD[53] that found a "U-shaped" association between timing of endoscopy and mortality among more acutely ill patients presenting with hemodynamically unstable UGIB. Based on this study, there was an increased mortality in patients who underwent endoscopy within 6 hours or after 24 hours from presentation, which emphasizes the importance of adequate early resuscitation and optimization of the patient's medical comorbidities before endoscopy, without, however, delaying endoscopy beyond 24 hours once the patient has been stabilized. Current practice guidelines agree that all patients with NVUGIB should undergo early endoscopy (within 24 hours of presentation) but only after adequate resuscitative measures are implemented to optimize clinical outcomes, potentially allowing early discharge of low-risk patients with subsequent reduction in health-care costs.[14–16]

- *Variceal bleeding:* The optimal timing of endoscopy in patients with variceal bleeding remains controversial due to the paucity of high-quality data. A recent meta-analysis that included 9 retrospective studies of patients with liver cirrhosis and variceal bleeding found lower overall mortality in patients in whom an endoscopy is performed within 12 hours compared with later but without any differences in rebleeding, length of stay, endoscopic hemostasis, and blood transfusion requirements.[54] Based on the limited evidence, current practice guidelines for variceal bleeding recommend performing endoscopy within 12 hours in patients with suspected variceal bleeding after adequate hemodynamic resuscitation.[18,27,38]

SUMMARY

UGIB continues to be an important cause for ED visits and still carries significant morbidity and mortality. Resuscitative measures form the basis for the initial management of patients presenting with UGIB; this review does not address the management of the rare patient with UGIB presenting with massive hemorrhage. The first and most important step in the management of UGIB, regardless of cause, is fluid resuscitation to correct intravascular volume losses and restoring hemodynamic stability. A restrictive blood transfusion strategy results in improved patient outcomes. An evidence-based approach to correcting coagulopathy should be used with highly restricted use of blood products and reversal agents in patients taking antithrombotics. Preendoscopic PPI administration in patients with NVUGIB may be considered to downgrade high-risk endoscopic lesions, whereas the use of antibiotics is essential in patients with underlying liver cirrhosis with, in addition, administration of vasoactive drugs in suspected variceal bleeding to improve outcomes and reduce mortality in these patients. Risk assessment using preendoscopic risk assessment scores is useful for patient triage, allowing early identification of low-risk patients who can be safely discharged home for an early outpatient management. Early endoscopy is appropriate for patients presenting with UGIB but should only be performed after adequate resuscitation and patient stabilization.

CLINICS CARE POINTS

- Early risk stratification using preendoscopic risk assessment scores, specifically the GBS, is recommended in patients presenting with UGIB. Low-risk patients (score ≤1 or 2) can be safely discharged for an early outpatient assessment.

- Fluid resuscitation is the first and one of the most crucial steps in the management of patients with UGIB to ensure hemodynamic stabilization and has been shown to decrease mortality.
- Despite the lack of improvement in important patient clinical outcomes, the use of preendoscopy PPIs can be considered in patients presenting with UGIB to downgrade high-risk lesion during endoscopy, reducing the need for endoscopic therapy.
- A restrictive blood transfusion strategy (with a threshold of 7 g/dL) is superior to a liberal blood transfusion strategy in patients presenting with stable UGIB. A more liberal approach might be appropriate for patients with underlying cardiovascular disease or hemodynamically unstable bleeding.
- Among patients with advanced chronic liver disease presenting with variceal bleeding, the administration of both vasoactive drugs and prophylactic antibiotics starting before the endoscopy is recommended to improve the clinical outcomes, including survival and rebleeding.
- Early endoscopy (within 24 hours) should be performed in patients with suspected NVUGIB, whereas patients with suspected variceal bleeding should undergo a gastroscopy within 12 hours of presentation. In either situation, endoscopy should only be performed after adequate resuscitation.

ACKNOWLEDGMENTS

A. Alali: Drafting and revision of the article; A. Barkun: drafting and revision of the article. Both authors approved the final version of the article.

CONFLICTS OF INTEREST

A.A. Alali and A.N. Barkun have no financial relationships relevant to this publication to disclose.

REFERENCES

1. Abougergi MS, Travis AC, Saltzman JR. The in-hospital mortality rate for upper GI hemorrhage has decreased over 2 decades in the United States: a nationwide analysis. Gastrointest Endosc 2015;81:882–8.e1.
2. Wuerth BA, Rockey DC. Changing epidemiology of upper gastrointestinal hemorrhage in the last decade: a nationwide analysis. Dig Dis Sci 2018;63:1286–93.
3. Simon TG, Travis AC, Saltzman JR. Initial assessment and resuscitation in nonvariceal upper gastrointestinal bleeding. Gastrointest Endosc Clin N Am 2015;25:429–42.
4. Callum J, Evans CCD, Barkun A, et al. Nonsurgical management of major hemorrhage. CMAJ (Can Med Assoc J) 2023;195:E773–81.
5. Garcia-Tsao G, Bosch J. Management of varices and variceal hemorrhage in cirrhosis. N Engl J Med 2010;362:823–32.
6. Loperfido S, Baldo V, Piovesana E, et al. Changing trends in acute upper-GI bleeding: a population-based study. Gastrointest Endosc 2009;70:212–24.
7. Alali AA, Barkun AN. An update on the management of non-variceal upper gastrointestinal bleeding. Gastroenterol Rep (Oxf) 2023;11:goad011.
8. Sengupta N, Feuerstein JD, Jairath V, et al. Management of patients with acute lower gastrointestinal bleeding: an updated ACG guideline. Am J Gastroenterol 2023;118:208–31.
9. Srygley FD, Gerardo CJ, Tran T, et al. Does this patient have a severe upper gastrointestinal bleed? JAMA 2012;307:1072–9.

10. Alharbi A, Almadi M, Barkun A, et al. Predictors of a variceal source among patients presenting with upper gastrointestinal bleeding. Can J Gastroenterol 2012; 26:187–92.
11. Kherad O, Restellini S, Almadi M, et al. Comparative evaluation of the abc score to other risk stratification scales in managing high-risk patients presenting with acute upper gastrointestinal bleeding. J Clin Gastroenterol 2023;57:479–85.
12. Alali AA, Boustany A, Martel M, et al. Strengths and limitations of risk stratification tools for patients with upper gastrointestinal bleeding: a narrative review. Expet Rev Gastroenterol Hepatol 2023;17(8):795–803, under review for publication.
13. Stanley AJ, Laine L, Dalton HR, et al. Comparison of risk scoring systems for patients presenting with upper gastrointestinal bleeding: international multicentre prospective study. BMJ 2017;356:i6432.
14. Laine L, Barkun AN, Saltzman JR, et al. ACG clinical guideline: upper gastrointestinal and ulcer bleeding. Am J Gastroenterol 2021;116:899–917.
15. Gralnek IM, Stanley AJ, Morris AJ, et al. Endoscopic diagnosis and management of nonvariceal upper gastrointestinal hemorrhage (NVUGIH): European Society of Gastrointestinal Endoscopy (ESGE) Guideline - Update 2021. Endoscopy 2021; 53:300–32.
16. Barkun AN, Almadi M, Kuipers EJ, et al. Management of nonvariceal upper gastrointestinal bleeding: guideline recommendations from the international consensus group. Ann Intern Med 2019;171:805–22.
17. Boustany A, Alali AA, Almadi M, et al. Pre-endoscopic scores predicting low risk patients with upper gastrointestinal bleeding: a systematic review and meta-analysis. J Clin Med 2023;12(16):5194, under review for publication.
18. Gralnek IM, Camus Duboc M, Garcia-Pagan JC, et al. Endoscopic diagnosis and management of esophagogastric variceal hemorrhage: European Society of Gastrointestinal Endoscopy (ESGE) Guideline. Endoscopy 2022;54:1094–120.
19. Bai Z, Li B, Lin S, et al. Development and Validation of CAGIB Score for Evaluating the Prognosis of Cirrhosis with Acute Gastrointestinal Bleeding: A Retrospective Multicenter Study. Adv Ther 2019;36:3211–20.
20. Josh O-P, Adrian JS. Update on the management of upper gastrointestinal bleeding. BMJ Medicine 2022;1:e000202.
21. Chaudhuri D, Bishay K, Tandon P, et al. Prophylactic endotracheal intubation in critically ill patients with upper gastrointestinal bleed: A systematic review and meta-analysis. JGH Open 2020;4:22–8.
22. Almashhrawi AA, Rahman R, Jersak ST, et al. Prophylactic tracheal intubation for upper GI bleeding: A meta-analysis. World J Metaanal 2015;3:4–10.
23. Baradarian R, Ramdhaney S, Chapalamadugu R, et al. Early intensive resuscitation of patients with upper gastrointestinal bleeding decreases mortality. Am J Gastroenterol 2004;99:619–22.
24. Odutayo A, Desborough MJ, Trivella M, et al. Restrictive versus liberal blood transfusion for gastrointestinal bleeding: a systematic review and meta-analysis of randomised controlled trials. Lancet Gastroenterol Hepatol 2017;2:354–60.
25. Villanueva C, Colomo A, Bosch A, et al. Transfusion strategies for acute upper gastrointestinal bleeding. N Engl J Med 2013;368:11–21.
26. Razzaghi A, Barkun AN. Platelet transfusion threshold in patients with upper gastrointestinal bleeding: a systematic review. J Clin Gastroenterol 2012;46: 482–6.
27. de Franchis R, Bosch J, Garcia-Tsao G, et al. Baveno VII - Renewing consensus in portal hypertension. J Hepatol 2022;76:959–74.

28. Abraham NS, Barkun AN, Sauer BG, et al. American College of Gastroenterology-Canadian Association of Gastroenterology Clinical Practice Guideline: Management of Anticoagulants and Antiplatelets During Acute Gastrointestinal Bleeding and the Periendoscopic Period. Am J Gastroenterol 2022;117:542–58.

29. Barkun AN, Douketis J, Noseworthy PA, et al. Management of Patients on Anticoagulants and Antiplatelets During Acute Gastrointestinal Bleeding and the Peri-Endoscopic Period: A Clinical Practice Guideline Dissemination Tool. Am J Gastroenterol 2022;117:513–9.

30. Mohanty A, Kapuria D, Canakis A, et al. Fresh frozen plasma transfusion in acute variceal haemorrhage: Results from a multicentre cohort study. Liver Int 2021;41:1901–8.

31. Kwon JO, MacLaren R. Comparison of Fresh-Frozen Plasma, Four-Factor Prothrombin Complex Concentrates, and Recombinant Factor VIIa to Facilitate Procedures in Critically Ill Patients with Coagulopathy from Liver Disease: A Retrospective Cohort Study. Pharmacotherapy 2016;36:1047–54.

32. Effects of a high-dose 24-h infusion of tranexamic acid on death and thromboembolic events in patients with acute gastrointestinal bleeding (HALT-IT): an international randomised, double-blind, placebo-controlled trial. Lancet 2020;395:1927–36.

33. Kanno T, Yuan Y, Tse F, et al. Proton pump inhibitor treatment initiated prior to endoscopic diagnosis in upper gastrointestinal bleeding. Cochrane Database Syst Rev 2022;1:Cd005415.

34. Tsoi KK, Lau JY, Sung JJ. Cost-effectiveness analysis of high-dose omeprazole infusion before endoscopy for patients with upper-GI bleeding. Gastrointest Endosc 2008;67:1056–63.

35. Siau K, Hearnshaw S, Stanley AJ, et al. British Society of Gastroenterology (BSG)-led multisociety consensus care bundle for the early clinical management of acute upper gastrointestinal bleeding. Frontline Gastroenterol 2020;11:311–23.

36. Wells M, Chande N, Adams P, et al. Meta-analysis: vasoactive medications for the management of acute variceal bleeds. Aliment Pharmacol Ther 2012;35:1267–78.

37. Seo YS, Park SY, Kim MY, et al. Lack of difference among terlipressin, somatostatin, and octreotide in the control of acute gastroesophageal variceal hemorrhage. Hepatology 2014;60:954–63.

38. Garcia-Tsao G, Abraldes JG, Berzigotti A, et al. Portal hypertensive bleeding in cirrhosis: Risk stratification, diagnosis, and management: 2016 practice guidance by the American Association for the study of liver diseases. Hepatology 2017;65:310–35.

39. Lee S, Saxinger L, Ma M, et al. Bacterial infections in acute variceal hemorrhage despite antibiotics-a multicenter study of predictors and clinical impact. United European Gastroenterol J 2017;5:1090–9.

40. Soares-Weiser K, Brezis M, Tur-Kaspa R, et al. Antibiotic prophylaxis of bacterial infections in cirrhotic inpatients: a meta-analysis of randomized controlled trials. Scand J Gastroenterol 2003;38:193–200.

41. Chavez-Tapia NC, Barrientos-Gutierrez T, Tellez-Avila F, et al. Meta-analysis: antibiotic prophylaxis for cirrhotic patients with upper gastrointestinal bleeding - an updated Cochrane review. Aliment Pharmacol Ther 2011;34:509–18.

42. Fernández J, Ruiz del Arbol L, Gómez C, et al. Norfloxacin vs ceftriaxone in the prophylaxis of infections in patients with advanced cirrhosis and hemorrhage. Gastroenterology 2006;131:1049–56, quiz 1285.

43. Rahman R, Nguyen DL, Sohail U, et al. Pre-endoscopic erythromycin administration in upper gastrointestinal bleeding: an updated meta-analysis and systematic review. Ann Gastroenterol 2016;29:312–7.
44. Winstead NS, Wilcox CM. Erythromycin prior to endoscopy for acute upper gastrointestinal haemorrhage: a cost-effectiveness analysis. Aliment Pharmacol Ther 2007;26:1371–7.
45. Vimonsuntirungsri T, Thungsuk R, Nopjaroonsri P, et al. The efficacy of metoclopramide of gastric visualization by endoscopy in pateints with active upper gastrointestinal bleeding: double-blind randomized controlled trial. Gastroenterology 2023;164(6). https://doi.org/10.1016/s0016-5085(23)01118-6.
46. Kessel B, Olsha O, Younis A, et al. Evaluation of nasogastric tubes to enable differentiation between upper and lower gastrointestinal bleeding in unselected patients with melena. Eur J Emerg Med 2016;23:71–3.
47. Garg SK, Anugwom C, Campbell J, et al. Early esophagogastroduodenoscopy is associated with better Outcomes in upper gastrointestinal bleeding: a nationwide study. Endosc Int Open 2017;5:E376–86.
48. Shih PC, Liu SJ, Li ST, et al. Weekend effect in upper gastrointestinal bleeding: a systematic review and meta-analysis. PeerJ 2018;6:e4248.
49. Cho SH, Lee YS, Kim YJ, et al. Outcomes and Role of Urgent Endoscopy in High-Risk Patients With Acute Nonvariceal Gastrointestinal Bleeding. Clin Gastroenterol Hepatol 2018;16:370–7.
50. Ahn DW, Park YS, Lee SH, et al. Clinical outcome of acute nonvariceal upper gastrointestinal bleeding after hours: the role of urgent endoscopy. Korean J Intern Med 2016;31:470–8.
51. Bai L, Jiang W, Cheng R, et al. Does early endoscopy affect the clinical outcomes of patients with acute nonvariceal upper gastrointestinal bleeding? a systematic review and meta-analysis. Gut Liver 2022;17(4):566–80.
52. Lau JYW, Yu Y, Tang RSY, et al. Timing of endoscopy for acute upper gastrointestinal bleeding. N Engl J Med 2020;382:1299–308.
53. Laursen SB, Leontiadis GI, Stanley AJ, et al. Relationship between timing of endoscopy and mortality in patients with peptic ulcer bleeding: a nationwide cohort study. Gastrointest Endosc 2017;85:936–44.e3.
54. Bai Z, Wang R, Cheng G, et al. Outcomes of early versus delayed endoscopy in cirrhotic patients with acute variceal bleeding: a systematic review with meta-analysis. Eur J Gastroenterol Hepatol 2021;33:e868–76.

Management of Anticoagulant and Antiplatelet Agents in Acute Gastrointestinal Bleeding and Prevention of Gastrointestinal Bleeding

Amany Elshaer, MBBS[a],
Neena S. Abraham, MD, MSCE, MACG, FASGE, AGAF[a,b],*

KEYWORDS

- Anticoagulation • Direct oral anticoagulants • Antiplatelet agents • Warfarin
- Dual antiplatelet therapy • Endoscopy • Bleeding prevention

KEY POINTS

- In patients presenting with gastrointestinal bleeding, provide adequate resuscitation and hemodynamic stabilization before endoscopy.
- For patients on antithrombotic agents, reversal agents may be considered in life-threatening hemorrhages.
- Preventive measures, including proton pump inhibitor use and eradication of *Helicobacter pylori*, should be implemented to reduce the risk of recurrent gastrointestinal bleeding.

INTRODUCTION

Gastrointestinal bleeding (GIB) is frequently encountered among patients prescribed antiplatelet and anticoagulant medications, as they are commonly prescribed to treat or prevent cardiovascular and cerebrovascular diseases.[1] Commonly used medications include vitamin K antagonists (VKAs) (warfarin and acenocoumarol), direct oral anticoagulants (apixaban, dabigatran, edoxaban, and rivaroxaban), $P2Y_{12}$ receptor inhibitors (clopidogrel, prasugrel, and ticagrelor), and acetylsalicylic acid (ASA). In patients on antithrombotic agents, GIB presents a dilemma where the physician must

a Department of Internal Medicine, Mayo Clinic, 13400 East Shea Boulevard, Scottsdale, AZ 85259, USA; b Division of Gastroenterology and Hepatology, Department of Medicine, Mayo Clinic, 13400 East Shea Boulevard, Scottsdale, AZ 85259, USA
* Corresponding author.
E-mail address: abraham.neena@mayo.edu

Gastrointest Endoscopy Clin N Am 34 (2024) 205–216
https://doi.org/10.1016/j.giec.2023.09.002
giendo.theclinics.com

balance managing acute bleeding and the associated risk of thrombosis. In this article, the authors will highlight the best practice recommendations for GIB, focusing on managing antithrombotic therapy safely and preventing rebleeding.

DISCUSSION
Initial Assessment: Evaluation and Risk Stratification

Acute GIB is overt GIB (either upper or lower) manifesting as melena, hematochezia, coffee ground emesis, or hematemesis in hospitalized patients or those under observation. Resuscitation is a priority during the patient's presentation. Concurrently, a thorough history and physical examination are needed to determine potential sources, assess the severity of bleeding, and evaluate the patient's risk of complications and underlying thromboembolic risk (**Table 1**). These clinical considerations influence the periendoscopic period's antiplatelet and anticoagulant drug management approach. It is critical to identify if the patient is experiencing a life-threatening hemorrhage, which is characterized by overt or apparent bleeding with severe hypotension or hypovolemic shock that requires pressors or surgery, is associated with $\geq$ 5 g/dL drop in hemoglobin (Hg), requires $\geq$ 5 units of packed red blood cells (pRBC), or is at risk of causing death.[2] It is important to differentiate between life-threatening and non–life-threatening bleeding to guide the pharmacologic management of acutely bleeding patients on antithrombotic agents (**Fig. 1**).

Hemodynamic resuscitation

In hemodynamically unstable patients, immediate fluid resuscitation should be initiated to restore organ perfusion and tissue oxygenation while taking the necessary steps to control active bleeding. The type of fluid (colloid vs crystalloid), amount (restrictive vs aggressive), and timing protocol have not been universally standardized.[3] Studies have shown no significant difference between using crystalloid versus colloid fluids for resuscitation.[4] Current evidence does not demonstrate increased survival rates with colloids compared to crystalloids, and guidelines suggest against the routine use of colloids in clinical practice due to higher costs.[4] Trials to assess the

Table 1
Patient-specific thromboembolic risk established by the International Society on Thrombosis and Hemostasis Guidance statement, BRIDGE trial , published guidelines, and expert opinion

Thromboembolic risk stratification			
High-risk characteristics	VTE	Atrial fibrillation	Mechanical heart valve
	Acute VTE within the past 90 d	CHADS$_2$ score: 5 or 6	Any mitral valve prosthesis
	Severe thrombophilia (Protein C, protein S or antithrombin deficiency, antiphospholipid antibodies)	CHA$_2$DS$_2$VASc score: $\geq$7; stroke or ischemic attack within the past 90 d	Old generation mechanical prosthesis (caged ball or tilting disc aortic valve)
	Previous VTE with temporary VKA interruption	Rheumatic valvular heart disease	Stroke or transient ischemic attack within the past 90 d

Abbreviations: CHADS$_2$, congestive heart failure, hypertension, age $\geq$75 years, diabetes mellitus, prior stroke or transient ischemic attack or thromboembolism (doubled); CHA$_2$DS$_2$VASc, congestive heart failure, hypertension, age $\geq$75 (doubled), diabetes, stroke (doubled), vascular disease, age 65–74, and sex category (female); VKA, Vitamin K antagonist; VTE, venous thromboembolism.

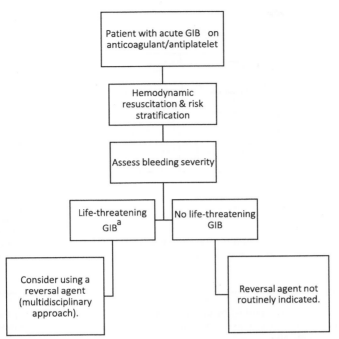

Fig. 1. Systematic approach to patients with acute gastrointestinal bleeding on antiplatelet or anticoagulant. GIB, gastrointestinal bleeding. [a]Life-threatening GIB is defined as overt or apparent bleeding with severe hypotension or hypovolemic shock that requires pressors or surgery, is associated with ≥ 5 g/dL drop in hemoglobin, requires ≥ 5 units of packed red blood cells, or is at risk of causing death[2].

volume of fluid required for resuscitation showed no difference in mortality between restrictive resuscitation (delayed or smaller volume of fluid) versus aggressive resuscitation (early or larger volume of fluid).[3] Thus, the main target of resuscitation is to normalize blood pressure and heart rate while minimizing bleeding before the endoscopic procedure.[3] Some patients require blood transfusions, which have been associated with a lower risk of rebleeding and death than no transfusion.[5-8] In upper GIB (UGIB) in patients without cardiovascular disease, a restrictive transfusion threshold for a Hg level of 7 g/dL improves survival and decreases rebleeding compared to a more liberal threshold (9 g/dL).[9] However, patients with a history of acute coronary syndrome, peripheral vascular disease, cerebrovascular disease, and massive bleeding were excluded from these studies. Therefore, these patients may benefit from a higher transfusion threshold of 9 to 10 g/dL.[10]

Management of Antithrombotic Medications in the Setting of Acute Bleeding

In patients presenting with GIB while on an anticoagulant, it is important to assess the bleeding severity, as it will guide further management and determine the consideration of using a reversal agent. The use of reversal agents is reserved for patients presenting with a life-threatening bleed (hypotension requiring pressors, a drop in Hg ≥ 5 g/dL, transfusion ≥ 5 units of pRBC, or at risk of causing death) (**Fig. 2**).[2]

The following sections summarize the most recent guidelines for managing antithrombotic medications in GIB (**Tables 2 and 3**).[2]

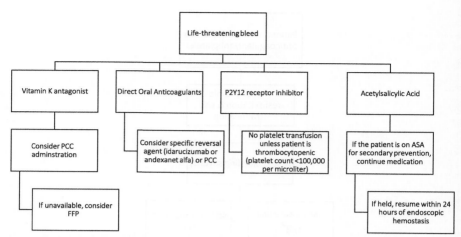

Fig. 2. Approach to antithrombotic medications in the setting of gastrointestinal bleeding. ASA, acetylsalicylic acid; FFP, fresh frozen plasma; PCC, prothrombin complex concentrate.

Table 2
Summary of evidence established by the American College of Gastroenterology-Canadian Association of Gastroenterology on the management of anticoagulants in the setting of acute gastrointestinal bleeding

	Anticoagulant management in the setting of acute gastrointestinal bleed	
Medication	**Approach to anticoagulant management**	**Level of recommendation**
Vitamin K antagonist: warfarin	Avoid routine FFP or vitamin K administration. However, in the setting of a life-threatening hemorrhage[a], PCC is preferred.	Conditional recommendation, low certainty of evidence.
Direct oral anticoagulants	Guidelines recommend against routine PCC administration, may be considered in the setting of a life-threatening hemorrhage.	Conditional recommendation, low certainty of evidence.
Thrombin inhibitor: dabigatran	Guidelines recommend against routine idarucizumab administration; it can be considered in the setting of life-threatening hemorrhage if dabigatran has been taken within 24 h.	Conditional recommendation, low certainty of evidence.
Factor Xa inhibitor: rivaroxaban, apixaban	Guidelines recommend against routine andexanet alfa administration. However, its use could be considered in the setting of life-threatening hemorrhage when the drug was taken within 24 h.	Conditional recommendation, low certainty of evidence.

Abbreviations: FFP, fresh frozen plasma; PCC, prothrombin complex concentrate.
   [a] Life-threatening hemorrhage is defined as overt or apparent bleeding with severe hypotension or hypovolemic shock that requires pressors or surgery, is associated with ≥ 5 g/dL drop in hemoglobin, requires ≥ 5 units of packed red blood cells, or is at risk of causing death.[2]

Table 3
Summary of evidence established by the American College of Gastroenterology-Canadian Association of Gastroenterology on the management of antiplatelet in the setting of acute gastrointestinal bleeding

Medication	Approach to antiplatelet management	Level of recommendation
Antiplatelet management in the setting of acute gastrointestinal bleed		
$P2Y_{12}$ receptor antagonist: clopidogrel, prasugrel, ticagrelor	Guidelines recommend against platelet transfusion unless thrombocytopenic (<100,000 g/dl)	Conditional recommendation, low certainty of evidence
Platelet cyclooxygenase-1 inhibitor: acetylsalicylic acid	If for secondary prevention, continue medication. If held, guidelines suggest resumption the day homeostasis is confirmed.	Conditional recommendation, low certainty of evidence.

Vitamin K antagonists

In patients presenting with a life-threatening GIB while on a VKA, options for reversal agents include prothrombin complex concentrate (PCC), fresh frozen plasma (FFP), and vitamin K. According to the joint American College of Gastroenterology (ACG)-Canadian Association of Gastroenterology guidelines,[2] administering PCC is preferred due to its efficacy in providing rapid and reliable correction of international normalized ratio (INR) and decreased volume of administration.[11–15] Compared to FFP, PCC was associated with a lower risk of thromboembolic complications[16] and reduced all-cause mortality.[17] FFP is not routinely recommended due to the low certainty of evidence to infer positive effects, cost, and possible risk of infection transmission.[2,11,15,18–20] However, it may be considered in patients experiencing life-threatening bleeding with a supratherapeutic INR in whom massive blood transfusion is undesirable or when PCC is unavailable.[2] Vitamin K administration (intramuscularly or intravenously) is not recommended due to its delayed onset of action in achieving rapid hemostasis and its limited value in the acute setting.[21] It may be administered in patients with a supratherapeutic INR if the aim is to reverse the VKA over an extended period or if the plan is to stop the VKA altogether.[2] The authors do not recommend the latter be done without consultation with the patient's hematologist or cardiologist.

Before the endoscopic procedure, temporary interruption of warfarin without heparin bridging is advised. Bridging with heparin has been linked to an increased risk of postprocedural bleeding without improved cardiac outcomes, as shown in the BRIDGE (Perioperative Bridging Anticoagulation in Patients with Atrial Fibrillation)[22] and PERIOP2 (Postoperative Low Molecular Weight Heparin Bridging Therapy for Patients Who Are at High Risk for Arterial Thromboembolism)[23] trials. However, periprocedural bridging may be appropriate in patients at high risk of thromboembolic events, such as those with atrial fibrillation and a $CHADS_2$ (congestive heart failure, hypertension, age $\geq$75 years, diabetes mellitus, prior stroke or transient ischemic attack or thromboembolism) score of 5 or 6, mechanical valves, or a history of prior thromboembolism during temporary VKA interruption (see **Table 1**). In these high-risk cases, consultation with a hematologist or cardiologist is advised for the periprocedural management of warfarin.[2] If interrupted, the timing of VKA resumption is guided by achieving adequate endoscopic hemostasis and the patient's estimated risk of thrombosis with temporary interruption of the VKA.

Direct oral anticoagulants

In patients presenting with GIB, holding the direct oral anticoagulant (DOAC) on admission and providing adequate resuscitation are recommended, as the kidneys quickly excrete the drug in patients without renal dysfunction. If the patient is experiencing a life-threatening hemorrhage, a reversal agent may be necessary. DOAC-specific reversal agents, such as idarucizumab for dabigatran and andexanet alfa for rivaroxaban or apixaban, are available to counter the effects of DOACs. However, the routine use of these agents for acute GIB is not supported due to their high cost, risk of thromboembolic consequences, and lack of clear benefits in all patients experiencing GIB.[24] PCC, idarucizumab, or andexanet alfa administration may be considered for patients who have taken DOACs within 24 hours and present with a life-threatening bleed.[2]

Due to the lack of published data in the GIB literature, there are no specific recommendations for restarting DOACs on the same day or the ideal period of delay to resumption after endoscopic hemostasis.[2] The decision to resume the medication should consider the onset of action of the DOAC, the patient's risk of thrombosis, the potential for delayed bleeding, patient preferences, and consultation with the patient's cardiologist or hematologist. Generally, it is safe to restart the DOAC the day after an endoscopic procedure with a low risk of postprocedural bleeding and within 48 hours of a procedure with a higher risk of postprocedural bleeding.[25]

Antiplatelet agents

For patients on dual antiplatelet therapy (ASA and a $P2Y_{12}$ inhibitor), holding the P2Y12 inhibitor agent and continuing ASA are recommended.[2] Given ASA's pharmacodynamic profile of irreversible inhibition of cyclooxygenase 1,[26,27] the interruption of ASA would have a minimal clinical impact during the acute bleeding episode due to the persistent antiplatelet effect. Additionally, studies have demonstrated a significant reduction in mortality and cardiovascular complications for patients who continued ASA.[28,29] If ASA was held, it should be resumed within 24 hours of successful endoscopic hemostasis in most patients. $P2Y_{12}$ inhibitor should be resumed within 5 days of endoscopic hemostasis in patients at high risk of stent thrombosis (stent placed within a year).[30] For patients taking ASA for primary prevention of cardiovascular disease, it should be permanently discontinued as studies have shown there is a minimal cardiovascular benefit and a significant risk of GIB.[2,31,32]

For patients presenting with GIB while on an antiplatelet, the 2022 ACG multidisciplinary guideline[2] does not recommend platelet transfusion as several studies demonstrate an increased mortality risk with platelet transfusion and a lack of clear benefit in the reduction of bleeding.[33] No current data are available to guide the transfusion threshold in thrombocytopenic patients. However, it is recommended to maintain a platelet count of greater than 30×10^9/L and a higher transfusion threshold of greater than 50×10^9/L if an invasive procedure is required.[34]

Timing of the Endoscopy

The ACG guideline conditionally recommends that patients admitted to the hospital or under observation for UGIB undergo endoscopy within 24 hours from the presentation.[35] In patients with hemodynamic instability and significant comorbidities (American Society of Anesthesiologists score 3–5), resuscitation and stabilization of other comorbidities should take precedence over endoscopy. Very early endoscopy could harm high-risk patients with limited benefit due to inadequate resuscitation.[35] In hemodynamically stable patients, endoscopic intervention is recommended as soon as possible within normal daytime hours to allow for early discharge and reduce the length of hospitalization.[36,37] The American Society of Gastrointestinal Endoscopy also suggests that endoscopic therapy should not be delayed in patients with an INR of less than 2.5 with serious GIB, as endoscopic hemostasis is effective even with a moderately elevated INR ($\leq$2.5).[38]

For lower GIB (LGIB), randomized controlled trials showed that early colonoscopy (<24 hours) was associated with a higher incidence of recurrent bleeding and hospital admissions compared to standard colonoscopy (within 24–72 hours).[39] Therefore, the most recent guideline published by Sengupta and colleagues recommends nonemergent inpatient colonoscopy for LGIB.[40] Urgent colonoscopy may be considered in certain high-risk patients with a high pretest probability to detect stigmata of recent hemorrhage and perform an endoscopic intervention.[40]

Prevention of Antithrombotic-Related Gastrointestinal Bleeding

Risk factors for bleeding
Understanding the risk factors predisposing patients to an increased risk of bleeding may facilitate the effective implementation of preventive measures. Regardless of the patient's cardiovascular condition and antithrombic drug strategy, advancing age is linked with the greatest risk of GIB at 1 year (up to 10% per year).[1] Additionally, combining antithrombotic agents further increases the risk of antithrombotic-related GIB.[1] The probability of bleeding increases to 17.5% per year if both risk factors are present (age >75 years and on several antithrombotic agents).[1] Therefore, awareness of these risk factors and reduction in the overall burden of antithrombotic medications in those at greatest risk are encouraged to prevent future GIB.

Proton pump inhibitors
Current guidelines recommend high-dose proton pump inhibitors (PPIs) to reduce the risk of bleeding and mortality after endoscopic hemostatic therapy.[41–43] The recommended dose is $\geq$ 80 mg per day for a minimum of 3 days, either continuously (80 mg bolus followed by 8 mg/hr) or intermittently (80 mg bolus followed by 40 mg twice daily).[35] The choice between continuous and intermittent dosing depends on cost and ease of administration. PPIs help prevent bleeding at preexisting lesions by suppressing acid production, promoting healing, and stabilizing blood clots.[44] After the initial 3-day high-dose PPI treatment, it is recommended to transition to oral PPI therapy twice daily for 2 weeks (days 4–14) to reduce rebleeding risk.[35]

Patients prescribed chronic antiplatelet or anticoagulant therapy should continue taking PPIs indefinitely, as studies have shown PPI prophylaxis reduces the risk of future bleeding.[45–48] PPIs were also shown in the OBERON (Esomeprazole for Prevention and Resolution of Upper Gastrointestinal Symptoms in Patients Treated with Low-Dose Acetylsalicylic Acid for Cardiovascular Protection) trial to protect the gastrointestinal tract and prevent gastroesophageal/dyspeptic symptoms in patients taking chronic ASA.[49]

Avoiding nonsteroidal anti-inflammatory drugs
In patients with a history of GIB, nonsteroidal anti-inflammatory drugs (NSAIDs) should be avoided as they increase the risk of both incident and recurrent bleeding.[50–52] As previously discussed, ASA for secondary prevention should be continued in patients with established cardiovascular disease, as its discontinuation is associated with increased mortality and cardiovascular and cerebrovascular complications.[28] In patients on chronic ASA therapy for secondary cardiac prevention, gastroprotection with a PPI is taken once daily on an empty stomach 30 to 60 minutes before breakfast to optimize the gastroprotective effect. ASA prescribed for primary cardiovascular

prevention is discouraged because of a lack of benefit and higher risk of GIB in most, and should be discontinued.[31,32]

Avoidance of concomitant antithrombotic administration

The concurrent use of anticoagulants and antiplatelets increases bleeding risk compared to monotherapy with either an anticoagulant or an antiplatelet drug.[1] To decrease the risk of future GIB, it is important to periodically review the rationale for prescription and re-evaluate the risk-to-benefit ratio of continued use for each patient. Reducing the overall burden of antithrombotic agents will decrease the risk of GIB complications.

Eradication of Helicobacter pylori

Testing for and treating *Helicobacter pylori* is indicated in patients with active peptic ulcer disease (PUD), a history of PUD (unless *H.pylori* cure has been documented), and in patients on long-term low-dose ASA or chronic treatment with NSAIDs to decrease the risk of bleeding.[53] In patients who do not require endoscopy, a urease breath test or stool antigen is highly sensitive and specific for *H pylori* testing. Invasive endoscopic testing (biopsy urease test or biopsy for histology) may be performed if the patient undergoes endoscopy for other symptom evaluation. Before noninvasive testing, the patient should be advised to stop PPI therapy for 2 weeks. The treatment regimen of choice will depend on the history of antibiotic exposure, local resistance patterns, allergies, local prevalence of *H pylori*, and cost. Due to the rising antibiotic resistance, testing for eradication at least 4 weeks after completing treatment is important.[53] Eradication could be confirmed with a urea breath test, stool antigen testing, or endoscopy-based testing. Serology use is not advised as antibodies persist following eradication.[54] Before testing for *H pylori* eradication, PPIs should be held for 2 weeks to decrease false negative test results.[53]

SUMMARY

The incidence of GIB among patients taking antithrombotic therapy can range from 4% to 17%, depending on the type of antithrombotic therapy (monotherapy vs combination therapy) and the patient's age. The first step in managing acute GIB is to provide adequate resuscitation before endoscopy. In patients with a life-threatening anticoagulant-related GIB (hypotension requiring pressors, transfusion $\geq$ 5 units of pRBC, a drop in Hg $\geq$ 5 g/dL, or at risk of causing death), the use of an anticoagulant reversal agent may be considered. Transfusion of platelets is not recommended in patients on antiplatelet agents due to an increased risk of mortality. Platelet transfusion can be considered if the patient is thrombocytopenic. Strategies such as PPI use, reducing concomitant antithrombotic use, avoiding NSAIDs, and eradicating *H pylori* infection should be considered to prevent future GIB.

CLINICS CARE POINTS

- A reversal agent may be considered in a life-threatening anticoagulant-related gastrointestinal hemorrhage. For warfarin, PCC is the preferred agent. PCC may also be considered for DOAC reversal. The routine administration of andexanet alfa for rivaroxaban and idarucizumab for dabigatran is not recommended.

- The transfusion of platelets is not recommended due to a higher risk of mortality unless the patient is significantly thrombocytopenic.

- ASA prescribed for secondary cardiac prevention should not be interrupted.

- Endoscopy should be performed after achieving adequate resuscitation.

- Measures to prevent antithrombotic-related GIB include the prescription of PPI; avoidance of concomitant antithrombotic administration, especially in the elderly population; avoidance of NSAIDs; and ensuring *H pylori* eradication in high-risk patients.

DISCLOSURE

The authors report no conflict of interest.

REFERENCES

1. Abraham NS, Noseworthy PA, Inselman J, et al. Risk of Gastrointestinal Bleeding Increases With Combinations of Antithrombotic Agents and Patient Age. Clin Gastroenterol Hepatol 2020;18(2):337–46.e19.
2. Abraham NS, Barkun AN, Sauer BG, et al. American College of Gastroenterology-Canadian Association of Gastroenterology Clinical Practice Guideline: Management of anticoagulants and antiplatelets during acute gastrointestinal bleeding and the periendoscopic period. Am J Gastroenterol 2022;117(4):542–58.
3. Kwan I, Bunn F, Roberts I. Timing and volume of fluid administration for patients with bleeding. Cochrane Database Syst Rev 2003;3. https://doi.org/10.1002/14651858.CD002245.
4. Perel P, Roberts I, Ker K. Colloids versus crystalloids for fluid resuscitation in critically ill patients. Cochrane Database Syst Rev 2013;2013(2). https://doi.org/10.1002/14651858.CD000567.PUB6.
5. Jairath V, Hearnshaw S, Brunskill SJ, et al. Red cell transfusion for the management of upper gastrointestinal haemorrhage. Cochrane Database Syst Rev 2010;9. https://doi.org/10.1002/14651858.CD006613.PUB3.
6. Blair SD, Janvrin SB, McCollum CN. Effect of early blood transfusion on gastrointestinal haemorrhage. Br J Surg 1986;73(10):783–5.
7. Elizalde JI, Moitinho E, García-Pagán JC, et al. Effects of increasing blood hemoglobin levels on systemic hemodynamics of acutely anemic cirrhotic patients. J Hepatol 1998;29(5):789–95.
8. Hearnshaw SA, Logan RFA, Palmer KR, et al. Outcomes following early red blood cell transfusion in acute upper gastrointestinal bleeding. Aliment Pharmacol Ther 2010;32(2):215–24.
9. Villanueva C, Colomo A, Bosch A, et al. Transfusion strategies for acute upper gastrointestinal bleeding. N Engl J Med 2013;368(1):11–21.
10. Strate LL, Gralnek IM. ACG Clinical Guideline: Management of Patients With Acute Lower Gastrointestinal Bleeding. Am J Gastroenterol 2016;111(4):459–74.
11. Sarode R, Milling TJ, Refaai MA, et al. Efficacy and safety of a 4-factor prothrombin complex concentrate in patients on vitamin K antagonists presenting with major bleeding: a randomized, plasma-controlled, phase IIIb study. Circulation 2013;128(11):1234–43.
12. Karaca MA, Erbil B, Ozmen MM. Use and effectiveness of prothrombin complex concentrates vs fresh frozen plasma in gastrointestinal hemorrhage due to warfarin usage in the ED. Am J Emerg Med 2014;32(6):660–4.
13. Lubetsky A, Hoffman R, Zimlichman R, et al. Efficacy and safety of a prothrombin complex concentrate (Octaplex®) for rapid reversal of oral anticoagulation. Thromb Res 2004;113(6):371–8.
14. Vigué B, Ract C, Tremey B, et al. Ultra-rapid management of oral anticoagulant therapy-related surgical intracranial hemorrhage. Intensive Care Med 2007;33(4):721–5.

15. Steiner T, Poli S, Griebe M, et al. Fresh frozen plasma versus prothrombin complex concentrate in patients with intracranial haemorrhage related to vitamin K antagonists (INCH): a randomised trial. Lancet Neurol 2016;15(6):566–73.

16. Brekelmans MPA, van Ginkel K, Daams JG, et al. Benefits and harms of 4-factor prothrombin complex concentrate for reversal of vitamin K antagonist associated bleeding: a systematic review and meta-analysis. J Thromb Thrombolysis 2017; 44(1):118–29.

17. Chai-Adisaksopha C, Hillis C, Siegal DM, et al. Prothrombin complex concentrates versus fresh frozen plasma for warfarin reversal. A systematic review and meta-analysis. Thromb Haemostasis 2016;116(5):879–90.

18. Makris M, Greaves M, Phillips WS, et al. Emergency oral anticoagulant reversal: the relative efficacy of infusions of fresh frozen plasma and clotting factor concentrate on correction of the coagulopathy. Thromb Haemostasis 1997;77(3):477–80.

19. Moustafa F, Stehouwer A, Kamphuisen P, et al. Management and outcome of major bleeding in patients receiving vitamin K antagonists for venous thromboembolism. Thromb Res 2018;171:74–80.

20. Boulis NM, Bobek MP, Schmaier A, et al. Use of factor IX complex in warfarin-related intracranial hemorrhage. Neurosurgery 1999;45(5):1113–9.

21. Holbrook A, Schulman S, Witt DM, et al. Evidence-based management of anticoagulant therapy: Antithrombotic Therapy and Prevention of Thrombosis, 9th ed: American College of Chest Physicians Evidence-Based Clinical Practice Guidelines. Chest 2012;141(2 Suppl):e152S–84S.

22. Douketis JD, Spyropoulos AC, Kaatz S, et al. Perioperative Bridging Anticoagulation in Patients with Atrial Fibrillation. N Engl J Med 2015;373(9):823–33.

23. Kovacs MJ, Wells PS, Anderson DR, et al. Postoperative low molecular weight heparin bridging treatment for patients at high risk of arterial thromboembolism (PERIOP2): double blind randomised controlled trial. BMJ 2021;373. https://doi.org/10.1136/BMJ.N1205.

24. Abramowicz M, Zuccotti G, Pflomm JM. Andexxa-an antidote for apixaban and rivaroxaban. JAMA, J Am Med Assoc 2018;320(4):399–400.

25. Douketis JD, Spyropoulos AC, Duncan J, et al. Perioperative Management of Patients With Atrial Fibrillation Receiving a Direct Oral Anticoagulant. JAMA Intern Med 2019;179(11):1469–78.

26. Santilli F, Rocca B, De Cristofaro R, et al. Platelet cyclooxygenase inhibition by low-dose aspirin is not reflected consistently by platelet function assays: implications for aspirin "resistance". J Am Coll Cardiol 2009;53(8):667–77.

27. Becker RC, Scheiman J, Dauerman HL, et al. Management of platelet-directed pharmacotherapy in patients with atherosclerotic coronary artery disease undergoing elective endoscopic gastrointestinal procedures. J Am Coll Cardiol 2009; 54(24):2261–76.

28. Sung JJY, Lau JYW, Ching JYL, et al. Continuation of low-dose aspirin therapy in peptic ulcer bleeding: a randomized trial. Ann Intern Med 2010;152(1):1–9.

29. Cheung J, Rajala J, Moroz D, et al. Acetylsalicylic acid use in patients with acute myocardial infarction and peptic ulcer bleeding. Can J Gastroenterol 2009;23(9): 619–23.

30. Eisenberg MJ, Richard PR, Libersan D, et al. Safety of short-term discontinuation of antiplatelet therapy in patients with drug-eluting stents. Circulation 2009; 119(12):1634–42.

31. McNeil JJ, Wolfe R, Woods RL, et al. Effect of Aspirin on Cardiovascular Events and Bleeding in the Healthy Elderly. N Engl J Med 2018;379(16):1509–18.

32. Gaziano JM, Brotons C, Coppolecchia R, et al. Use of aspirin to reduce risk of initial vascular events in patients at moderate risk of cardiovascular disease (ARRIVE): a randomised, double-blind, placebo-controlled trial. Lancet (London, England) 2018;392(10152):1036–46.

33. Platelet transfusions during coronary artery bypass graft surgery are associated with serious adverse outcomes. https://oce.ovid.com/article/00007885-200408000-00005. Accessed January 29, 2023.

34. Padhi S, Kemmis-Betty S, Rajesh S, et al, Guideline Development Group. Blood transfusion: summary of NICE guidance. BMJ 2015;351. https://doi.org/10.1136/BMJ.H5832.

35. Laine L, Barkun AN, Saltzman JR, et al. ACG Clinical Guideline: Upper Gastrointestinal and Ulcer Bleeding. Am J Gastroenterol 2021;116(5):899–917.

36. Bjorkman DJ, Zaman A, Fennerty MB, et al. Urgent vs. elective endoscopy for acute non-variceal upper-GI bleeding: an effectiveness study. Gastrointest Endosc 2004;60(1):1–8.

37. Lee JG, Turnipseed S, Romano PS, et al. Endoscopy-based triage significantly reduces hospitalization rates and costs of treating upper GI bleeding: a randomized controlled trial. Gastrointest Endosc 1999;50(6):755–61.

38. Acosta RD, Abraham NS, Chandrasekhara V, et al. The management of antithrombotic agents for patients undergoing GI endoscopy. Gastrointest Endosc 2016;83(1):3–16.

39. Van Rongen I, Thomassen BJW, Perk LE. Early Versus Standard Colonoscopy: A Randomized Controlled Trial in Patients With Acute Lower Gastrointestinal Bleeding: Results of the BLEED Study. J Clin Gastroenterol 2019;53(8):591–8.

40. Sengupta N, Feuerstein JD, Jairath V, et al. Management of Patients With Acute Lower Gastrointestinal Bleeding: An Updated ACG Guideline. Am J Gastroenterol 2023;118(2):208–31.

41. Zargar SA, Javid G, Khan BA, et al. Pantoprazole infusion as adjuvant therapy to endoscopic treatment in patients with peptic ulcer bleeding: prospective randomized controlled trial. J Gastroenterol Hepatol 2006;21(4):716–21.

42. Wei KL, Tung SY, Sheen CH, et al. Effect of oral esomeprazole on recurrent bleeding after endoscopic treatment of bleeding peptic ulcers. J Gastroenterol Hepatol 2007;22(1):43–6.

43. JY L, JJ S, KK L, et al. Effect of intravenous omeprazole on recurrent bleeding after endoscopic treatment of bleeding peptic ulcers. N Engl J Med 2000;343(5):130–2.

44. Abraham NS, Hlatky MA, Antman EM, et al. ACCF/ACG/AHA 2010 Expert Consensus Document on the Concomitant Use of Proton Pump Inhibitors and Thienopyridines: A Focused Update of the ACCF/ACG/AHA 2008 Expert Consensus Document on Reducing the Gastrointestinal Risks of Antiplatelet Therapy and NSAID Use. Circulation 2010;122(24):2619–33.

45. Ray WA, Chung CP, Murray KT, et al. Association of Proton Pump Inhibitors With Reduced Risk of Warfarin-Related Serious Upper Gastrointestinal Bleeding. Gastroenterology 2016;151(6):1105–12.e10.

46. Lin KJ, Hernándezdíaz S, García Rodríguez LA. Acid suppressants reduce risk of gastrointestinal bleeding in patients on antithrombotic or anti-inflammatory therapy. Gastroenterology 2011;141(1):71–9.

47. Chan EW, Lau WCY, Leung WK, et al. Prevention of Dabigatran-Related Gastrointestinal Bleeding With Gastroprotective Agents: A Population-Based Study. Gastroenterology 2015;149(3):586–95.

48. Barkun AN, Almadi M, Kuipers EJ, et al. Management of Nonvariceal Upper Gastrointestinal Bleeding: Guideline Recommendations From the International Consensus Group. Ann Intern Med 2019;171(11):805.

49. Scheiman JM, Herlitz J, Veldhuyzen Van Zanten SJ, et al. Esomeprazole for prevention and resolution of upper gastrointestinal symptoms in patients treated with low-dose acetylsalicylic acid for cardiovascular protection: the OBERON trial. J Cardiovasc Pharmacol 2013;61(3):250–7.

50. Yuhara H, Corley DA, Nakahara F, et al. Aspirin and non-aspirin NSAIDs increase risk of colonic diverticular bleeding: A systematic review and meta-analysis. J Gastroenterol 2014;49(6):992–1000.

51. Aoki T, Nagata N, Niikura R, et al. Recurrence and mortality among patients hospitalized for acute lower gastrointestinal bleeding. Clin Gastroenterol Hepatol 2015;13(3):488–94.e1.

52. Nagata N, Niikura R, Aoki T, et al. Impact of discontinuing non-steroidal anti-inflammatory drugs on long-term recurrence in colonic diverticular bleeding. World J Gastroenterol 2015;21(4):1292–8.

53. Chey WD, Leontiadis GI, Howden CW, et al. ACG Clinical Guideline: Treatment of *Helicobacter pylori* Infection. Am J Gastroenterol 2017;112(2):212–38.

54. Cutler AF, Prasad VM, Santogade P. Four-year trends in *Helicobacter pylori* IgG serology following successful eradication. Am J Med 1998;105(1):18–20.

Endoscopic Diagnosis, Grading, and Treatment of Bleeding Peptic Ulcer Disease

Nimish Vakil, MD*

KEYWORDS

- Peptic ulcer disease • Gastrointestinal hemorrhage • Proton pump inhibitor
- H pylori • Over-the-scope clips • Hemostatic powders

KEY POINTS

- Endoscopic therapy is indicated in Forrest 1a, 1b, and 2a lesions.
- Patients with Forrest 2b lesions may do well with proton-pump inhibitor therapy alone.
- Intravenous proton-pump inhibitor therapy reduces the need for endoscopic intervention at index endoscopy.
- Failure to treat *Helicobacter pylori* results in rebleeding.
- Over-the-scope clips and hemostatic sprays are new developments that may affect future management.

INTRODUCTION

An accurate endoscopic diagnosis and grading can direct appropriate therapy in bleeding peptic ulcer disease. The initial goal is to stabilize the patient and has been covered elsewhere. An accurate endoscopic diagnosis and classification allows appropriate patients to be discharged early and identifies high-risk patients who need hospital care and patients who are at risk for rebleeding and bleeding relayed morbidity and mortality. Endoscopic grading prevents unnecessary endoscopic intervention in patients who do not need it and allows selection of the appropriate endoscopic tool in patients needing intervention. Several recent guidelines summarize the available evidence and offer guidance for clinical practice.[1–5] Despite advances in pharmacotherapy and endoscopic therapy, the mortality rate remains at 10%.[6] Optimizing endoscopic intervention in gastrointestinal bleeding could reduce mortality in the years to come.

TIMING OF ENDOSCOPY

The pressure to perform endoscopy in unstable patients with peptic ulcer bleeding has been replaced by a more measured process that has improved outcomes for patients.

Competing interests: Consultant Phathom Pharmaceuticals, Isothrive.
University of Wisconsin School of Medicine and Public Health, Madison, WI, USA
* W231N1440 Corporate Ct, Waukesha, WI 53186.
E-mail address: nvakil@wisc.edu

Gastrointest Endoscopy Clin N Am 34 (2024) 217–229
https://doi.org/10.1016/j.giec.2023.09.003
giendo.theclinics.com

Endoscopy may be performed emergently (<6 hours), early (6–24 hours), and electively (beyond 24 hours). In a meta-analysis of studies available in 2001, we concluded that the evidence although limited in quality suggested that endoscopy performed within 24 hours of admission should become a standard of care.[7] We also recommended that a randomized controlled trial of urgent endoscopy was needed to guide management further. This need has recently been met in a randomized controlled trial of patients who presented with acute upper gastrointestinal tract bleeding and were at high risk for further bleeding or death based on a Glasgow-Blatchford score greater than 12.[8] Patients were randomized to urgent (within 6 hours) or early endoscopy (6–24 hours) after gastroenterology consultation. The primary end point was death from any cause within 30 days of admission. Urgent endoscopy was not associated with a lower mortality than endoscopy performed 6 to 24 hours after gastroenterology consultation. Further bleeding within 30 days occurred in 11% of patients in the urgent endoscopy group and in 8% in the early-endoscopy group (not significantly different). The study was performed at a single university hospital with a large experience in gastrointestinal (GI) bleeding. Their results may not be generalizable to a community hospital setting. Another large retrospective study evaluated patients at all public hospitals in Hong Kong undergoing therapy for GI bleeding[9]; 6474 adult patients who presented with acute upper GI bleeding between 2013 and 2019 and received therapeutic endoscopy within 48 hours were recruited. Patients were classified based on the timing of endoscopy following admission: urgent (≤6 hours), early (6–24 hours), and late (24–48 hours). One thousand eight patients had urgent endoscopy and had significantly higher 30-day all-cause mortality, repeat endoscopy and intensice care unit (ICU) admission rates compared with the 3865 patients who underwent early endoscopy; 1601 patients had late endoscopy and this group also had worse outcomes compared with early endoscopy, with higher 30-day mortality, in-hospital mortality, and 30-day transfusion rates.

INTRAVENOUS PROTON PUMP INHIBITOR THERAPY BEFORE ENDOSCOPY

The ESGE recommends a bolus (80 mg) followed by a continuous infusion (8 mg/h) of proton-pump inhibitor in patients presenting with upper GI bleeding who are awaiting endoscopy.[2] The authors of the American College of Gastroenterology (ACG) guideline were unable to reach a conclusion regarding pre-endoscopic proton-pump inhibitor therapy.[4] However, they recommend high-dose proton pump inhibitor (PPI) therapy given continuously or intermittently for 3 days after successful endoscopic hemostatic therapy of a bleeding ulcer. Intravenous PPI therapy is typically started in the emergency room in most US hospitals in patients with upper GI bleeding. A Cochrane meta-analysis of six randomized controlled trials that included 2223 patients showed that administering PPIs before endoscopy significantly decreases the finding of high-risk stigmata of ulcer bleeding at the index endoscopy and the need for endoscopic hemostasis drops to 8.6% compared 11.7% without PPI therapy (odds ratio 0.68, 95%CI 0.50–0.93).[10] PPIs had has no effect on rebleeding rates or the need for surgery. Mortality was unchanged. In patients with low-risk lesions, intravenous PPI therapy can be discontinued immediately after endoscopy. In contrast, patients with high-risk lesions who undergo endoscopic therapy and receive intravenous PPI therapy for 3 days should receive twice daily PPI therapy for 2 weeks.

PROKINETICS BEFORE ENDOSCOPY

The American College of Gastroenterology and the European Society of Gastrointestinal endoscopy guidelines recommend the use of erythromycin intravenously before endoscopy to simulate gastric emptying.[2,4] Stimulating gastric emptying clears blood and clots from the endoscopic field and enhances visualization and may improve the accuracy of endoscopic therapy. The usual dose is 250 mg administered intravenously 30 to 120 minutes before endoscopy.

ENDOSCOPIC CLASSIFICATION OF PEPTIC ULCER BLEEDING

The Forrest Classification (**Table 1**) is the most widely used and validated classification system for peptic ulcer bleeding. Forrest 1a lesions have the highest risk of rebleeding, and therefore, this classification provides prognostic information that guides therapy.[11] Lesions with active oozing, spurting, and a non-bleeding visible vessel should receive endoscopic therapy. Management strategies are based on the Forrest Classification and are described further below.

ENDOSCOPIC HEMOSTATIC THERAPY IN PATIENTS WITH ACTIVE BLEEDING (OOZING AND SPURTING) OR NON-BLEEDING VISIBLE VESSELS (FORREST 1A, 1B, AND 2A LESIONS)

A meta-analysis of studies that compared endoscopic therapy versus no therapy in patients with active bleeding found a significant reduction in further bleeding in patients who had active bleeding (relative risk 0.29, number needed to treat = 2) and also in patients with non-bleeding visible vessels (relative risk = 0.49, number needed to treat = 5).[12]

The ACG guidelines evaluate the evidence for endoscopic treatments and report that the most robust evidence is for contact thermal devices such as bipolar coagulation or heater probe.[4] Low-quality evidence suggested efficacy for clips, argon plasma coagulation, and soft monopolar electrocoagulation. Oozing and spurting are variously defined in the literature. In some studies, they are grouped together, but others separate oozing lesions from spurting lesions.

ENDOSCOPIC THERAPY FOR ULCERS WITH ADHERENT CLOTS (FORREST 2B LESIONS)

There is uncertainty about whether endoscopic therapy is warranted or needed in patients with adherent clots who are receiving PPI therapy. The ACG guideline could not reach a recommendation for endoscopic therapy in an ulcer with adherent clot despite

Table 1
Forrest classification and risk stratification

Forrest Grade	Endoscopic Finding
High-Risk lesions	
Ia	Active bleeding spurting or pulsatile
IIa	Non-bleeding visible vessel
IIb	Adherent clot
Intermediate-risk	
Ib	Oozing hemorrhage
IIc	Flat spot, dark pigmentation
Low-risk	
III	Clean base

Other high-risk factors for rebleeding. Large ulcers (>2 cm), location on posterior wall of duodenal bulb or high on the lesser curve of the stomach, large diameter visible vessel.

vigorous irrigation.[4] European guidelines offer two options: clot removal with endoscopic hemostasis if high-risk stigmata are found or medical management with high-dose intravenous proton-pump inhibitor therapy.[2] A randomized controlled trial from Hong Kong comparing intravenous PPI therapy to endoscopic intervention in this group of patients found no rebleeding in the intravenous PPI group, suggesting that endoscopic therapy may not be warranted.[13]

ENDOSCOPIC MODALITIES FOR TREATMENT OF PEPTIC ULCER BLEEDING
Injectable Agents

Epinephrine injection and injection of absolute alcohol have both been studied in ulcer bleeding. Rebleeding rates are high when epinephrine is used alone, and therefore, it is most often used in combination with other therapies as described below.[14] Current guidelines recommend against the use of epinephrine as the sole treatment of peptic ulcer bleeding.[2,4] A meta-analysis comparing injection therapy alone to thermal therapy and mechanical clips concluded that injection therapy alone was inferior to both thermal therapy and mechanical clips in achieving hemostasis.[15] For patients with actively bleeding ulcers, the European Society for Gastrointestinal Endoscopy (ESGE) recommends injection with epinephrine and additional therapy with mechanical or thermal devices or injection of a sclerosant.[2] Epinephrine is not recommended as monotherapy because of the high incidence of rebleeding when it is used alone. Some endoscopists use epinephrine in active bleeding to slow the flow of blood and improve visualization, but the submucosal bleb may make clip application difficult. Other endoscopists therefore inject epinephrine after clip placement to prevent further bleeding. A meta-analysis of 17 studies evaluated epinephrine injection in combination with mechanical clips or thermal therapy.[14] The addition of mechanical clips after epinephrine injection significantly reduced the rate of rebleeding and the need for surgery. Epinephrine in conjunction with thermal therapy also reduced the rate of rebleeding significantly, and there was trend toward a reduction in need for surgery.[14] Sclerosant use provided no additional benefit when used with a second modality and had significant side effects. Injection of absolute alcohol to stop bleeding has shown efficacy and is endorsed by the ACG guideline and the ESGE guideline, whereas the use of polidocanol is not recommended.[16]

Thermal Therapies

Contact thermal devices

Thermal treatments include contact devices such as bipolar coagulation probe and heater probe, which is no longer being manufactured. These devices are designed to compress the walls of the vessel in the base of the ulcer bringing the walls of the vessel into apposition. The thermal energy then fuses the walls of the vessel together preventing rebleeding. Thermal energy also promotes clot formation and may coagulate smaller vessels around the major vessel that may contribute to blood loss. Moderate pressure is required to bring the vessel walls into apposition and this can be a disadvantage in patients with deep ulcers where the pressure can lead to perforation. In vitro studies suggest that applying firm pressure for longer periods at low wattage settings is the optimal strategy with bipolar probes.[17] A meta-analysis comparing mechanical clips to thermal coagulation found no significant difference between these modalities in achieving hemostasis.[15]

Monopolar hemostatic forceps with soft coagulation

The technique of soft coagulation was developed to control bleeding after endoscopic submucosal dissection. Soft coagulation uses a lower voltage than bipolar devices and may therefore reduce the risk of perforation. This technique has been studied in the management of peptic ulcer bleeding. Two randomized controlled trials have shown that it is superior to the heater probe in initial hemostasis and prevention of recurrent bleeding.[18,19]

In a randomized controlled trial of patient with Forrest 1a, 1b, and 2a lesions, monopolar hemostatic forceps with soft coagulation were superior to mechanical clips in achieving initial hemostasis and were associated with a shorter procedure time and less recurrent bleeding.[20] Monopolar hemostatic forceps with soft coagulation were non-inferior to argon plasma coagulation in a randomized controlled trial.[21] A meta-analysis of five randomized controlled trials and one observational study suggested found that monopolar forceps with soft coagulation were superior to clips, argon plasma coagulation and the heater probe with higher initial rates of hemostasis, lower rebleeding rates.[22] A relative disadvantage is the high cost of the monopolar forceps.

Noncontact devices

Argon plasma coagulation is the prototype of noncontact agents. Argon is an inert gas that is converted into ionized argon gas by an electrode at the tip of the probe that is passed through the channel of the endoscope. High-energy monopolar current is carried through the argon gas to coagulate tissue.[23] Although the lack of contact is an advantage with small superficial vessels, this technique may be less effective for larger vessels. A randomized controlled trial compared argon plasma coagulation combined with epinephrine injection to heater probe with epinephrine injection and found no significant difference between the two modalities.[24] Another randomized controlled trial compared soft coagulation with epinephrine injection to argon plasma coagulation with epinephrine injection and found no difference in outcomes between the two treatment modalities.[25]

Mechanical clips: through-the-scope clips

Mechanical clips on a delivery catheter are passed through the biopsy channel of the endoscope. The characteristics of different mechanical clips are described in **Table 2**. Through the scope, mechanical clips are effective in stopping bleeding but are difficult to apply when the ulcer base is fibrosed. Some locations are difficult to access with the clips, and these include ulcers located in the fundus on the posterior wall of the duodenum and at the junction of the first and second portion of the duodenum. A meta-analysis evaluated mechanical clips compared with other endoscopic modalities in the management of upper GI bleeding.[26] Through the scope, clips were more effective than epinephrine injection but when compared with thermal therapies, no significant differences in mortality or rebleeding were seen. The evidence is limited by small study size and wide confidence intervals around the point estimates. The ACG guideline provided a conditional recommendation for clip use in ulcer bleeding.[4]

Mechanical clips: over-the-endoscope clips

Over-the-endoscope clips are devices that are attached to the end of the endoscope. **Table 3** describes the characteristics of available over-the-endoscope clips. The mode of action is similar to endoscopic banding. The vessel is drawn into the cup of the device using suction and the clip is deployed. Over-the-endoscope clips have a wider diameter and greater compressive force than through-the-scope clips. These clips were initially developed to close perforations but are now increasingly used in the management of gastrointestinal bleeding.

A meta-analysis of 10 studies, 4 of which were randomized controlled trials compared over-the-endoscope clips with standard endoscopic therapy in patients with high-risk upper GI bleeding and concluded that over-the-endoscope clips had lower 7- and

Table 2
Through-the-scope mechanical clips for endoscopic hemostasis

Name of Clip	Manufacturer Material	Width of Clip	Minimal Channel Size	Ability to Rotate	Compressive Strength of Closed Clip
Resolution 360 and Resolution Ultra	Boston Scientific Steel/cobalt	11 mm and 17 mm	2.8 mm	+++	+++
Instinct Plus	Cook Medical Steel/nitinol	16 mm	2.8 mm	+++	+++
Quick Clip Pro	Olympus Elgiloy	11 mm	2.8 mm	+	+
Dura Clip	ConMed Stainless steel	11 mm and 16 mm	2.8 mm	++	+
Sure Clip	MicroTech Stainless steel	8, 11, 16, and 17 mm	2.8 mm	+	+
Mantis Clip*	Boston Scientific Stainless steel	11 mm	2.8 mm		

* Primarily designed for closure of large defects.

Table 3 Over-the-scope mechanical clips for endoscopic hemostasis					
Name	**Manufacturer**		**Sizes**		
OTSC Clip System	Ovecso	Mini	11 mm	12 mm	14 mm
Endoscope diameter		8.5–10 mm	8.5–11 mm	10.5–12 mm	11.5–14 mm
Depth of cap and clip	3 mm	Not available	11 mm, Type a & t	12 mm Type a & t	14 mm Type a & t
	6 mm	6 mm, Type a, t	11 mm, Type a, t	12 mm, Type a, t, gc	14 mm, Type a, t
Final deployed diameter		14.6 mm	16.5 mm	17.5 mm	21 mm

Name	**Manufacturer**	**Sizes**	
Padlock Clip System	Steris	Small	Large
Endoscope diameter		9.5–11 mm	11.3–14 mm
Final deployed diameter		19 mm	19 mm

Type a: Clip with blunt teeth has a primarily compressive effect.
Type t: Clip with teeth that have small spikes with a compressing and anchoring effect.
Type gc: Elongated teeth with spikes for closure of gastric wall defects.

30-day rebleeding rates with a shorter procedure time and a higher likelihood of success.[26] The precise role of over-the-endoscope clips in the primary treatment of peptic ulcer bleeding remains uncertain, but over-the-scope clips deserve consideration in patients with recurrent ulcer bleeding and in patients with large ulcers with a fibrotic base or locations that make through-the-scope mechanical clips difficult to deploy.

A multicenter randomized controlled trial compared over-the-scope clips with standard endoscopic therapy. Persistent bleeding was significantly higher (14%) in patients treated with standard therapy compared with over-the-scope clips (6%).[27] Over-the-scope clips may therefore have an advantage over standard therapy in the setting of recurrent bleeding after initial hemostasis. Over-the-scope clips were recently compared with standard clips as primary therapy at the index endoscopy in a randomized controlled trial in patients at high risk for rebleeding.[28] Successful endoscopic hemostasis with no evidence of rebleeding was significantly better (91.7%) in the over-the-scope group compared with standard treatment group (73%), most of whom were treated with standard clips. The precise role of over-the-scope clips in the management of upper GI bleeding awaits clarification, but these devices are likely to a major role in the future in recurrent bleeding and perhaps as initial therapy in high-risk patients.

Topical hemostatic sprays

Topical hemostatic sprays are a novel method of treating bleeding lesions in the GI tract (**Table 4**). These sprays do not require precise localization of the bleeding lesion and can be used in situations where the bleeding is massive and the precise site of bleeding cannot be identified. These sprays are also useful in diffuse bleeding such as in malignant ulcers where a precise site for bleeding cannot be identified. The disadvantages of these sprays are that rebleeding can be a problem when the material sloughs off.

TC-325. TC-325 is the best studied hemostatic spray.[29] A meta-analysis of 16 studies reported a high initial hemostasis rate of 94%, but the pooled rebleeding rate at 3 days

Table 4
Hemostatic powders used in GI hemorrhage

Commercial Name Manufacturer, Country	Composition	Mode of Action
Hemospray Cook Medical, USA	Mineral powder delivered through a catheter with a carbon dioxide cartridge to propel powder	Forms an adhesive layer when it comes into contact with fluid. The adhesive layer provides mechanical compression and promotes hemostasis
EndoClot (manufactured by EPI, Santa Clara and distributed by Olympus) USA	Starch-derived polysaccharides delivered through a catheter with an air compressor to propel powder	The powder absorbs water concentrating platelets and clotting factors promoting clotting
Nexpowder Medtronic, USA	Succinic anhydride (ε-poly-L-lysine) and oxidized dextran	Forms mucoadhesive hydrogel to create mechanical barrier on bleeding site
CGEP-003 CGBio, South Korea Korea	Natural polymer with epidermal growth factor	Forms adhesive gel to create mechanical barrier and promote local wound healing pathways
ABS Ankaferd, Turkey	Five herbal extracts	Forms encapsulated protein matrix, leading to erythrocyte aggregation

was 10% and the 30-day rebleeding rate was 18%.[30] Several unusual complications have been reported including perforation, thromboembolic events likely due to embolization of the powder, and impaction of the endoscope due to a coagulum adhering the tip to the mucosa.[31] In a randomized controlled trial of upper GI bleeding, most of whom had gastroduodenal ulcers, Lau and colleagues compared standard endoscopic treatment with TC-325 as initial therapy. The primary outcome was control of bleeding more than 30 days. Initial hemostasis at the index endoscopy was higher with the hemostatic spray and control of bleeding more than the 30-day period was similar in both groups as was the rate of rebleeding. The American College of Gastroenterology guideline suggests that endoscopic hemostatic therapy with TC-325 can be considered with actively bleeding ulcers.[4]

EndoClot. Data on EndoClot are more limited. A study of patients with upper and lower GI bleeding reported an initial hemostasis rate of 64%.[32] A small non-randomized comparison of EndoClot to TC-325 suggests that their efficacy is comparable.[33]

Nexpowder. Much of the information on this powder comes from Korean studies. In a study of 56 patients with non-variceal bleeding from several lesions, including a small group of peptic ulcers, immediate hemostasis was achieved in 96.4% and 30-day rebleeding was surprisingly low at 3.7%.[34] Larger studies in other populations are needed to confirm the low rebleeding rate.

CGEP-003 and ABS Ankaferd are not available in the United States.

DOPPLER-GUIDED THERAPY FOR GASTROINTESTINAL BLEEDING

A through-the-scope Doppler probe can be used to locate the vessel as it makes its way to the ulcer base. The device does not require specialized training in endoscopic ultrasound and identifying the vessel allows therapy to be targeted to the vessel. The

Doppler probe can also be used to demonstrate that flow has decreased or stopped after endoscopic therapy.

A recent systematic review evaluated the evidence and reported that the Doppler endoscopic probe may be better than visual inspection the ulcer alone reducing rebleeding rates and decreasing the need for surgery.[35] The ESGE guideline does not recommend the routine use of the Doppler probe in GI bleeding.[2] Its greatest role may be in patients who have recurrent bleeding after successful initial therapy.

ENDOSCOPIC SUTURING

Endoscopic suturing devices are used to close defects in the GI tract but have also been studied in bleeding. A small international study of 10 patients, most of whom had failed initial endoscopic therapy for bleeding ulcers underwent endoscopic suturing. Immediate hemostasis was 100% and there was no early or late rebleeding.[36] These devices are not widely available and require specialized training and are best used by experts in referral centers.

POST-ENDOSCOPIC MANAGEMENT
Second-Look Endoscopy

Routine second-look endoscopy is not recommended and is reserved for patients with evidence of rebleeding or if the adequacy of initial treatment remains in question.[2]

Proton-Pump Inhibitor Therapy

There is no evidence that continuing intravenous PPI therapy beyond 72 hours offers any additional benefit. Patients are transitioned to oral PPI therapy after 72 hours, and treatment is generally continued for 28 days. A single randomized controlled trial has looked at the dose of PPI therapy after the initial 3-day intravenous infusion.[37] High-dose twice-daily PPI therapy (esomeprazole 40 mg twice a day) reduced rebleeding in high-risk patients compared with once daily therapy. Based on this study, the ACG guideline recommends the use of twice-daily PPI therapy for 2 weeks in patients who received endoscopic therapy for GI bleeding and also in patients with adherent clots who do not receive endoscopic therapy.[4]

Helicobacter pylori Testing and Treatment

Helicobacter pylori testing is recommended at the time of initial endoscopy. Recent studies show that many patients are never tested for H pylori particularly if they were admitted to the ICU at initial hospitalization and these patients have a high rate of rebleeding and death at 1 year.[38] The rapid urease test may be falsely negative in patients with significant amounts of blood in the stomach.[39] A positive test is reliable and should prompt treatment for H pylori before the patient is discharged from the hospital. Histology with immunostaining for H pylori can increase the diagnostic yield in this setting. Serology has been suggested as a supplement to biopsy testing. The rationale is that although serology has a high rate of false positives, serology is not affected by blood in the upper GI tract and a negative serology test provides reassurance that therapy directed at H pylori infection is not needed. Finally, testing can be performed 2 weeks or longer after the episode of bleeding with discontinuation of PPIs for 2 weeks using the urea breath test or the stool antigen test.[40] The problem with delaying diagnosis and treatment for H pylori infection is that many patients do not return for follow-up. Untreated H pylori infection is a significant cause for recurrent bleeding and a missed diagnosis of this infection puts the patient at risk for another bleeding episode and adds to the societal costs of care.[41]

REBLEEDING

Rebleeding is a significant complication of initial endoscopic treatment of ulcer bleeding. A large nationwide study of peptic ulcer bleeding in Denmark from 2006 to 2014 showed that the rebleeding rate was 10.8% and the death rate was 10.2% with rebleeding increasing the mortality rate by greater than twofold.[42] Predictors for rebleeding were endoscopic high-risk stigmata of bleeding, bleeding from duodenal ulcers, and presentation with hemodynamic instability. Among patients with all three risk factors, 24% rebled, 50% with rebleeding failed endoscopic therapy, and 23% died. Patients with these clinical features deserve careful monitoring in the hospital.

ARTIFICIAL INTELLIGENCE AND PEPTIC ULCER BLEEDING

Artificial intelligence and machine learning have the potential to improve outcomes in peptic ulcer bleeding. Although we are in the early stages of the use of artificial intelligence in ulcer bleeding, initial studies suggest that this technology will be of benefit and may play a role in management decisions in the future. Shung and colleagues conducted a large international study to develop a machine learning model to predict the need for transfusion or endoscopic intervention or 1 month mortality.[43] Only non-endoscopic data (demographics, laboratory) were used in the model. The model performed better than established scales (Glasgow-Blatchford score, Rockall Score, and AIM 65) and was a reliable predictor of low-risk patients who could be safely discharged. Preliminary studies based on still images of bleeding ulcers suggest that image analysis may benefit novice endoscopists to evaluate the endoscopic features of an ulcer.

SUMMARY

Peptic ulcer bleeding is a major cause for hospital admissions and has a significant mortality. Endoscopic interventions reduce the risk of rebleeding in high-risk patients and several options are available including injection therapies, thermal therapies, mechanical clips, hemostatic sprays, and endoscopic suturing. Proton-pump inhibitors and *H pylori* treatment are important adjuncts to endoscopic therapy. Endoscopic therapy is indicated in Forrest 1a, 1b, and 2a lesions. Patients with Forrest 2b lesions may do well with proton-pump inhibitor therapy alone but can also be managed by removal of the clot and targeting endoscopic therapy to the underlying lesion. Intravenous PPI therapy reduces the likelihood of endoscopic intervention. Treatment of *H pylori* infection reduces the risk of recurrent bleeding.

CLINICS CARE POINTS

- Endoscopic therapy is indicated in Forrest 1a, 1b, and 2a lesions.
- Patients with Forrest 2b lesions may do well with proton-pump inhibitor therapy alone.
- A variety of endoscopic techniques are available and their use depends on local expertise.
- Intravenous proton-pump inhibitor therapy is indicated in all patients with high-risk lesions.
- High-dose PPI therapy should be continued for 2 weeks in patients who receive endoscopic therapy.
- *H pylori* testing should be performed at initial endoscopy.
- If inconclusive, testing for *H pylori* should be repeated.
- Failure to treat *H pylori* results in rebleeding.

CONFLICT OF INTEREST

None.

REFERENCES

1. Mullady DK, Wang AY, Waschke KA. AGA clinical practice update on endoscopic therapies for non-variceal upper gastrointestinal bleeding: expert review. Gastroenterology 2020;159(3):1120–8. Epub 2020 Jun 20.
2. Gralnek IM, Stanley AJ, Morris AJ, et al. Endoscopic diagnosis and management of nonvariceal upper gastrointestinal hemorrhage (NVUGIH): European Society of Gastrointestinal Endoscopy (ESGE) Guideline- Update 202. Endoscopy 2021; 53(3):300–32.
3. Barkun AN, Almadi M, Kuipers EJ, et al. Management of nonvariceal upper gastrointestinal bleeding: guideline recommendations from the international consensus group. Ann Intern Med 2019;171(11):805–22.
4. Laine L, Barkun AN, Saltzman JR, et al. ACG clinical guideline: upper gastrointestinal and ulcer bleeding. Am J Gastroenterol 2021;116(5):899–917.
5. Kim JS, Kim BW, Kim DH, et al. Guidelines for nonvariceal upper gastrointestinal bleeding. Gut Liver 2020;14(5):560–70.
6. Laine L, Yang H, Chang SC, et al. Trends for incidence of hospitalization and death due to GI complications in the United States from 2001 to 2009. Am J Gastroenterol 2012;107:1190–5.
7. Spiegel BM, Vakil NB, Ofman JJ. Endoscopy for acute nonvarical upper gastrointestinal tract hemorrhage: is sooner better? A systematic review Arch Intern Med 2001;161(11):1393–404.
8. Lau JYW, Yu Y, Tang RSY, et al. Timing of endoscopy for acute upper gastrointestinal bleeding. N Engl J Med 2020;382(14):1299–308.
9. Guo CLT, Wong SH, Lau LHS, et al. Timing of endoscopy for acute upper gastrointestinal bleeding: a territory-wide cohort study. Gut 2022;71(8):1544–50. Epub 2021 Sep 21. PMID: 34548338.
10. Kanno T, Yuan Y, Tse F, et al. Proton pump inhibitor treatment initiated prior to endoscopic diagnosis in upper gastrointestinal bleeding. Cochrane Database Syst Rev 2022;1(1):CD005415.
11. de Groot NL, van Oijen MG, Kessels K, et al. Reassessment of the predictive value of the Forrest classification for peptic ulcer rebleeding and mortality: can classification be simplified? Endoscopy 2014;46(1):46–52. Epub 2013 Nov 11.PMID: 24218308.
12. Laine L, McQuaid KR. Endoscopic therapy for bleeding ulcers: an evidence-based approach based on meta-analyses of randomized controlled trials. Clin Gastroenterol Hepatol 2009;7:33–47.
13. Sung JJ, Chan FK, Lau JY, et al. The effect of endoscopic therapy in patients receiving omeprazole for bleeding ulcers with nonbleeding visible vessels or adherent clots: a randomized comparison. Ann Intern Med 2003;139:237–43.
14. Shi K, Shen Z, Zhu G, et al. Systematic review with network meta-analysis: dual therapy for high-risk bleeding peptic ulcers. BMC Gastroenterol 2017;17(1):55. https://doi.org/10.1186/s12876-017-0610-0.
15. Sung JJ, Tsoi KK, Lai LH, et al. Endoscopic clipping versus injection and thermocoagulation in the treatment of non-variceal upper gastrointestinal bleeding: a meta-analysis. Gut 2007;56(10):1364–73.

16. Nishiaki M, Tada M, Yanai H, et al. Endoscopic hemostasis for bleeding peptic ulcer using a hemostatic clip or pure ethanol injection. Hepato-Gastroenterology 2000;47(34):1042–4.

17. Laine L. Determination of the optimal technique for bipolar electrocoagulation treatment. An experimental evaluation of the BICAP and Gold probes. Gastroenterology 1991;100:107–12.

18. Nunoue T, Takenaka R, Hori K, et al. A randomized trial of monopolar soft-mode coagulation versus heater probe thermocoagulation for peptic ulcer bleeding. J Clin Gastroenterol 2015;49:472–6.

19. Soon M, Wu S, Chen Y, et al. Monopolar coagulation versus conventional endoscopic treatment for high-risk peptic ulcer bleeding: a prospective, randomized study. Gastrointest Endosc 2003;58:323–9.

20. Toka B, Eminler AT, Karacaer C, et al. Comparison of monopolar hemostatic forceps with soft coagulation versus hemoclip for peptic ulcer bleeding: a randomized trial (with video). Gastrointest Endosc 2019;89(4):792–802.

21. Kim JW, Jang JY, Lee CK, et al. Chang YW Comparison of hemostatic forceps with soft coagulation versus argon plasma coagulation for bleeding peptic ulcer. Endoscopy 2015;47(8):680–7.

22. Kamal F, Khan MA, Tariq R, et al. Systematic review and meta-analysis: monopolar hemostatic forceps with soft coagulation in the treatment of peptic ulcer bleeding. Eur J Gastroenterol Hepatol 2020;32(6):678–85.

23. ASGE technology committee, Parsi MA, Schulman AR, Aslanian HR, et al, ASGE Technology Committee Chair. Devices for endoscopic hemostasis of nonvariceal GI bleeding (with videos). VideoGIE 2019;4(7):285–99. PMID: 31334417.

24. Chau CH, Siu WT, Law BK, et al. Randomized controlled trial comparing epinephrine injection plus heat probe coagulation versus epinephrine injection plus argon plasma coagulation for bleeding peptic ulcers. Gastrointest Endosc 2003;57(4):455–61.

25. Kim JW, Jang JY, Lee CK, et al. Comparison of hemostatic forceps with soft coagulation versus argon plasma coagulation for bleeding peptic ulcer–a randomized trial. Endoscopy 2015;47(8):680–7.

26. Bapaye J, Chandan S, Naing L, et al. Safety and efficacy of over-the-scope clips versus standard therapy for high-risk nonvariceal upper GI bleeding: systematic review and meta-analysis Gastrointest. Endosc 2022;96:712–20.

27. Schmidt A, Gölder S, Goetz M, et al. Over-the-scope clips are more effective than standard endoscopic therapy for patients with recurrent bleeding of peptic ulcers. Gastroenterology 2018;155(3):674–86.

28. Meier B, Wannhoff A, Denzer U, et al. Over-the-scope-clips versus standard treatment in high-risk patients with acute non-variceal upper gastrointestinal bleeding: a randomised controlled trial (STING-2). Gut 2022;71(7):1251–8.

29. Chahal D, Lee JGH, Ali-Mohamad N, et al. High rate of re-bleeding after application of Hemospray for upper and lower gastrointestinal bleeds. Dig Liver Dis 2020;52(7):768–72.

30. Chahal D, Sidhu H, Zhao B, et al. Efficacy of Hemospray (TC-325) in the treatment of gastrointestinal bleeding: an updated systematic review and meta-analysis. J Clin Gastroenterol 2021;55(6):492–8.

31. Jiang SX, Chahal D, Ali-Mohamad N, et al. Hemostatic powders for gastrointestinal bleeding: a review of old, new, and emerging agents in a rapidly advancing field. Endosc Int Open 2022;10(8):E1136–46.

32. Prei JC, Barmeyer C, Bürgel N, et al. EndoClot polysaccharide hemostatic system in nonvariceal gastrointestinal bleeding: results of a prospective multicenter observational pilot study. J Clin Gastroenterol 2016;50. e95–e100.
33. Vitali F, Naegel A, Atreya R, et al. Comparison of Hemospray ® and EndoclotTM for the treatment of gastrointestinal bleeding. World J Gastroenterol 2019;25: 1592–602.
34. Park J-S, Kim HK, Shin YW, et al. Novel hemostatic adhesive powder for nonvariceal upper gastrointestinal bleeding. Endosc Int Open 2019;7:E1763–7.
35. Chapelle N, Martel M, Bardou M, et al. Role of the endoscopic Doppler probe in nonvariceal upper gastrointestinal bleeding: Systematic review and meta-analysis. Dig Endosc 2023. https://doi.org/10.1111/den.14356.
36. Agarwal A, Benias P, Brewer Gutierrez OI, et al. Endoscopic suturing for management of peptic ulcer-related upper gastrointestinal bleeding: a preliminary experience. Endosc Int Open 2018;6(12):E1439–44.
37. Cheng HC, Wu CT, Chang WL, et al. Double oral esomeprazole after a 3-day intravenous esomeprazole infusion reduces recurrent peptic ulcer bleeding in high-risk patients: a randomised controlled study. Gut 2014;63(12):1864–72.
38. Hung KW, Knotts RM, Faye AS, et al. Factors associated with adherence to *Helicobacter pylori* testing during hospitalization for bleeding peptic ulcer disease. Clin Gastroenterol Hepatol 2020;18(5):1091–8.
39. Laine L, Nathwani R, Naritoku W. The effect of GI bleeding on *Helicobacter pylori* diagnostic testing: a prospective study at the time of bleeding and 1 month later. Gastrointest Endosc 2005;62:853–9.
40. Graham DY, Opekun AR, Hammoud F, et al. Studies regarding the mechanism of false negative urea breath tests with proton pump inhibitors. Am J Gastroenterol 2003;98(5):1005–9.
41. Guo CG, Cheung KS, Zhang F, et al. Delay in retreatment of *Helicobacter pylori* infection increases risk of upper gastrointestinal bleeding. Clin Gastroenterol Hepatol 2021;19(2):314–22.
42. Laursen SB, Stanley AJ, Laine L, et al. Rebleeding in peptic ulcer bleeding - a nationwide cohort study of 19,537 patients. Scand J Gastroenterol 2022;57(12): 1423–9. Epub 2022 Jul 19.PMID: 35853234.
43. Shung DL, Au B, Taylor RA, et al. Validation of a machine learning model that outperforms clinical risk scoring systems for upper gastrointestinal bleeding. Gastroenterology 2020;158:160–7.

The Role of Endoscopy for Primary and Secondary Prophylaxis of Variceal Bleeding

Andrew S. Ma, MD, Paul J. Thuluvath, MD, FRCP*

KEYWORDS

- Esophageal • Gastric • Varices • Cirrhosis • Prophylaxis

KEY POINTS

- Variceal hemorrhage portends poor survival in patients with cirrhosis.
- Screening for varices should be performed in all high-risk patients with cirrhosis.
- Validated methods for primary and secondary prevention of esophageal variceal hemorrhage include beta blockers and variceal band ligation.
- Treatment options for gastric variceal hemorrhage include injection sclerotherapy and balloon-occluded retrograde transvenous obliteration.

INTRODUCTION

Cirrhosis is the fifth-leading cause of adult deaths with a 2-year mortality rate of 26.4% based on a population study conducted during an 11-year period.[1] Up to 7% of patients with cirrhosis develop some form of decompensation, including acute gastroesophageal variceal bleeding, each year.[2] Esophageal variceal bleeding is an unpredictable complication of cirrhosis with an associated mortality of 20% to 40% with each bleeding episode.[3] The mortality rate is directly related to the severity of liver disease with a very high mortality (>70%) in patients with Child C cirrhosis.[3]

Cirrhosis causes structural changes and alterations in the microcirculation of the liver resulting in increased vascular resistance, causing an elevation in portal pressure.[4] Portal hypertension (PHTN) is defined as an increase in the pressure of the portal vein and its branches.[5] This can be measured by calculating the hepatic venous pressure gradient (HVPG), which is the difference between the hepatic venous pressure and the wedged (usually using an occlusion balloon) hepatic venous pressure. An HVPG greater than 5 mm of Hg is diagnostic of PHTN but complications of PHTN rarely occur when the HVPG is less than 10 mm of Hg. Of patients with cirrhosis

Institute for Digestive Health and Liver Disease Mercy Medical Center, Professional Office Building, 7th Floor 345 St. Paul Place, Baltimore, MD 21202, USA
* Corresponding author.
E-mail address: pthuluv@mdmercy.com

Gastrointest Endoscopy Clin N Am 34 (2024) 231–248
https://doi.org/10.1016/j.giec.2023.09.012
1052-5157/24/© 2023 Elsevier Inc. All rights reserved.

giendo.theclinics.com

whose HVPG remains less than 10 mm Hg to 12 mm Hg, approximately 10% will develop decompensation within 4 years.[6] Once the HVPG exceeds 10 mm Hg to 12 mm Hg, it is considered clinically significant portal hypertension (CSPH) and portends an increased risk of decompensating events including variceal hemorrhage, ascites, and hepatic encephalopathy.[7] A reduction in HVPG by at least 20% from baseline or to less than 12 mm Hg with pharmacologic therapy is associated with a reduced risk of variceal hemorrhage or spontaneous bacterial peritonitis.[8] Once patients develop decompensated cirrhosis, their 1-year mortality rate is 20.2% with a median survival of 1.8 years.[9,10] Decompensation from variceal hemorrhage, ascites, or hepatic encephalopathy is a major turning point in survival outcomes in those with cirrhosis irrespective of the underlying cause of their liver disease.

Gastroesophageal varices form when increased portal pressure stimulates growth factors in the splanchnic circulation to form portosystemic collaterals. Collaterals that develop from the left gastric vein become visible within the distal esophagus, forming what are known as esophageal varices.[11] Less commonly, other branches of the gastric vein can also become engorged and form gastric varices. The prevalence of gastroesophageal varices in cirrhosis varies depending on the severity of liver disease. In a study evaluating data from 68 practices comprising 1688 esophagogastroduodenoscopy (EGDs) performed for variceal screening, the incidence of esophageal varices was found to be 42.7% in patients with Child-Pugh A cirrhosis and 71.9% in those with Child-Pugh B or C cirrhosis.[12]

Patients who do not have varices on index endoscopy develop varices at a rate of up to 8% each year.[13] Once small varices develop, 2% of patients with compensated cirrhosis will see an increase in size to large varices within 1 year and 16% will experience enlargement of varices within 3 years. This is much higher for patients with Child-Pugh B or C cirrhosis because 22% will experience enlargement from small to large varices within 1 year and 51% at 3 years. Although beta blockers have demonstrated efficacy in reducing portal pressures, they have been found to be ineffective in preventing the development or enlargement of varices.[14]

Excessive wall tension within varices leads to rupture with subsequent hemorrhage but there are no reliable biochemical markers to predict variceal bleeding. Variceal bleeding is most likely to occur when the HVPG is greater than 12 mm Hg but it is not practical to repeat HVPG on a regular interval in those with cirrhosis.[15] Therefore, surrogate markers such as variceal size and characteristics (such as red signs) or severity of liver disease are used to estimate the risks of variceal hemorrhage. Each year, 4% to 15% of patients with esophageal varices will suffer from spontaneous hemorrhage, which portends a 6-week mortality of up to 25%.[16–18] When bleeding itself does not lead to death, it is associated with complications such as sepsis, spontaneous bacterial peritonitis, or renal failure.[19] Once variceal bleeding has occurred, 60% of patients will experience recurrence of bleeding within 1 year.[20] As such, both prevention of index bleeding (primary prophylaxis) and prevention of recurrence of bleeding after an episode of index bleeding (secondary prophylaxis) are critical for patient survival. Therapy to prevent bleeding from esophageal varices is based on 2 primary aspects: reducing portal pressure and eradicating the varices that have already formed. The evidence and indications for these therapies will be discussed below.

PRIMARY PROPHYLAXIS

Various liver societies, including the American Association for the Study of Liver Diseases (AASLD), the European Association for the Study of the Liver (EASL), and the

Asian Pacific Association for the Study of the Liver (APASL), have published practice guidelines (**Table 1**) regarding the diagnosis and management of esophageal varices based on evidence and expert opinion.[21–23] To screen for esophageal varices, the AASLD and EASL recommend that all patients who do not meet exclusion criteria (liver stiffness <20 kPa and platelet count >150,000/mL) undergo endoscopy once diagnosed with cirrhosis.[21,22] In a cross-sectional study evaluating methods for predicting CSPH, liver stiffness combined with platelet count or spleen size was found to have greater than 80% accuracy in predicting the presence of CSPH when verified by HVPG.[24] The APASL does not permit for such exclusions and instead recommends endoscopy for all patients with newly diagnosed cirrhosis without exception.[23] Relatively lower costs in Asia may partly explain the discordance in the recommendation.

Screening and Risk Stratification

If the index endoscopy reveals esophageal varices, it is imperative to characterize their extent and stratify the risk of bleeding. One classification system that decreases intraobserver and interobserver variability comes from the Japanese Research Society for Portal Hypertension system.[25] Within this system, varices are graded on a scale from F0 to F3 by evaluating their extent (distance from the gastroesophageal junction) and size (F0: none; F1: small and without tortuosity; F2: tortuous and comprising <50% of the esophageal lumen; F3: very large and tortuous) (**Fig. 1**). Size is directly related to bleeding: F3 varices have a 68% chance of hemorrhage, F2 varices have a 32% chance, and F1 varices have a 15% chance.[26–28] In addition to size, signs that are associated with increased risk for bleeding include red wale markings and cherry-red spots (76% chance of hemorrhage) as well as blue discoloration (80% chance).[26]

Varices that extend beyond the gastroesophageal junction into the stomach are classified as either gastro-oesophageal varice 1 (GOV1) (along the lesser curvature) or GOV2 (along the gastric fundus).[29]

For the purposes of consensus recommendations, it is worth noting that differing classification systems are recommended by various liver societies. The AASLD favors simplicity of classification, defining small varices as those with a diameter of less than 5 mm while all varices of greater than 5 mm in diameter are classified as large.[21] "Large" varices encompass those that were formerly classified as medium due to a lack of distinction in their management.[30] The APASL uses this same system but the EASL defines varices as either small or large based on whether they collapse with insufflation.[23,30]

For patients with compensated cirrhosis, the AASLD recommends (see **Table 1**) that those without varices should have a surveillance period of 2 years if experiencing ongoing liver injury although this can be extended to every 3 years if the liver injury is quiescent.[21] The EASL recommends that if no varices are present on screening endoscopy but the cause of liver injury persists, screening endoscopy should still be performed every year.[22] Conversely, the APASL recommends 2-year intervals for all patients without varices on index endoscopy.[23] If index endoscopy reveals small varices and the cause of liver injury remains persistent, the AASLD and APASL recommend annual endoscopy with the AASLD adding that this can be extended to every other year if the insult has been removed.[21,23] However, once patients have been started on nonselective beta blockers (NSBBs), guidelines from the Baveno VII consensus workshop recommend discontinuing routine screening endoscopies.[7] For patients who develop decompensated cirrhosis, the AASLD and EASL recommend annual EGD for variceal screening, whereas the APASL recommends screening "more frequently" than every 2 years.[21–23]

Table 1
Summary of consensus recommendations from expert societies for screening and surveillance of esophageal varices

	AASLD (2017)	EASL/Baveno VII (2018/2021)	APASL (2008/2011)
Screening EGD	At time of diagnosis of cirrhosis, unless platelet count >150,000/cc and liver stiffness >20 kPa At time of decompensation of cirrhosis	At time of diagnosis of cirrhosis, unless platelet count >150,000/cc and liver stiffness >20 kPa At time of decompensation of cirrhosis Not indicated if already taking NSBBs for the prevention of decompensation	At time diagnosis of cirrhosis
Surveillance EGD	Compensated, with small varices and ongoing liver injury: every year Compensated, with no or small varices but with ongoing liver injury: every 2 y Compensated, without varices or ongoing liver injury: every 3 y Not indicated if receiving NSBB or carvedilol for primary prophylaxis	Decompensated: every year Ongoing liver injury: every year	Compensated, with small varices: every year Compensated, without varices: every 2 y Decompensated: more frequently than every 2 y

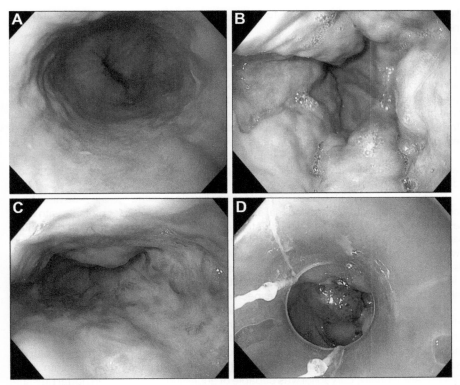

Fig. 1. Esophageal varices. (*A*) Small, F1 varices; (*B*) large, F3 varices; (*C*) red wale sign and cherry-red spots; and (*D*) treatment with band ligation.

The rationale for primary prophylaxis is to prevent the first bleeding episode and the associated mortality in high-risk subjects, and the options include variceal band ligation, NSBB, or a combination of both. The pros and cons of all those will be discussed herein.

Endoscopic Variceal Ligation

Endoscopic therapies for the treatment of esophageal varices include variceal ligation and injection sclerotherapy. The latter has fallen out of favor because multiple studies have demonstrated that variceal ligation has lower associated rates of mortality, risk of recurrent hemorrhage, and risk of adverse events.[31–33] Variceal ligation was first introduced in 1986, and since then, developments have been made that allow for the delivery of multiple bands without the need for an overtube.[34,35] Several high-quality studies have demonstrated the efficacy of variceal ligation compared with no therapy for primary prophylaxis with decreased risk of hemorrhage, blood transfusion, and overall mortality.[36]

Additionally, a meta-analysis evaluating 601 patients with cirrhosis from 5 single-center RCTs demonstrated that prophylactic variceal ligation significantly reduces the risk of variceal bleeding as well as associated and all-cause mortality within an average follow-up of 19 months when compared with untreated controls.[37] Relative risks for the first variceal bleed (0.36, 0.26–0.50), bleeding-related mortality (0.20, 0.11–0.39), and all-cause mortality (0.55, 0.43–0.71) favored prophylactic band ligation and the number needed to treat for each outcome was 4.1, 6.7, and 5.3, respectively.

Beta Blockers

The medications that have demonstrated the greatest benefit for prophylaxis against variceal bleeding are traditional NSBBs (propranolol and nadolol) and carvedilol. Beta blockers reduce cardiac output as well as splanchnic blood flow resulting in the reduction of portal pressure. A review of 4 RCTs evaluated the efficacy of traditional NSBBs (propranolol and nadolol, n = 286) against placebo (n = 303) for primary prophylaxis of esophageal variceal bleeding in varices that were classified as medium-large or F2-F3.[38] The results demonstrated a significant reduction in occurrence of GI bleeding within 2 years (78% with NSBBs, 65% with placebo) although there was no significant difference in overall survival.

Beta blockers have also been studied for small varices, although the data have been conflicting. A placebo-controlled trial evaluating nadolol (n = 83) for patients with small esophageal varices without high-risk stigmata against placebo (n = 62) in preventing enlargement of varices with a mean follow-up of 36 months suggested that nadolol was effective in reducing progression (20% vs 51%, $P < .001$) without difference in survival.[39] However, a subsequent trial evaluating the effect of propranolol (n = 77) against placebo (n = 73) in preventing growth of varices found a similar risk of progression within 2 years (11% vs 16%, respectively).[40]

The evidence for carvedilol is robust. A meta-analysis comprising 4 RCTs evaluated the effect of carvedilol (n = 181) against no treatment (n = 92) or variceal ligation (n = 79) in reducing the risk of decompensation and mortality in patients with compensated cirrhosis.[41] Carvedilol resulted in a decreased risk of developing decompensated cirrhosis (subdistribution HR [SHR] 0.506) and lower risk of death (SHR 0.417). Additionally, carvedilol was capable of achieving a reduction in portal pressure by at least 20% or to less than 12 mm Hg in up to 56% of patients that did not have such a response to propranolol.[42]

Dosing parameters are affected by the presence of ascites because the majority of RCTs evaluating beta blockers excluded patients with refractory ascites. In a single-center observational study, the median survival for patients with cirrhosis and ascites who received beta blockers to prevent variceal hemorrhage was compared with those who did not receive beta blockers.[43] One hundred fifty-one patients were included and were found to have a significantly decreased median survival when taking beta blockers (5 vs 20 months). The role of beta blockers in the presence of significant ascites remains a controversial topic.

Comparative Analysis of Variceal Band Ligations and Beta Blockers

Given the demonstrated benefit of both variceal ligation and beta blockers for the prevention of variceal hemorrhage, numerous studies have been performed to determine the optimal therapy for primary prophylaxis. A meta-analysis evaluated 8 RCTs comprising 596 patients to compare variceal ligation against traditional NSBBs.[44] The data demonstrated an insignificant difference in variceal obliteration between the 2 (91.6% vs 94.5%, respectively). Variceal ligation did significantly reduce the rate of first variceal bleed with a relative risk reduction of 43% with an number needed to treat (NNT) of 11. Neither therapy demonstrated superiority in reducing all-cause mortality.

A subsequent meta-analysis evaluated 12 RCTs comparing variceal ligation with beta blockers (primarily traditional NSBBs, although one included carvedilol) in a total of 1023 patients and found no significant difference in GI bleeding (16.4% vs 20.5%), bleeding-related deaths, or all-cause deaths (29.1% vs 26.4%).[45] There were similar rates of complications in both groups: 30.3% of patients who underwent variceal liga-tion experienced events such as dysphagia or chest pain and 35.8% of patients that received beta blockers reported symptoms such as dizziness, symptomatic hypoten-sion, and symptomatic bradycardia. Another meta-analysis evaluated 19 RCTs comparing variceal ligation with traditional NSBBs for primary prevention of esopha-geal variceal hemorrhage.[46] In total, there were 1504 patients who underwent 1 of the 2 therapies with nearly identical mortality (24% with EVL and 23% with beta blockers). Additionally, both variceal ligation (RR 0.69) and non-selective beta blockers (RR 0.67) reduced upper GI bleeding and variceal hemorrhage at a similar rate.

Carvedilol has also been compared with variceal ligation in a multicenter RCT for prophylaxis of grade II or larger esophageal varices and was found to have a lower rate of first variceal bleed (10% vs 23%) without notable differences in mortality or bleeding-related mortality.[47]

Combination Therapy for Variceal Band Ligations and Beta Blockers

Given the demonstrated benefit of both beta blockers and variceal ligation for primary prophylaxis for variceal hemorrhage, an RCT compared traditional NSBBs with vari-ceal ligation against ligation alone for primary prophylaxis.[48] In this study, 144 patients were randomized to either arm and demonstrated similar rates of bleeding and mor-tality. They did also note reported side effects of propranolol in 22% of patients requiring discontinuation in 8% while noting no reported serious complications from variceal ligation. A meta-analysis evaluated the effects of a combination of beta blockers and variceal ligation on preventing bleeding from high-risk varices.[49] Twelve RCTs (n = 1571) were included and the results demonstrated no significant improve-ment in reducing variceal bleeding, total upper GI bleeding, or mortality. Currently, combination therapy is not recommended for primary prophylaxis.

Cost Effectiveness of Variceal Band Ligations and Beta Blockers

Markov modeling has been used to examine the cost-effectiveness of screening and prophylaxis for variceal bleeding. In one study, 6 different strategies were compared: (1) universal screening with beta blockers for prophylaxis of varices; (2) universal screening with ligation of varices; (3) screening of high-risk patients with beta blockers if varices are present; (4) screening of high-risk patients followed by ligation of varices; (5) empiric beta blockers for all patients; and (6) no prophylaxis for any patients.[50] The primary outcome was the cost associated with first variceal bleeding for each strategy, analyzed from a third-party payer perspective. Strategy 6 was the least expensive, whereas strategies 2 and 3 were the most expensive (approximately US$175,000 for the prevention of each additional bleed). Strategy 5 estimated a cost of US$12,408 for the prevention of each additional variceal bleed and was recommended as the most cost-effective method. Additional studies have also suggested universal beta blockers while another found screening followed by beta blockers in compensated cirrhosis or universal beta blockers in decompensated cirrhosis to be cost-effective.[51,52]

It is worth noting that these analyses were highly sensitive to factors such as cost of endoscopy, prevalence of esophageal varices, bleeding risk, and choice of treatment. There do not exist randomized clinical trials comparing these methods and as will be discussed below, there are not expert consensuses that recommend against screening or using beta blockers over variceal ligation.

Consensus Recommendations on Primary Prophylaxis

Guidelines for the management of esophageal varices (see **Tables 1**; **2**) have been put forth by multiple hepatology societies including the AASLD, EASL, and APASL.[7,21–23]

Table 2
Summary of consensus recommendations from expert societies for primary and secondary prophylaxis for esophageal varices

	AASLD (2017)	EASL/Baveno VII (2018/2021)	APASL (2008/2011)
Primary prophylaxis	Small varices, with high-risk stigmata: NSBBs Small varices, with decompensated cirrhosis: NSBBs Medium/large varices: NSBB, carvedilol, or EVL[a]	Small varices with red wale marks or Child-Pugh C cirrhosis: NSBBs[b] Medium-large varices: NSBBs or EVL Compensated cirrhosis with high-risk varices but contraindications to NSBBs: EVL Small varices without high risk in decompensated cirrhosis: NSBBs or carvedilol High-risk varices in decompensated cirrhosis: NSBBs or carvedilol preferred over EVL	Small varices with compensated disease: NSBBs Small varices with red signs or decompensated disease: NSBBs Medium varices: NSBBs or EVL Large varices: NSBB with EVL or HVPG monitoring High-risk varices: EVL at time of screening
Secondary prophylaxis	NSBB with EVL, repeat EVL every 1–4 wk until eradication, then again in 3–6 mo, and again every 6–12 mo TIPS for refractory bleeding	Combination of NSBBs/carvedilol and EVL TIPS for bleeding refractory to NSBBs/carvedilol and EVL	

[a] EVL should be performed every 2 wk until eradication, then 3 to 6 mo, and then every 6 to 12 mo.
[b] High doses of NSBBs should be avoided in patients with severe ascites.

As noted in the earlier section, there is no uniform classification system for varices shared by all 3 societies. Additionally, the term "nonselective beta blockers" also varies—the AASLD and APASL use NSBB to refer to traditional NSBBs (propranolol and nadolol) while the EASL includes carvedilol under its definition of NSBBs.

Should the index screening endoscopy demonstrate small varices, the AASLD does not recommend prophylaxis unless there are high-risk features (red spots, red wale sign) or the patient has decompensated cirrhosis. For these cases, the AASLD suggests NSBBs as EVL may be challenging for small varices. However, the EASL and APASL both note that for small varices without high-risk features, NSBBs "may be" used for primary prophylaxis. The EASL adds that if beta blockers are started for small varices with high-risk features, no further screening is indicated but that if the patients are intolerant of or have contraindications to beta blockers, they should undergo EVL.

For patients found to have medium-to-large esophageal varices, the AASLD, EASL, and APASL all recommend beta blockers or EVL based on patient preference and characteristics (**Table 2**). For varices that are treated with EVL, the AASLD recommends that endoscopy be repeated every 2 to 8 weeks until confirmation of eradication. Once eradicated, endoscopy should be repeated within 3 to 6 months, then again, every 6 to 12 months afterward. If varices are large, the APASL recommends NSBBs, preferably with monitoring of HVPG or VBL but does not specify the frequency. When there are high-risk features, the APASL recommends prophylactic EVL.

Traditional nonselective beta blockers include propranolol (starting dose 20–40 mg PO twice daily) and nadolol (20–40 mg PO daily). The dosage should be adjusted every 2 to 3 days to achieve treatment goals, which are a resting heart rate of 55 to 60 beats per minute but not resulting in a systolic blood pressure of less than 90 mm Hg. The maximum dose for propranolol in patients without ascites is 320 mg daily; in patients with ascites, the maximum recommended dose is reduced to 160 mg daily. For nadolol, the maximum doses for patients without and with ascites are 160 mg/d and 80 mg/d, respectively.

For carvedilol the recommended starting dose is 6.25 mg once daily, which can then be increased to 6.25 mg twice daily after 3 days of therapy up to a maximum dose of 12.5 mg daily while avoiding reduction of a systolic blood pressure to less than 90 mm Hg. The AASLD does not provide dosing parameters based on the presence of ascites. Should patients experience clinical deterioration (hypotension, sepsis, spontaneous bacterial peritonitis, and renal failure), the EASL adds that beta blockers be held until recovery.

Once patients have been started on beta blockers for primary prophylaxis, the AASLD and EASL note that further surveillance endoscopies are no longer necessary unless the patient previously had compensated cirrhosis and develops decompensated disease.

Choice of Therapy for Primary Prophylaxis

Because clinical studies and expert recommendations do not have a preferential choice of treatment of primary prophylaxis, it is important for the clinician to discuss with the patient the therapies available as a form of shared medical decision-making. Endoscopic variceal ligation can be performed in the same session as endoscopy for variceal screening, provided that the endoscopy suite is in an appropriately equipped facility. Variceal ligation can be associated with more severe immediate complications such as dysphagia, chest pain, esophageal ulcerations, and posttreatment bleeding although these are often short-lived.

In comparison, beta blockers are noninvasive and require less coordination and expertise but may result in side effects such as fatigue, dizziness, or light-headedness that prevent appropriate uptitration. Up to 15% of patients may have contraindications for beta blockers while another 15% report side effects that result in discontinuation.[53] However, because beta blockers treat PHTN itself, they also may prevent other sequelae of PHTN as shown by a double-blinded, multicenter RCT that evaluated the effects of beta blockers on preventing clinical decompensation. A total of 201 patients received intravenous propranolol, and those with a decrease in HVPG of at least 10% were randomized to either carvedilol or placebo. This study found that in patients that received carvedilol, there was a significantly decreased incidence of development of ascites (16%) compared with placebo (27%) but no difference in bleeding or death during a period of 3 years.[54]

The published studies showed that band ligation and beta blockers have similar efficacy but there is a paucity of RCTs in those with very high risk of bleeding (large varices with red signs and very advanced cirrhosis). The treatment selection should be based on patient's preference, severity of varices and cirrhosis, tolerance or relative contraindications to beta blockers, anesthesia risks associated with repeated endoscopic procedures, practice setting, costs and probability of compliance with daily medications or repeated endoscopic sessions. For optimal outcomes, there should be a transparent and well-informed discussion between patients (including their immediate families) and the physician before a decision is made on primary prophylaxis.

SECONDARY PROPHYLAXIS
Initial Management

For patients that survive their first episode of variceal hemorrhage, measures must be taken to prevent recurrent bleeding. This is referred to as secondary prophylaxis. These patients have up to a 60% risk of rebleeding within the first year after variceal hemorrhage and a mortality rate of up to 33%.[55] Risk factors associated with increased likelihood of rebleeding include HVPG greater than 20 mm Hg, alcoholic liver disease, and infections.

Given the demonstrated benefits of both beta blockers and EVL, a meta-analysis consists of 5 studies with 476 patients evaluated EVL alone or combined with beta blockers and in some cases, isosorbide mononitrate. This demonstrated that the addition of traditional NSBBs to EVL decreased variceal rebleeding (RR 0.44) compared with pharmacologic or endoscopic therapy alone for a follow-up period of at least 15 months.[56] A subsequent meta-analysis evaluated 48 RCTs comprising 4415 patients with cirrhosis with variceal bleeding, assessing the benefits of carvedilol, EVL with beta blockers, beta blockers with isosorbide mononitrate, or transjugular intrahepatic portosystemic shunting (TIPS) in preventing rebleeding from esophageal varices for at least 6 and up to 55 months.[57] Carvedilol had the highest overall survival (87.4%) but this was not statistically significant when compared with the other therapies. TIPS was superior in reducing rebleeding (98.8%) but did not influence overall mortality.

Societal Guidelines

After patients have recovered from variceal hemorrhage, the AASLD and EASL recommend (see **Table 2**) a combination of beta blockers with variceal ligation unless they have undergone TIPS, in which case they require neither.[21,22] The AASLD does not include carvedilol but after the Baveno VII conference, the EASL added that carvedilol is a reasonable alternative. The parameters for NSBBs are the same for primary prophylaxis for starting dose, rate of titration, heart rate and blood pressure limits, and maximum dosage. For endoscopic variceal ligation, the AASLD recommends that it be performed every 1 to 4 weeks until varices are eradicated. Once eradicated, a surveillance EGD should be performed within 3 to 6 months and repeated every 6 to 12 months. The APASL does not provide recommendations for secondary prophylaxis. Should patients experience bleeding refractory to both NSBBs and EVL, both the AASLD and EASL recommend TIPS.

GASTRIC VARICES

Classification Gastric Varices

PHTN can also result in the formation of gastric varices, which are incident in up to 20% of patients with cirrhosis.[56] Gastric varices are most commonly described using the Sarin classification (**Fig. 2**) system: GOVs represent esophageal varices that extend into the stomach and are denoted as GOV1 (extending below the cardia into the lesser curvature) or GOV2 (extension into the fundus).[29]

GOV1 varices comprise approximately 75% of all gastric varices. There are also isolated gastric varices (IGVs) that originate independent of esophageal varices, classified as IGV1 (located in the fundus) or IGV2 (located outside the fundus). Varices that form along the lesser curvature originate from the left gastric vein, whereas varices in the fundus originate from short gastric or posterior gastric veins.

Compared with esophageal variceal hemorrhage, gastric variceal hemorrhage can prove more difficult to control and is associated with greater mortality (up to 45%).[57] A retrospective study evaluated risk factors associated with gastric variceal hemorrhage in 132 patients with cirrhosis and gastric fundal varices. The findings portending greatest risk of bleeding included varix size, presence of red spots, severity of

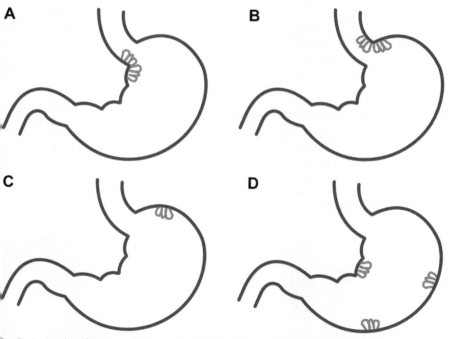

Fig. 2. Sarin classification of GOV and IGV. (*A*) GOV1: Esophageal varices extending to the lesser curvature; (*B*) GOV2: Esophageal varices extending into the fundus; (*C*) IGV1: Gastric varix located in the fundus; and (*D*) IGV2: Gastric varix located outside the fundus. (*Credit:* VectorStock.)

liver disease (by Child-Pugh classification), and type of varix (without therapy, IGV1: 78%, GOV2: 55%, and GOV1: 28%).[58]

Primary Prophylaxis of Gastric Varices

Varices along the lesser curve (GOV1) could be managed similar to esophageal varices if they bleed. There are only limited data on primary prophylaxis of gastric varices. Both sclerotherapy and variceal ligation have been used for gastric varices since the 1980s. There exists little head-to-head data but sclerotherapy via cyanoacrylate injection (**Fig. 3**) has proven to be the favored method owing to lower rates of rebleeding and fewer sessions required for obliteration.[59] Variceal band ligation could be performed for GOV1 but not recommended for GOV2. Adverse events associated with cyanoacrylate injection include bleeding from the injection site as well as embolization to distant sites with associated complications such as stroke or pulmonary embolism.[60]

There is a paucity of RCTs evaluating primary prophylaxis for gastric varices. In the only prospective RCT, 79 patients with cirrhosis and GOV2 or IGV1 varices were randomized to receive cyanoacrylate injection (n = 30), beta blockers (n = 29), or no treatment (n = 30) with primary endpoints being bleeding from gastric varices or death within a median follow-up of 26 months.[61] The probability of bleeding was significantly lower for patients who received cyanoacrylate injection (13%), followed by beta blockers (28%), then placebo (45%). The difference in survival between cyanoacrylate injection and beta blockers was not statistically significant (93% vs 83%), although both were significantly more effective than placebo (74%).

As such, expert recommendations for primary prophylaxis of gastric variceal hemorrhage are less comprehensive. For GOV2 or IGV1 varices, the AASLD and EASL suggest NSBBs while the APASL limits this recommendation to GOV2/IGV1 varices with high-risk stigmata (red spots, >5 mm in size, or Child-Pugh B/C cirrhosis). Neither the AASLD, EASL, nor APASL recommend cyanoacrylate injection for the prevention of initial gastric variceal hemorrhage, citing a paucity of data. For GOV1 varices, the AASLD and EASL recommend the same methods for primary prophylaxis as with esophageal varices.

Secondary Prophylaxis of Gastric Varices

As with primary prophylaxis, there are no robust data to guide secondary prophylaxis of gastric variceal hemorrhage. In one RCT, 67 patients who had bled from GOV2 or IGV1 varices were randomized to receive either cyanoacrylate injection (n = 33) or NSBBs (n = 34) to prevent rebleeding and death.[62] There was a significantly lower probability of gastric variceal rebleeding in the sclerotherapy group (15% vs 55%) as well as a lower mortality rate within a median follow-up period of 26 months (3%

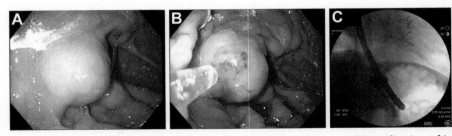

Fig. 3. (*A*) Gastric varix; (*B*) varix after injection of cyanoacrylate; and (*C*) verification of injection under fluoroscopy.

vs 25%). Another RCT compared cyanoacrylate injection alone (n = 48) to a combination of sclerotherapy with NSBB (n = 47) after initial gastric variceal hemorrhage and did not find any difference in rebleeding or mortality after a mean follow-up period of 20.3 months.[63] The gastric varices could be injected under fluoroscopic guidance, to confirm that there is no major collateral shunting into the lungs, with or without endoscopic ultrasound assistance.

Additional data suggest that rebleeding from gastric varices may be more appropriately treated through catheter-based angiographic methods. One trial evaluated the efficacy of serial cyanoacrylate injection (n = 37) against TIPS (n = 35) for secondary prophylaxis during a median follow-up of 33 months, demonstrating a significantly lower rate of rebleeding after TIPS (11% vs 34%).[64] Cyanoacrylate injection has also been evaluated against balloon-occluded retrograde transvenous obliteration (BRTO) for secondary prophylaxis.[65] Thirty-two patients, each with either GOV2 or IGV1 varices, were randomized to sclerotherapy or BRTO. The group that underwent BRTO had a significantly higher probability of remaining free of all-cause rebleeding at up to 2 years after therapy (92.6% vs 65.2%) though mortality rates were similar for both groups.

Worldwide, variceal glue injection is the most widely used modality, followed by TIPS and BRTO. There are only very limited data to make an evidence-based recommendation. The AASLD recommends a combination of NSBBs with EVL or cyanoacrylate injection for secondary prophylaxis after GOV1 hemorrhage. For secondary prophylaxis after IGV1 hemorrhage, the AASLD recommends TIPS or BRTO but notes that when access to such therapies is limited, cyanoacrylate injection is an option. The EASL recommends consideration of TIPS in combination with selective embolization or BRTO for secondary prophylaxis of gastric variceal hemorrhage, whereas the APASL does not make recommendations.

DISCUSSION

Cirrhosis is associated with a high morbidity and mortality, predominantly due to the consequences of PHTN. Because the pathophysiology of PHTN is very complex involving multiple organs, the medical treatment of complications of PHTN is very limited. One of the unpredictable consequences of PHTN is bleeding from esophageal or gastric varices, which may lead to multiorgan failures, especially in the presence of advanced cirrhosis, and death. Death from uncontrolled hemorrhage is very rare these days in most centers.

Upper endoscopy remains the standard for screening for varices because this allows for diagnosis, stratification of risk for hemorrhage, and therapy. The frequency of screening varies based on the presence of varices, high-risk findings, and ongoing liver injury. Expert societal recommendations differ in the nuances of prophylaxis but the mainstays that have both been demonstrated to reduce the risk of bleeding are beta blockers and EVL, with neither being demonstrated to be superior or preferred. As such, the choice should be tailored to the patient. EVL should be repeated periodically until varices are eradicated, whereas beta blockers should be uptitrated while avoiding bradycardia and hypotension. Once patients have bled, secondary prophylaxis consists of a combination of both therapies and, if refractory, consideration of TIPS.

Esophageal varices can extend into the stomach, and in some patients, gastric varices can originate in isolation. There do not exist validated screening methods for gastric varices beyond the guidelines for esophageal varices. Data are less robust for prophylaxis for bleeding from gastric varices, with expert recommendations suggesting beta blockers without a firm recommendation for endoscopy with cyanoacrylate injection.

There are no recommendations for secondary prophylaxis though methods that have been effective include sclerotherapy, TIPS, and BRTO.

Most importantly, early recognition of liver disease, the optimal management of the precipitating causes of liver disease, early identification of complications resulting from PHTNs and appropriate prophylactic treatments will improve short-term and intermediate-term outcomes of patients with cirrhosis.

CLINICS CARE POINTS

- Endoscopy is indicated for variceal screening in those with cirrhosis unless patients are considered low risk (in the absence of clinical or imaging evidence of PHTN, platelet counts >150,000/cc or liver stiffness <20 kPa).

- Surveillance intervals for esophageal varices are governed by the size of varices on initial screening and the severity of liver disease.

- Primary prophylaxis for esophageal varices includes beta blockers (nonselective beta blockers or carvedilol) or variceal band ligation; the modality of primary prophylaxis used should be tailored to the patient as well as the expertise of the responsible physician.

- Once patients have suffered from variceal hemorrhage, they should undergo serial ligation until eradication while also receiving beta blockers (secondary prophylaxis).

- There are no consensus recommendations for primary prophylaxis of gastric varices. Secondary prophylaxis options include cyanoacrylate injection (off-label use), BRTO or TIPS with coil embolization.

DISCLOSURES

The authors have no financial conflicts of interests and did not receive funding from any sources for this article.

REFERENCES

1. Scaglione S, Kliethermes S, Cao G, et al. The Epidemiology of cirrhosis in the United States: A Population-based Study. J Clin Gastroenterol 2015;49(8):690–6.
2. D'Amico G, Garcia-Tsao G, Pagliaro L. Natural history and prognostic indicators of survival in cirrhosis: a systematic review of 118 studies. J Hepatol 2006;44(1):217–31.
3. Dy SM, Cromwell DM, Thuluvath PJ, et al. Hospital experience and outcomes for esophageal variceal bleeding. Int J Qual Health Care 2003;15(2):139–46.
4. Iwakiri Y, Groszmann RJ. Vascular endothelial dysfunction in cirrhosis. J Hepatol 2007;46(5):927–34.
5. Miñano C, Garcia-Tsao G. Clinical pharmacology of portal hypertension. Gastroenterol Clin N Am 2010;39(3):681–95.
6. Ripoll C, Groszmann R, Garcia-Tsao G, et al. Hepatic venous pressure gradient predicts clinical decompensation in patients with compensated cirrhosis. Gastroenterology 2007;133(2):481–8.
7. de Franchis R, Bosch J, Garcia-Tsao G, et al, Baveno VII Faculty. Baveno VII - Renewing consensus in portal hypertension. J Hepatol 2022;76(4):959–74 [published correction appears in J Hepatol. 2022 Apr 14;].
8. Turnes J, Garcia-Pagan JC, Abraldes JG, et al. Pharmacological reduction of portal pressure and long-term risk of first variceal bleeding in patients with cirrhosis. Am J Gastroenterol 2006;101(3):506–12.

9. Zipprich A, Garcia-Tsao G, Rogowski S, et al. Prognostic indicators of survival in patients with compensated and decompensated cirrhosis. Liver Int 2012;32(9): 1407–14.

10. D'Amico G, Pasta L, Morabito A, et al. Competing risks and prognostic stages of cirrhosis: a 25-year inception cohort study of 494 patients. Aliment Pharmacol Ther 2014;39(10):1180–93.

11. Philips CA, Arora A, Shetty R, et al. A Comprehensive review of portosystemic collaterals in cirrhosis: historical aspects, anatomy, and classifications. Int J Hepatol 2016;2016:6170243.

12. Kovalak M, Lake J, Mattek N, et al. Endoscopic screening for varices in cirrhotic patients: data from a national endoscopic database. Gastrointest Endosc 2007; 65(1):82–8.

13. Merli M, Nicolini G, Angeloni S, et al. Incidence and natural history of small esophageal varices in cirrhotic patients. J Hepatol 2003;38(3):266–72.

14. Groszmann RJ, Garcia-Tsao G, Bosch J, et al. Beta-blockers to prevent gastroesophageal varices in patients with cirrhosis. N Engl J Med 2005;353(21): 2254–61.

15. Maruyama H, Yokosuka O. Pathophysiology of portal hypertension and esophageal varices. Int J Hepatol 2012;2012:895787.

16. North Italian Endoscopic Club for the Study and Treatment of Esophageal Varices. Prediction of the first variceal hemorrhage in patients with cirrhosis of the liver and esophageal varices. A prospective multicenter study. N Engl J Med 1988;319(15):983–9.

17. D'Amico G, Luca A. Natural history. Clinical-haemodynamic correlations. Prediction of the risk of bleeding. Bailliere Clin Gastroenterol 1997;11(2):243–56.

18. Reverter E, Tandon P, Augustin S, et al. A MELD-based model to determine risk of mortality among patients with acute variceal bleeding. Gastroenterology 2014; 146(2):412–9.e3.

19. Tandon P, Abraldes JG, Keough A, et al. Risk of bacterial infection in patients with cirrhosis and acute variceal hemorrhage, based on child-pugh class, and effects of antibiotics. Clin Gastroenterol Hepatol 2015;13(6):1189–96.e2.

20. Bosch J, García-Pagán JC. Prevention of variceal rebleeding. Lancet 2003; 361(9361):952–4.

21. Garcia-Tsao G, Abraldes JG, Berzigotti A, et al. Portal hypertensive bleeding in cirrhosis: Risk stratification, diagnosis, and management: 2016 practice guidance by the American Association for the study of liver diseases. Hepatology 2017; 65(1):310–35.

22. European Association for the Study of the Liver. EASL clinical practice guidelines for the management of patients with decompensated cirrhosis. J Hepatol 2018; 69(2):406–60.

23. Sarin SK, Kumar A, Angus PW, et al. Primary prophylaxis of gastroesophageal variceal bleeding: consensus recommendations of the Asian Pacific Association for the Study of the Liver. Hepatol Int 2008;2(4):429–39.

24. Berzigotti A, Seijo S, Arena U, et al. Elastography, spleen size, and platelet count identify portal hypertension in patients with compensated cirrhosis. Gastroenterology 2013;144(1):102–11.e1.

25. Idezuki Y. General rules for recording endoscopic findings of esophagogastric varices (1991). Japanese Society for Portal Hypertension. World J Surg 1995; 19(3):420–3.

26. Beppu K, Inokuchi K, Koyanagi N, et al. Prediction of variceal hemorrhage by esophageal endoscopy. Gastrointest Endosc 1981;27(4):213–8.

27. Abraldes JG, Bureau C, Stefanescu H, et al. Anticipate investigators. Noninvasive tools and risk of clinically significant portal hypertension and varices in compensated cirrhosis: The "Anticipate" study. Hepatology 2016;64(6):2173–84.

28. Lebrec D, De Fleury P, Rueff B, et al. Portal hypertension, size of esophageal varices, and risk of gastrointestinal bleeding in alcoholic cirrhosis. Gastroenterology 1980;79(6):1139–44.

29. Sarin SK, Lahoti D, Saxena SP, et al. Prevalence, classification and natural history of gastric varices: a long-term follow-up study in 568 portal hypertension patients. Hepatology 1992;16(6):1343–9.

30. de Franchis R, Pascal JP, Ancona E, et al. Definitions, methodology and therapeutic strategies in portal hypertension. a consensus development workshop, Baveno, Lake Maggiore, Italy, April 5 and 6, 1990. J Hepatol 1992;15(1–2):256–61.

31. Van Ruiswyk J, Byrd JC. Efficacy of prophylactic sclerotherapy for prevention of a first variceal hemorrhage. Gastroenterology 1992;102(2):587–97.

32. Laine L, Cook D. Endoscopic ligation compared with sclerotherapy for treatment of esophageal variceal bleeding. A meta-analysis. Ann Intern Med 1995;123(4):280–7.

33. Dai C, Liu WX, Jiang M, et al. Endoscopic variceal ligation compared with endoscopic injection sclerotherapy for treatment of esophageal variceal hemorrhage: a meta- analysis. World J Gastroenterol 2015;21(8):2534–41.

34. Van Stiegmann G, Cambre T, Sun JH. A new endoscopic elastic band ligating device. Gastrointest Endosc 1986;32(3):230–3.

35. Saeed ZA. The Saeed Six-Shooter: a prospective study of a new endoscopic multiple rubber- band ligator for the treatment of varices. Endoscopy 1996;28(7):559–64.

36. Lo GH, Lai KH, Cheng JS, et al. Prophylactic banding ligation of high-risk esophageal varices in patients with cirrhosis: a prospective, randomized trial. J Hepatol 1999;31(3):451–6.

37. Imperiale TF, Chalasani N. A meta-analysis of endoscopic variceal ligation for primary prophylaxis of esophageal variceal bleeding. Hepatology 2001;33(4):802–7.

38. Poynard T, Calès P, Pasta L, et al. Beta-adrenergic-antagonist drugs in the prevention of gastrointestinal bleeding in patients with cirrhosis and esophageal varices. An analysis of data and prognostic factors in 589 patients from four randomized clinical trials. Franco- Italian Multicenter Study Group. N Engl J Med 1991;324(22):1532–8.

39. Merkel C, Marin R, Angeli P, et al. A placebo-controlled clinical trial of nadolol in the prophylaxis of growth of small esophageal varices in cirrhosis. Gastroenterology 2004;127(2):476–84.

40. Sarin SK, Mishra SR, Sharma P, et al. Early primary prophylaxis with beta-blockers does not prevent the growth of small esophageal varices in cirrhosis: a randomized controlled trial. Hepatol Int 2013;7(1):248–56.

41. Villanueva C, Torres F, Sarin SK, et al. Carvedilol reduces the risk of decompensation and mortality in patients with compensated cirrhosis in a competing-risk meta-analysis. J Hepatol 2022;77(4):1014–25.

42. Reiberger T, Ulbrich G, Ferlitsch A, et al. Carvedilol for primary prophylaxis of variceal bleeding in cirrhotic patients with haemodynamic non-response to propranolol. Gut 2013;62(11):1634–41.

43. Serste T, Melot C, Francoz C, et al. Deleterious effects of beta-blockers on survival in patients with cirrhosis and refractory ascites. Hepatology 2010;52(3):1017–22.

44. Khuroo MS, Khuroo NS, Farahat KL, et al. Meta-analysis: endoscopic variceal ligation for primary prophylaxis of oesophageal variceal bleeding. Aliment Pharmacol Ther 2005;21(4):347–61.

45. Li L, Yu C, Li Y. Endoscopic variceal ligation versus pharmacological therapy for variceal bleeding in cirrhosis: a meta-analysis. Can J Gastroenterol 2011;25(3): 147–55.

46. Gluud LL, Krag A. Banding ligation versus beta-blockers for primary prevention in oesophageal varices in adults. Cochrane Database Syst Rev 2012;8:CD004544.

47. Tripathi D, Ferguson JW, Kochar N, et al. Randomized controlled trial of carvedilol versus variceal band ligation for the prevention of the first variceal bleed. Hepatology 2009;50(3):825–33.

48. Sarin SK, Wadhawan M, Agarwal SR, et al. Endoscopic variceal ligation plus propranolol versus endoscopic variceal ligation alone in primary prophylaxis of variceal bleeding. Am J Gastroenterol 2005;100(4):797–804.

49. Bai M, Qi X, Yang M, et al. Combined therapies versus monotherapies for the first variceal bleeding in patients with high-risk varices: a meta-analysis of randomized controlled trials. J Gastroenterol Hepatol 2014;29(3):442–52.

50. Spiegel BM, Targownik L, Dulai GS, et al. Endoscopic screening for esophageal varices in cirrhosis: Is it ever cost effective? Hepatology 2003;37(2):366–77.

51. Saab S, DeRosa V, Nieto J, et al. Costs and clinical outcomes of primary prophylaxis of variceal bleeding in patients with hepatic cirrhosis: a decision analytic model. Am J Gastroenterol 2003;98(4):763–70.

52. Arguedas MR, Heudebert GR, Eloubeidi MA, et al. Cost-effectiveness of screening, surveillance, and primary prophylaxis strategies for esophageal varices. Am J Gastroenterol 2002;97(9):2441–52.

53. Longacre AV, Imaeda A, Garcia-Tsao G, et al. A pilot project examining the predicted preferences of patients and physicians in the primary prophylaxis of variceal hemorrhage. Hepatology 2008;47(1):169–76.

54. Villanueva C, Albillos A, Genescà J, et al. β blockers to prevent decompensation of cirrhosis in patients with clinically significant portal hypertension (PREDESCI): a randomised, double-blind, placebo-controlled, multicentre trial. Lancet 2019; 393(10181):1597–608.

55. Puente A, Hernández-Gea V, Graupera I, et al. Drugs plus ligation to prevent rebleeding in cirrhosis: an updated systematic review. Liver Int 2014;34(6):823–33.

56. Miao Z, Lu J, Yan J, et al. Comparison of Therapies for Secondary Prophylaxis of Esophageal Variceal Bleeding in Cirrhosis: A Network Meta-analysis of Randomized Controlled Trials. Clin Therapeut 2020;42(7):1246–75.e3.

57. Zhou Y, Qiao L, Wu J, et al. Comparison of the efficacy of octreotide, vasopressin, and omeprazole in the control of acute bleeding in patients with portal hypertensive gastropathy: a controlled study. J Gastroenterol Hepatol 2002;17(9):973–9.

58. Kim T, Shijo H, Kokawa H, et al. Risk factors for hemorrhage from gastric fundal varices. Hepatology 1997;25(2):307–12.

59. Lo GH, Lai KH, Cheng JS, et al. A prospective, randomized trial of butyl cyanoacrylate injection versus variceal ligation in the management of bleeding gastric varices. Hepatology 2001;33(5):1060–4.

60. Roesch W, Rexroth G. Pulmonary, cerebral and coronary emboli during bucrylate injection of bleeding fundic varices. Endoscopy 1998;30(8):S89–90.

61. Mishra SR, Sharma BC, Kumar A, et al. Primary prophylaxis of gastric variceal bleeding comparing cyanoacrylate injection and beta-blockers: a randomized controlled trial. J Hepatol 2011;54(6):1161–7.

62. Mishra SR, Chander Sharma B, Kumar A, et al. Endoscopic cyanoacrylate injection versus beta-blocker for secondary prophylaxis of gastric variceal bleed: a randomised controlled trial. Gut 2010;59(6):729–35.

63. Hung HH, Chang CJ, Hou MC, et al. Efficacy of non-selective β-blockers as adjunct to endoscopic prophylactic treatment for gastric variceal bleeding: a randomized controlled trial. J Hepatol 2012;56(5):1025–32.

64. Lo GH, Liang HL, Chen WC, et al. A prospective, randomized controlled trial of transjugular intrahepatic portosystemic shunt versus cyanoacrylate injection in the prevention of gastric variceal rebleeding. Endoscopy 2007;39(8):679–85.

65. Luo X, Xiang T, Wu J, et al. Endoscopic cyanoacrylate injection versus balloon-occluded retrograde transvenous obliteration for prevention of gastric variceal bleeding: a randomized controlled trial. Hepatology 2021;74(4):2074–84.

Endoscopic Treatment of Acute Esophageal and Gastric Variceal Bleeding

Kendra Jobe, MD[a], Zachary Henry, MD, MSc[b],*

KEYWORDS

- Esophageal varices • Gastric varices • Cyanoacrylate injection • Band ligation

KEY POINTS

- Initial diagnosis of bleeding esophageal varices should be based upon witnessed active bleeding or presence of high-risk stigmata in the absence of alternative causes of acute upper gastrointestinal bleeding.
- Both the initial and definitive endoscopic management of esophageal variceal bleeding should be band ligation. In patients where this cannot adequately control bleeding or in high-risk patients as defined by underlying liver function, early endovascular intervention with transjugular intrahepatic portosystemic shunt should be considered after initial endoscopy with band ligation.
- Initial diagnosis of gastric variceal bleeding requires adequate clearance of the fundus during the initial endoscopy. When a high-risk mark (typically a flat, white area) is identified on a gastric varix, this should be considered diagnostic of bleeding.
- Initial therapy of bleeding gastric varices is best accomplished with endoscopic cyanoacrylate injection. When this is not available, balloon tamponade followed by cross-sectional imaging is best employed as a bridge to definitive therapy.
- Definitive endoscopic therapy of bleeding gastric varices should utilize cyanoacrylate injection with or without the use of endoscopic ultrasound guidance.

INTRODUCTION

Acute variceal bleeding is a serious complication of portal hypertension (HTN) with high associated morbidity and mortality. Although variceal bleeding occurs in patients with non-cirrhotic portal HTN, most of the diagnosis, risk stratification, and management of acute variceal bleeding have been defined in patients with cirrhosis and so that will be the focus of this article. Varices develop at a rate of 7% to 8% per year and are present in 30% to 40% of patients with compensated cirrhosis and up to

[a] Department of Medicine, University of Virginia School of Medicine, 1215 Lee Street, PO Box 800708, Charlottesville, VA 22908-0708, USA; [b] Division of Gastroenterology & Hepatology, University of Virginia School of Medicine, 1215 Lee Street, PO Box 800708, Charlottesville, VA 22908-0708, USA
* Corresponding author.
E-mail address: zhenry@virginia.edu

Gastrointest Endoscopy Clin N Am 34 (2024) 249–261
https://doi.org/10.1016/j.giec.2023.09.004
1052-5157/24/© 2023 Elsevier Inc. All rights reserved.

85% of patients with decompensated cirrhosis.[1-3] Esophageal varices (EV) are much more prevalent than gastric varices (GV) and have a higher incidence of bleeding; however, GV bleeding is often more severe.[4] Variceal bleeding occurs at a rate of 10% to 15% per year and is associated with a 6-week mortality of up to 25%.[5-8] Risk of bleeding for both esophageal and gastric varices is affected by the severity of underlying liver disease, the size of the varices, and the presence of high-risk stigmata (red wale marks and platelet plugs).[5,9,10] Six-week mortality is considered the primary endpoint from which to assess therapeutic interventions for variceal bleeding and is primarily affected by severity of underlying liver disease and the treatment at the time of bleeding.[11] Longer term survival after a variceal bleed is also affected by the severity of underlying liver disease, that is, the presence of additional decompensating symptoms such as ascites or encephalopathy. The 5-year mortality for a patient who suffers variceal bleeding as their initial decompensating event is only 20% but in the setting of additional portal hypertensive complications this can be as high as 80%.[6,11,12]

INITIAL MANAGEMENT

Patients with acute variceal bleeding will present with hematemesis, coffee-ground emesis, or melena in the setting of known or suspected portal HTN but at the time of presentation the source of bleeding will remain unknown and so initial medical management of these patients should follow standardized recommendations[11-13] as discussed in the first article of this issue (reference to Dr Barkun's article here). The primary goals of the initial medical management for suspected portal hypertensive bleeding revolve around hemodynamic stabilization and reduction of portal pressure. Some key points in this paradigm include adequate cardiopulmonary resuscitation to stabilize hemodynamics and control of the airway prior to initial endoscopy with a close eye to avoid over-resuscitation with blood products.[11-14] It is important to begin vasoactive medications, such as octreotide, to reduce portal pressure and decrease rates of early re-bleeding. In addition, antibiotic prophylaxis should be started immediately as it has been shown to not only reduce rates of infection but also reduce rates of re-bleeding.[11,15] Per both American and European guidelines, upper endoscopy should be performed as soon as possible but at a minimum within 12 hours of presentation. If a patient is unstable, they should be stabilized as mentioned earlier prior to endoscopy.[11,12] Regardless of current recommendations, comparisons between urgent endoscopy (within 6 hours) and early endoscopy (within 12–24 hours) have not shown a mortality benefit or significant differences in rates of early re-bleeding but given the need to facilitate definitive treatment plans for variceal bleeding earlier endoscopy (within 12 hours) is likely better.[16]

MANAGEMENT OF ESOPHAGEAL VARICES BLEEDING

The initial endoscopic examination is used for both risk stratification and diagnosis of EV and in many cases will also serve as the final therapeutic intervention given the effectiveness of band ligation. Definitive evidence of EV bleeding can be discerned by witnessing active bleeding from a varix or from the presence of a platelet plug, the so-called nipple sign (Fig. 1A). In absence of these findings, EV bleeding should be presumed in the presence of EV with or without red wales (Fig. 1B) and blood in the stomach at time of endoscopy where no alternative source of upper GI bleeding can be identified.[11,12] This recommendation is based on the relatively high incidence of EV bleeding in patients with underlying cirrhosis as compared to other causes of upper gastrointestinal (GI) bleeding in this population.

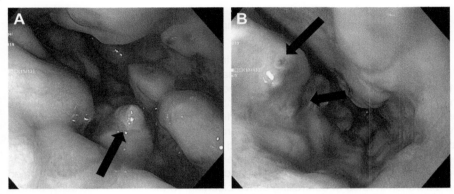

Fig. 1. High-Risk Stigmata on Esophageal Varices. (*A*) Large esophageal varices (EV) with an adherent platelet plug—black arrow; (*B*) Large EV with red wales present—black arrows.

Based on current recommendations from both the American Association for the Study of Liver Diseases and European Association for the Study of the Liver, the first-line therapy for acute esophageal variceal bleeding should be band ligation.[11,12] Bands should initially be deployed distally, at the gastro-esophageal (GE) junction, with progression proximally toward the mid-esophagus. Based on the inflow to EV from the left gastric vein, starting band ligation distally allows for decompression of the more proximal varices. Band ligation works by causing immediate hemostasis and then subsequent necrosis and fibrosis, which prevents penetrating veins infiltrating into the esophageal lumen. Variceal ligation is effective at controlling acute bleeding in 90% of cases but can be complicated by ulceration at the site of banding, esophageal rupture, esophageal stricture, dysphagia, and rebleeding.[17,18]

The Process of Band Ligation.

- Many acute variceal bleeds will present with hematemesis or at a minimum coffee ground emesis and often it is best to have the patient intubated prior to endoscopy to protect the airway. In addition, the process of band ligation can sometimes induce re-bleeding from EV and thus having the airway protected is paramount.
- During the initial pass with the endoscope, it is best to measure the z-line (GE junction) both on insertion and removal of the endoscope. If there is a large volume of bleeding, this will aid in identifying the best place to start band ligation when the lumen is obscured.
- On reintubation, with the banding cap in place, it is best to start banding as close to the GE junction as possible and often best to start between the 2 o'clock and 6 o'clock positions as this most often correlates with the lesser curve of the stomach and therefore the inflow of pressure from the left gastric vein.
- Bands should be place in spiral pattern moving proximally. Placing bands proximal to the lower third of the esophagus is unlikely to provide further benefit as the middle and upper thirds of the esophagus most often drain directly into the superior vena cava via the azygous system.
- When placing bands, it is important to suction the varix into the cap and hold it in place until a band is adequately deployed. During an acute variceal bleed, the pressure behind the varix is very high and suction will most likely induce bleeding. If the varix is dropped without placing a band, the bleeding can be severe and may conceal the lumen of the esophagus making further attempts at banding more difficult.

- During an acute bleed, direct visualization of the band passing into place over the varix may be obstructed and so it is important to get used to the feel of the band being deployed as well.

Alternative therapy includes endoscopic injection of sclerosing agents such as sodium tetradecyl sulfate, ethanolamine oleate, plain ethanol, and sodium morrhuate.[17,19] These agents can be injected directly into the varix to cause thrombosis or into the paravariceal space to cause tamponade but are associated with severe esophageal ulcers, increased risk of perforation, and esophageal strictures.[20-22] When compared to band ligation, sclerotherapy has higher rates of re-bleeding, lower rates of variceal eradication, and increased risk of complications but no clear difference in long-erm mortality.[22,23] In one interesting meta-analysis, band ligation was compared to combination therapy with band ligation and sclerotherapy. This revealed no difference in rates of controlling active bleeding, re-bleeding, or mortality, but did show a significantly higher rate of esophageal stricture in the group that received sclerotherapy in addition to band ligation.[24] Given the success of band ligation and the increased risk of complications with sclerotherapy, European and American GI/ Hepatology societial recommendations have removed its use from their guidelines.[11,12] There are reports of using endoscopic cyanoacrylate injection (ECI) in patients with acute EV bleeding which show good rates of initial hemostasis and relatively low rates of re-bleeding at 6 weeks but these were not controlled studies and it is unclear why the patients were selected for ECI over band ligation in these instances.[25,26] There are no randomized controlled trials comparing ECI to band ligation for management of EV bleeding and given thewidespread expertise with band ligation, the authors favor this over ECI.

In cases of severe bleeding where band ligation cannot be performed safely, then sclerotherapy or direct injection of cyanoacrylate may be reasonable alternatives to control the acute bleed until a more definitive treatment plan can be determined. Alternatively, balloon tamponade can be used as a temporizing measure with a reported 80% to 90% success rate in achieving hemostasis but can come with a high adverse event rate, most importantly esophageal necrosis if the balloon is left inflated for too long.[19] Esophageal stent placement has been compared to tamponade and shown to be superior in regards to controlling active bleeding with hemostasis rates greater than 90% but no difference noted in mortality.[27] Given the risk-benefit profile of the potential therapeutic options for acute EV bleeding, the authors recommend using band ligation as first-line therapy. If this cannot be done then, therapy with esophageal stent placement or ECI has the lowest reported complication rates. In general, the authors would recommend avoiding use of sclerotherapy or balloon tamponade in these patients unless there is no other option to control the acute bleed.

After the initial endoscopy, definitive therapy for EV is heavily influenced by the patient's underlying liver function as evidenced by the association between Child–Pugh score and risk of re-bleeding and death.[28] Based on this increased risk population, further studies suggested that performing early transjugular intrahepatic portosystemic shunt (TIPS) with polytetrafluoroethylene-covered stents after initial therapy with band ligation reduces the risk of re-bleeding and improves mortality.[29] Additionally, TIPS should also be considered as a salvage therapy when endoscopic intervention fails and refractory bleeding occurs—this will be discussed later in this issue.[11]

MANAGEMENT OF GASTRIC VARICEAL BLEEDING

The initial management of gastric variceal bleeding is the same as that for any suspected portal hypertensive bleeding—the differences in care are not evident until the initial diagnostic endoscopy. While GV along the lesser curve are the most prevalent form, it is the GV along the posterior wall and greater curvature of the cardiofundal region (Sarin class GOV2 and IGV1 – aka cardiofundal GV) that are most likely to bleed.[4] In many cases, the gastric fundus will be obscured with a mixture of fresh blood and clot that makes identifying cardiofundal GV difficult; however, spending the time to clear the fundus is very important as many patients may have both EV and GV present. Using a promotility agent, such as erythromycin, prior to endoscopy and/or using a therapeutic endoscope may improve visualization of the fundus during the initial endoscopy.[12,13]

Once the fundus is clear and GV identified, a standardized classification system should be used to risk stratify the gastric varix. Typically, this is done using the Sarin classification (**Fig. 2**) which describes GV based upon their location as well as their relationship to EV. While this system can be informative and is widely used, it does not impart any real risk stratification and so the authors recommend using a simplified approach based upon publications from Japan and Korea.[9,10] Similar to that for EV, these classification systems add information about the size of the varix, presence of

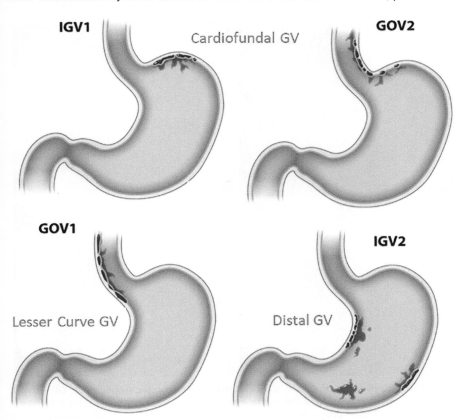

Fig. 2. Classification System of Gastric Varices Based on Location. The Sarin classification with an overlying simplified scheme based on location of the gastric varices (GV) in the stomach. Intra-gastric varices 1 (IGV1) and gastro-oesophageal varices 2 (GOV2) are grouped together as cardiofundal gastric varices. Gastro-oesophageal varices 1(GOV1) are also called lesser curve gastric varices. Intra-gastric varices 2 (IGV2) are also called distal varices—these are incredibly rare and are not discussed in this review.

high-risk stigmata, and severity of portal HTN as stratified by the Child–Pugh classification (**Fig. 3**). High-risk stigmata on a GV may appear differently than those for EV. This is typically seen as a platelet plug on EV (see **Fig. 1**A), but in the stomach the high-risk mark often looks like a flat or depressed area on the varix (see **Fig. 3**A). The presence of this high-risk mark or active bleeding seen at the time of endoscopy should be considered diagnostic for GV bleed.

During the initial endoscopy, a temporizing therapy should be applied until further evaluation with cross-sectional imaging can occur for a discussion of more definitive management.[13] The one occasion when the initial therapy may ultimately be the definitive therapy is for GV along the lesser curve of the stomach, so-called GOV1 by the Sarin classification. These varices often have similar vascular structure to EV(ie, an inflow from the left gastric vein) and can be treated with band ligation. For cardiofundal GV (GOV2, IGV1), endoscopic cyanoacrylate injection (ECI) is the initial treatment of choice and has been shown to be safe and effective.[30–32] However, this is often difficult to perform in the acute setting as there is no Food and Drug administration (FDA) approved, ready-made kit for ECI and most gastroenterologists in the United States

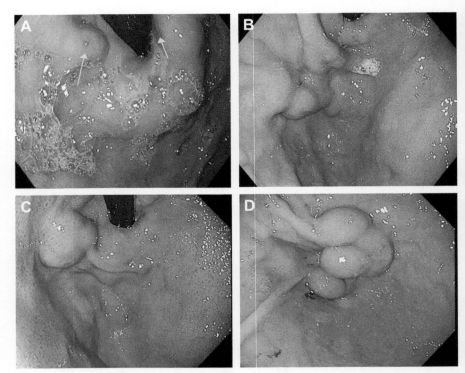

Fig. 3. Risk Stratification of Gastric Varices Based on Endoscopic Appearance. (*A*) GVwith high-risk stigmata as seen by a flat white mark with surround erythema. This is different than the classic platelet plug seen with EV. The *yellow arrow* on the left of box A is pointing to the high risk mark. The other arrow is simply pointing to the z-line. (*B*) Serpiginous varices in the cardiofundal region with diameter less than 10 mm—considered low risk. (*C*) Larger, nodular varices on the posterior wall of the cardiofundal region with diameter 10 to 20 mm—considered moderate to high risk. (*D*) Very large, tumorous-appearing varices with diameter greater than 20 mm on the greater curvature of the fundus—considered very high risk.

are not trained in its use. Furthermore, the preparation required for ECI can be cumbersome and time consuming, which is not always conducive for controlling acute bleeding—see **Fig. 4** for a detailed description of ECI.

Therefore, alternative options for emergent therapy include band ligation, balloon tamponade, endoscopic clip placement, thrombin injection, hemostatic powder, and sclerotherapy with alcohol-based sclerosants. In head-to-head studies, band ligation is feasible but inferior to ECI for acute and long-term management of GV, aside from those located along the lesser curve.[30,31] Unlike EV which are longitudinal cords of veins that can be easily suctioned into a banding device, cardiofundal GV are often large, tumorous-appearing vessels. Placing bands on these large vessels often leads to early ulceration and a much more severe re-bleeding event. In instances where band ligation is used to acutely control bleeding, the authors recommend urgent evaluation with cross-sectional imaging and definitive therapy to the GV as soon as possible. Endoscopic clip placement, thrombin injection, hemostatic powder, and alcohol-based sclerotherapy are not recommended due to lack of controlled data and, in the case of sclerotherapy, severe, acute re-bleeding due to creation of deep ulcerations over the varix.[33-36] When ECI cannot be performed, the safest technique to stabilize a cardiofundal GV bleed is to use balloon tamponade, but only inflating the gastric balloon. This creates direct compression to the varix to stop bleeding and allows time for multi-disciplinary discussion but the balloon should not be left inflated for greater than 16 hours and so definitive intervention should occur as soon as possible. A more in depth review of placing a balloon for tamponade is included in a prior publication.[37]

After the diagnostic endoscopy and initial temporizing therapy, contrasted cross-sectional imaging with either computed tomography (CT) or MRI must be obtained to better assess the underlying vasculature of the GV and to assess for the presence of porto-systemic shunts and thromboses. After obtaining these images, a multi-disciplinary conversation should occur between interventional radiologists, hepatologists/gastroenterologists, and in some cases advanced endoscopists.[13] Whether definitive treatment is endoscopic or endovascular, the patient's co-morbid portal hypertensive complications also need to be taken into account. Most endoscopic therapies will only treat the GV at the level of the stomach and will therefore have little impact on other portal HTN complications, but endovascular therapies may worsen or improve these co-morbid complications (ref to endovascular treatment chapter) (**Table 1**).

The ideal situation to pursue endoscopic therapy for definitive treatment of GV is in the absence of a large porto-systemic shunt where there is limited possibility for embolization, and efficacy of endovascular treatments is limited. In this setting, ECI is superior to other forms of endoscopic therapy[30,31]; however, once ECI is performed, it should be continued every 4 weeks with retreatment as needed, similar to band ligation for EV bleeding.[13] A step-by-step description of ECI via a standard gastroscope has previously been published.[13] The risks associated with ECI are rare when performed by trained endoscopists comfortable with the procedure and include thromboembolism in patients with an underlying porto-systemic shunt (up to 2%), infection (<3%), needle impaction (<1%), and bleeding (<1%).[38,39] Over the last 20 years, the use of endoscopic ultrasound for cyanoacrylate injection, with or without injection of a metallic coil, has been employed in an attempt to reduce the risks of embolization, better visualize the full varix, and ensure complete occlusion of the variceal complex in the gastric wall.[40,41] Unfortunately, due to heterogeneity of ECI techniques both with and without *endoscopic ultrasound* (EUS) guidance, definitive conclusions cannot be made about any one technique's superiority or cost effectiveness. Moving forward,

Recommended Method for Endoscopic Cyanoacrylate Injection

Preparation

1. Draw 15-20 cc neutral oil (such as olive oil) in 60 cc slip tip syringe
2. Connect endoscopic injector needle (19-23g) to 3-way stop cock[a]
3. Draw up 5 cc sterile water into a 5-10 cc syringe (prepare 2-4 syringes)[b]
4. Connect sterile water to side port of 3-way stop cock
5. Draw up 1-2 mL cyanoacrylate (CA) into a 5 cc syringe (prepare 2-4 syringes)[c]
6. Cap CA syringes and place on ice to prevent polymerization of CA[d]

Endoscopy

1. Use of standard gastroscope may be sufficient, but consider using a sigmoidoscope for increased flexibility needed in the cardia/fundus[e]
2. Best approach for cardiofundal varices is via retroflexion; for lesser curve or distal GV a forward view may be best
3. Use of endoscopic ultrasound will negate the need for retroflexion as the varix can be visualized using ultrasonography

Injection

1. Connect CA syringe at end of 3-way stop cock
2. Inject 1.5 cc of sterile water through injector needle while outside of scope to ensure patency[f]
3. Inject 5 cc of oil into working channel of endoscope[g]
4. Insert injector needle through working channel
5. In the gastric body test the needle mechanism by injecting 1.0-1.2 mL CA into the catheter (this will prime the injector needle with CA)[h]
6. Once in position, probe the GV with blunt injector catheter tip (needle in), away from bleeding site[i]
7. With the endoscope 3-5 cm away from the GV, put needle out and insert into GV[j]
8. As soon as needle is in the GV, inject CA, typically over 4-5 seconds
9. Once CA completely injected, switch stop cock to sterile water syringe and begin injecting the rest of the contents
10. After 2 cc of sterile water injected, remove needle from GV while still injecting the final amounts of water – this allows for all CA to be out of the catheter prior to removal and can help avoid needle impaction into the varix[k]
11. Once needle is retracted, remove injector catheter from working channel
12. Monitor injection site for 5-10 seconds before assessing other areas for injection[l]

Clean up

1. Once the endoscope is removed wash the working channel using a brush soaked in acetone[m]
2. Once the working channel is clear inspect the outside of the endoscope and scrub any CA residue with an acetone soaked gauze or sponge
3. Endoscopes should then be processed per standard protocols.
4. If endoscope withdrawn between injections to clean/remove CA residue, ensure endoscope is completely dry of acetone prior to re-intubation of the esophagus

Table 1
Gastric variceal intervention and its impact on portal hypertensive complications

	Endoscopic Cyanoacrylate Injection	Transjugular Intrahepatic Portosystemic Shunt	Balloon-Occluded Retrograde Transvenous Obliteration
Esophageal Varices	No change	Improves	Worsens
Ascites	No change	Improves	Worsens
Encephalopathy	No change	Worsens	Improves
Model for End-Stage Liver Disease (MELD) Score	No change	Either	Either

multi-centered randomized-controlled trials will be needed to discern the most efficient modality of cyanoacrylate delivery. Currently, treatment decisions should be made based upon local expertise and experience until such time that clinical trials identify a preferred method.

Due to the significant heterogeneity of vascular inflow and outflow with GV, multiple endovascular therapies have been identified for the management of bleeding GV. The largest randomized control trial (RCT) to compare ECI to TIPS was performed in 2001 and suggested that TIPS was superior in regards to short-term re-bleeding but there

◄───

Fig. 4. Recommended method for endoscopic cyanoacrylate (CA) therapy (derived from supplemental figure 1 in reference 13). [a]The authors do not recommend using an injector needle less than 23 gauge as the CA is increasingly difficult to inject through smaller gauge needles. [b]Sterile water should be used over normal saline as saline may interact with cyanoacrylate and cause rapid polymerization within the injector catheter. All of your materials and instruments should be tested in an ex vivo setting prior to ever performing endoscopic cyanoacrylate injection (ECI) in a patient to ensure early polymerization in the injector catheter will not occur. [c]Two mL aliquot allows a good volume of cyanoacrylate (CA) to be injected without increasing the risk of embolization, needle impaction, or need for many repeated injections. The use of mixing agents, such as lipiodol, is not recommended since they delay polymerization times and may increase risks of embolization. [d]Placing the syringe of CA on ice helps prevent polymerization of the glue within the syringe prior to injection. Once the glue is drawn into syringes, proceed with the endoscopy as soon as possible to avoid this. [e]A flexible sigmoidoscope (not often used in modern practice) has increased flexibility compared to a gastroscope and allows for easier access to the posterior wall of the cardia and fundus for CA injection. [f]This is to ensure the injector needle is patent and working correctly before you insert into the working channel. A 23 gauge injector needle holds approximately 1.3 to 1.5 mL of fluid within the catheter—you should inject just enough to see water leaves the tip of the needle. [g]Oil is used to coat the working channel to prevent CA coating the interior of the endoscope. [h]Injecting 1.2 mL into the catheter clears most of the sterile water from your injector catheter and primes it with CA so that once you begin injection, CA is immediately in contact with the inside of the vessel. [i]The authors recommend injecting away from a suspected site of bleeding to avoid inducing bleeding with needle insertion. This also allows the CA to polymerize over the high-risk area inside the vessel. [j]This distance is recommended to avoid "splash-back" of CA on the endoscope. [k]Ideally, this will clear the injector needle of any remaining CA and help avoid needle impaction into the GV while removing the needle. [l]Some oozing from the site is expected but is typically minimal and self-limited. [m]Acetone (nail polish remover) is a strong astringent that will help break up polymerized CA.

was no difference in survival and TIPS had a significantly increased risk of hepatic encephalopathy (HE) over the long term. Unfortunately, this study included both GVs along the lesser curve (GOV1) and true cardiofundal GV (GOV2). TIPS was superior to ECI only for the patients with GOV1 and not for those with GOV2. This suggests that ECI may be superior to TIPS for cardiofundal GV given similar efficacy but decreased morbidity with ECI.[42] Retrospective studies have suggested that balloon-occluded retrograde transvenous obliteration (BRTO) may be superior to ECI but have not shown a difference in mortality.[43] In 2021, the first true RCT between these 2 modalities was published suggesting while both therapies demonstrate good immediate control of bleeding, BRTO was superior in regards to long-term re-bleeding. Interestingly, there were no differences in mortality or adverse events between the groups, including rates of embolization in a population where all included study patients had a porto-systemic.[32] Further studies comparing ECI to BRTO are necessary as different ECI techniques, primarily those utilizing EUS to occlude the entire varix, may show equivalent rates of long-term re-bleeding with less procedural-related morbidity. In depth discussion of endovascular treatments for variceal bleeding is addressed later in this issue.

COMBINED MANAGEMENT OF ESOPHAGEAL VARICEAL AND GASTRO VARICEAL BLEEDING

In some cases, the source of bleeding is not clear on the initial endoscopy, that is, there is both the presence of high-risk GV and high-risk EV without overt bleeding from either one. Ideally, in this scenario, ECI would be performed for the GV followed by band ligation of the EV. This allows for local control of both entities and can still be followed by endovascular therapies if required. In addition, it allows for ongoing endoscopic follow-up to both at 4-week intervals as suggested by current guidelines.[11–13] Band ligation of the EV without addressing the underlying GV may preclude endoscopic access to the GV in the short term and therefore prevent ECI if deemed necessary. Generally, acute interventions to the GV will not interfere with management of EV with the exception of balloon tamponade. If there is no ability to perform both ECI to the GV and EV band ligation, then the authors recommend addressing EV bleeding first since this is much more likely to be the source of bleeding than a gastric varix. Regardless, cross-sectional imaging should still be obtained and a multi-disciplinary discussion has to determine if an alternative therapy (endovascular) may be available for management of the GV. Otherwise, it would be best to wait 3 to 5 days after initial band ligation of the EV before addressing the GV endoscopically.

SUMMARY

In summary, acute variceal bleeding is a serious and possibly life-threatening complication of cirrhosis and portal HTN. For bleeding EV, there is a large amount of data to show that band ligation is the best therapy though in instances where this cannot be performed alternative therapies with ECI or esophageal stent placement may be adequate measures until more definitive treatment can be performed, such as with TIPS. For gastric varices, acute therapy during the initial endoscopy as well as definitive therapy is not well defined. ECI has been shown to be effective in both situations but is not widely available for use in the United States and may be inferior to endovascular treatments such as BRTO. The addition of EUS for ECI may improve outcomes but has not yet shown superiority to standard ECI and further study is needed. Ultimately, management of these conditions should be based upon local expertise and available resources. When needed, patients should be transferred to tertiary care centers for multi-disciplinary care and follow-up.

CLINICS CARE POINTS

- During the initial endoscopy, it is important to clear the fundus of blood to ensure there are no underlying gastric varices.
- Band ligation of esophageal varices should start at the gastroesophageal junction and work proximally toward the middle esophagus
- The best initial therapy of bleeding GV is endoscopic cyanoacrylate injection.
- After the initial endoscopic temporizing therapy for gastric varices, contrasted cross-sectional imaging with CT or MRI must be obtained for further evaluation and planning of definitive management.

CONFLICTS OF INTEREST

K. Jobe – none; Z. Henry – none.

REFERENCES

1. Pagliaro L, D'Amico G, Pasta L, et al. Portal hypertension in cirrhosis: natural history. In: Bosch J, Groszmann RJ, editors. Portal hypertension. Pathophysiology and treatment. Oxford, UK: Blackwell Scientific; 1994. p. 72–92.
2. Kovalak M, Lake J, Mattek N, et al. Endoscopic screening for varices in cirrhotic patients: data from a national endoscopic database. Gastrointest Endosc 2007; 65:82–8.
3. Groszmann RJ, Garcia-Tsao G, Bosch J, et al. Beta-blockers to prevent gastroesophageal varices in patients with cirrhosis. N Engl J Med 2005;353:2254–61.
4. Sarin SK, Lahoti D, Saxena SP, et al. Prevalence, classification and natural history of gastric varices: a long-term follow-up study in 568 portal hypertension patients. Hepatology 1992 Dec;16(6):1343–9.
5. North Italian Endoscopic Club for the Study and Treatment of Esophageal Varices. Prediction of the first variceal hemorrhage in patients with cirrhosis of the liver and esophageal varices. A prospective multicenter study. N Engl J Med 1988;319:983–9.
6. D'Amico G, Pasta L, Morabito A, et al. Competing risks and prognostic stages of cirrhosis: a 25-year inception cohort study of 494 patients. Aliment Pharmacol Ther 2014;39(10):1180–93.
7. Reverter E, Tandon P, Augustin S, et al. A MELD-based model to determine risk of mortality among patients with acute variceal bleeding. Gastroenterology 2014; 146:412–9.
8. Amitrano L, Guardascione MA, Manguso F, et al. The effectiveness of current acute variceal bleed treatments in unselected cirrhotic patients: refining short-term prognosis and risk factors. Am J Gastroenterol 2012;107:1872–8.
9. Kim T, Shijo H, Kokawa H, et al. Risk factors for hemorrhage from gastric fundal varices. Hepatology 1997;25:307–12.
10. Hashizume M, Kitano S, Yamaga H, et al. Endoscopic classification of gastric varices. Gastrointest Endosc 1990;36:276–80.
11. Garcia-Tsao G, Abraldes JG, Berzigotti A, et al. Portal hypertensive bleeding in cirrhosis: Risk stratification, diagnosis, and management: 2016 practice

guidance by the American Association for the study of liver diseases. Hepatology 2017;65(1):310–35.

12. de Franchis R, Bosch J, Garcia-Tsao G, et al, Baveno VII Faculty. Baveno VII - Renewing consensus in portal hypertension. J Hepatol 2022;76(4):959–74.

13. Henry Z, Patel K, Patton H, et al. AGA clinical practice update on management of bleeding gastric varices: expert review. Clin Gastroenterol Hepatol 2021;19(6): 1098–107.

14. Villanueva C, Colomo A, Bosch A, et al. Transfusion strategies for acute upper gastrointestinal bleeding. N Engl J Med 2013;368(1):11–21.

15. Hou MC, Lin HC, Liu TT, et al. Antibiotic prophylaxis after endoscopic therapy prevents rebleeding in acute variceal hemorrhage: a randomized trial. Hepatology 2004;39(3):746–53.

16. Lau JYW, Yu Y, Tang RSY, et al. Timing of endoscopy for acute upper gastrointestinal bleeding. N Engl J Med 2020;382(14):1299–308.

17. Nett A, Binmoeller KF. Endoscopic management of portal hypertension-related bleeding. Gastrointest Endosc Clin N Am 2019;29(2):321–37. https://doi.org/10.1016/j.giec.2018.12.006.

18. Zuckerman MJ, Elhanafi S, Mendoza Ladd A. Endoscopic treatment of esophageal varices. Clin Liver Dis 2022;26(1):21–37. https://doi.org/10.1016/j.cld.2021.08.003.

19. Al-Obaid LN, Bazarbashi AN, Ryou M. Variceal bleeding: beyond banding. Dig Dis Sci 2022;67(5):1442–54.

20. Sarin SK, Nanda R, Sachdev G, et al. Intravariceal versus paravariceal sclerotherapy: a prospective, controlled, randomised trial. Gut 1987;28:657–62.

21. Sarin SK, Kumar A. Sclerosants for variceal sclerotherapy: a critical appraisal. Am J Gastroenterol 1990;85:641–9.

22. Dai C, Liu WX, Jiang M, et al. Endoscopic variceal ligation compared with endoscopic injection sclerotherapy for treatment of esophageal variceal hemorrhage: a meta-analysis. World J Gastroenterol 2015;21:2534–41.

23. Laine L, Cook D. Endoscopic ligation compared with sclerotherapy for treatment of esophageal variceal bleeding. A meta-analysis. Ann Intern Med 1995;123(4): 280–7.

24. Singh P, Pooran N, Indaram A, et al. Combined ligation and sclerotherapy versus ligation alone for secondary prophylaxis of esophageal variceal bleeding: a meta-analysis. Am J Gastroenterol 2002;97(3):623–9.

25. Cipolletta L, Zambelli A, Bianco MA, et al. Acrylate glue injection for acutely bleeding oesophageal varices: A prospective cohort study. Dig Liver Dis 2009; 41(10):729–34.

26. Ribeiro JP, Matuguma SE, Cheng S, et al. Results of treatment of esophageal variceal hemorrhage with endoscopic injection of n-butyl-2-cyanoacrylate in patients with Child-Pugh class C cirrhosis. Endosc Int Open 2015;3(6):E584–9.

27. Escorsell À, Pavel O, Cárdenas A, et al, Variceal Bleeding Study Group. Esophageal balloon tamponade versus esophageal stent in controlling acute refractory variceal bleeding: a multicenter randomized, controlled trial. Hepatology 2016; 63:1957–67.

28. Abraldes JG, Villanueva C, Banares R, et al. Hepatic venous pressure gradient and prognosis in patients with acute variceal bleeding treated with pharmacologic and endoscopic therapy. J Hepatol 2008;48:229–36.

29. Garcia-Pagan JC, Caca K, Bureau C, et al. Early TIPS (Transjugular Intrahepatic Portosystemic Shunt) Cooperative Study Group. Early use of TIPS in patients with cirrhosis and variceal bleeding. N Engl J Med 2010;362:2370–9.

30. Qiao W, Ren Y, Bai Y, et al. Cyanoacrylate injection versus band ligation in the endoscopic management of acute gastric variceal bleeding: meta-analysis of randomized, controlled studies based on the PRISMA statement. Medicine (Baltim) 2015;94(41):e1725.
31. Ríos Castellanos E, Seron P, Gisbert JP, et al. Endoscopic injection of cyanoacrylate glue versus other endoscopic procedures for acute bleeding gastric varices in people with portal hypertension. Cochrane Database Syst Rev 2015;(5): CD010180.
32. Luo X, Xiang T, Wu J, et al. Endoscopic cyanoacrylate injection versus balloon-occluded retrograde transvenous obliteration for prevention of gastric variceal bleeding: a randomized controlled trial. Hepatology 2021;74(4):2074–84.
33. Sarin SK. Long-term follow-up of gastric variceal sclerotherapy: an eleven-year experience. Gastrointest Endosc 1997;46:8–14.
34. Arantes V, Albuquerque W. Fundal variceal hemorrhage treated by endoscopic clip. Gastrointest Endosc 2005;61:732.
35. Holster IL, Poley J, Kuipers EJ, et al. Controlling gastric variceal bleeding with endoscopically applied hemostatic powder (HemosprayTM). J Hepatol 2012; 57:1397–8.
36. Yang WL, Tripathi D, Therapondos G, et al. Endoscopic use of human thrombin in bleeding gastric varices. Am J Gastroenterol 2002;97:1381–5.
37. Zachary H. Henry. Treatment of gastro-fundal varices (including a discussion of BRTO). Current Hepatology Reports 2018;17(3):184–92.
38. Cheng LF, Wang ZQ, Li CZ, et al. Low incidence of complications from endoscopic gastric variceal obturation with butyl cyanoacrylate. Clin Gastroenterol Hepatol 2010;8(9):760–6.
39. Caldwell SH, Hespenheide EE, Greenwald BD, et al. Enbucrilate for gastric varices: extended experience in 92 patients. Aliment Pharmacol Ther 2007;26(1): 49–59.
40. Mohan BP, Chandan S, Khan SR, et al. Efficacy and safety of endoscopic ultrasound-guided therapy versus direct endoscopic glue injection therapy for gastric varices: systematic review and meta-analysis. Endoscopy 2020;52(4): 259–67.
41. Baig M, Ramchandani M, Puli SR. Safety and efficacy of endoscopic ultrasound-guided combination therapy for treatment of gastric varices: a systematic review and meta-analysis. Clin J Gastroenterol 2022;15(2):310–9.
42. Lo GH, Liang HL, Chen WC, et al. A prospective, randomized controlled trial of transjugular intrahepatic portosystemic shunt versus cyanoacrylate injection in the prevention of gastric variceal rebleeding. Endoscopy 2007;39(8):679–85.
43. Stein DJ, Salinas C, Sabri S, et al. Balloon retrograde transvenous obliteration versus endoscopic cyanoacrylate in bleeding gastric varices: comparison of rebleeding and mortality with extended follow-up. J Vasc Intervent Radiol 2019; 30(2):187–94.

Role of Endoscopy in the Diagnosis, Grading, and Treatment of Portal Hypertensive Gastropathy and Gastric Antral Vascular Ectasia

Ali Khalifa, MD, Don C. Rockey, MD*

KEYWORDS

- Gastrointestinal bleeding • Iron deficiency anemia • Endoscopic management
- Liver cirrhosis • Portal hypertension

KEY POINTS

- Gastric antral vascular ectasia (GAVE) and portal hypertensive gastropathy (PHG) most commonly present with chronic iron deficiency anemia second to chronic gastrointestinal (GI) bleeding but can also cause overt GI bleeding.
- Although GAVE and PHG are distinct clinically, and in particular in endoscopic appearance and location, they may represent overlapping processes in patients with cirrhosis.
- When clinical and endoscopic features make GAVE and PHG difficult to differentiate, gastric biopsy and histologic assessment is helpful and is recommended.
- Distinguishing between GAVE and PHG is important because treatment approaches for each differ.
- Treatment of GAVE is primarily endoscopic, whereas treatment of PHG is primarily directed underlying portal hypertension.
- Treatment approaches for PHG and GAVE are constantly evolving and it is likely that more targeted and effective therapies will emerge over time.

INTRODUCTION

Gastric antral vascular ectasia (GAVE) and portal hypertensive gastropathy (PHG) are unique gastric lesions.[1] Despite being unique disease entities, they have been hypothesized to have a relatively similar pathophysiology and additionally often have a similar

Digestive Disease Research Center, Medical University of South Carolina, Charleston, South Carolina, USA
* Corresponding author. Department of Internal Medicine, Medical University of South Carolina, 96 Jonathan Lucas Street, Suite 803, MSC 623, Charleston, SC 29425.
E-mail address: rockey@musc.edu

Gastrointest Endoscopy Clin N Am 34 (2024) 263–274
https://doi.org/10.1016/j.giec.2023.09.013
giendo.theclinics.com

clinical presentation.[2] Differentiating between these 2 entities is important because their management and, ultimately, clinical outcomes vary.

GAVE is an infrequent yet significant cause of acute and occult cause of upper gastrointestinal bleeding (UGIB). Studies indicate that it accounts for approximately 2% to 4% of gastrointestinal (GI) bleeding episodes in most populations.[3] Although the first documented description of GAVE dates to 1953 and was not extensively investigated for another 25 years, the exact pathophysiology and underlying cause remain poorly understood, rendering it an idiopathic condition.[3] Furthermore, there is currently no universally agreed-upon approach for managing GAVE.

In contrast, it has been postulated that elevated portal pressure (whether cirrhotic or noncirrhotic portal hypertension) drives the pathogenesis of PHG.[4] It has been suggested that the prevalence of PHG among patients with cirrhosis is 20% to 75%, with a higher prevalence among patients with decompensated disease—likely secondary to increasing portal pressure.[5] Despite such a hypothesized correlation/causation of PHG and portal hypertension, the exact pathophysiology remains poorly understood. Therefore, the best proof that portal hypertension is required for the development of PHG is studies that demonstrate an improvement of PHG after shunt surgery or transjugular intrahepatic portosystemic shunt (TIPS) placement.

Given that PHG and GAVE have some characteristics in common (potential for similar endoscopic appearances, a potential link to portal hypertension, and so forth), there is potential for misdiagnosis and thus, inappropriate management. The goal of this review is to highlight key clinical and endoscopic features of GAVE and PHG and to review their management.

CLINICAL PRESENTATION

Either PHG or GAVE can present with overt GI bleeding or with evidence of chronic bleeding (in particular iron deficiency anemia [IDA]). These lesions may also be asymptomatic without evidence of bleeding (and can be identified incidentally during endoscopy).[6] Patients with PHG are most likely to be asymptomatic; thus PHG is typically found incidentally by esophagogastroduodenoscopy (EGD) done for variceal screening or for UGIB.[7] PHG most commonly presents with IDA secondary to chronic and occult blood loss (chronic GI bleeding is defined as a decrease of hemoglobin of 2 g/dL within a 6-month time period without evidence of overt bleeding and not attributed to nonsteroidal anti-inflammatory drugs usage) and, less commonly (2%–12%), as acute UGIB with or without hemodynamic instability.[8–11]

Similarly, patients with GAVE may be asymptomatic, or have IDA, or acute GI bleeding.[12] Most patients with GAVE are asymptomatic and GAVE is noted incidentally.[13] Symptomatic patients with GAVE typically present with IDA second to occult bleeding or with acute UGIB.[13] It has been suggested that among patients with cirrhosis, GAVE-related acute bleeding is much less common than that from PHG.[10] Overt UGIB due to GAVE bleeding was shown in one study to be more common in patients without cirrhosis than in patients with cirrhosis (86% vs 25%).[14]

ENDOSCOPIC EVALUATION

PHG and GAVE can often be differentiated based on appearance and location. PHG is usually found in the stomach fundus and body, whereas GAVE is most commonly antral. Nevertheless, PHG lesions have been reported to extend to the antrum, whereas GAVE lesions may extend toward the gastric body and fundus, where red spots may coalesce proximally and distally covering the entire stomach.[15]

Endoscopically, PHG is characterized by the presence of a fine white mosaic-like (or reticular-like) pattern separated by pinkish mucosa (snakeskin appearance). PHG lesions are most commonly found in the proximal stomach (ie, fundus or body).[15] The Baveno scoring system for PHG (and GAVE) was suggested in 1996, and it uses point calculations to define PHG as mild (≤3 points) versus severe (≥4 points).[16] In 2013, it was proposed to use binary criteria for the diagnosis of PHG (including mosaic-like pattern, red-point lesions, and cherry-red spots with no subdivisions or classification systems).[17] These binary criteria were associated with a high rate of interobserver reliability. Therefore, PHG is commonly classified as "mild" or "severe"—with "mild" denoting the snakeskin mosaic pattern and "severe" denoting a flat or bulging red or brown spots.[17] Notably, on some occasions, PHG may present with flat or raised red lesions that may resemble GAVE lesions.[18]

In contrast, GAVE may have a variety of endoscopic features, including the following: (1) watermelon stomach—the classic GAVE endoscopic morphology, described as flat (sometimes raised) red stripes spiraling away from the pylorus toward the antrum, (2) honeycomb stomach—characterized by the similar red lesions spread out in a diffuse pattern, or (3) nodular GAVE—characterized by the presence of nodules and is often more challenging to endoscopically distinguish from other benign antral nodules.[19] In one study, all GAVE patients with cirrhosis had a punctate pattern at the time of endoscopy, whereas most patients (86%) without cirrhosis had a striped pattern.[14] Given the various clinical phenotypes of GAVE, a recent study evaluated the likelihood of GAVE type misclassification on endoscopic assessment.[19] The study concluded that GAVE was misclassified in up to 40% of patients, with hepatologists and gastroenterologists having similar misclassification rates. The correlation of different clinical patterns of GAVE with a specific disease association is not fully clear.

RADIOGRAPHIC FEATURES

Although PHG and GAVE are typically identified endoscopically, they may also be identified radiographically. PHG may manifest on barium studies because thickened nodular folds in the gastric fundus mimicking gastric varices and gastritis induced thickened gastric folds.[20] Thus, PHG should be suspected when such a radiological finding is detected in patients with known portal hypertension. Similarly, enhancement on the inner layer of gastric walls on computed tomography (CT) imaging may reflect gastric congestion, and thus PHG should be suspected when this finding is detected on CT scans in patients with portal hypertension. Additionally, capsule endoscopy may identify PHG; several studies demonstrated a sensitivity and specificity for the detection of PHG of 69% to 74% and 83% to 99%, respectively.[21,22] However, characteristic findings of GAVE on CT include prominent scalloped antral folds radiating to the pylorus and thickening of the gastric antrum.[23] Furthermore, on endoscopic ultrasound, GAVE seems as hyperechoic focal thickening of the inner layers of the gastric wall.[24]

HISTOPATHOLOGICAL EVALUATION

The histopathologic evaluation may be helpful when the clinical diagnosis is unclear, especially in patients with cirrhosis presenting with nonvariceal upper GI bleeding who have reddish gastric lesions identified endoscopically.[15] PHG is characterized histologically by dilated mucosal and submucosal veins as well as dilated capillaries on an edematous noninflamed background.[25] PHG is also characterized by hypertrophied gastric glands, capillary congestion, and neutrophilic cellular infiltration.[26] In addition, gastric atrophy and intestinal metaplasia have also been reported.[27] In contrast, GAVE is characterized histologically by a noninflamed mucosa with reactive epithelial hyperplasia and vascular ectasia (mildly dilated lamina propria and congested thrombosed capillaries) as well as a reactive fibromuscular hyperplasia (second to spindle cell proliferation and fibrohyalinosis).[28] A recent study compared virtual chromoendoscopy (named "I-scan") to high-definition white light endoscopy (HDWLE) for real-time endoscopic diagnosis of GAVE and PHG.[29] The study demonstrated that I-scan was superior to HDWLE in GAVE patients and had a similar accuracy in detecting PHG. Further, I-scan was less likely to yield an accurate diagnosis of GAVE among patients with elevated creatinine or those on hemodialysis. Such an endoscopic approach is attractive because it would eliminate any risk of biopsy in decompensated patients with cirrhosis who may be at an increased bleeding risk.

MANAGEMENT

Patients with PHG or GAVE and evidence of active bleeding or IDA warrant treatment. The definition of treatment response for GAVE has been defined as follows: (1) resolution of the GI bleeding (includes clinical/endoscopic evidence that bleeding has stopped, with no further requirements for blood transfusion, and stable laboratory parameters (eg, hemoglobin and hematocrit), (2) complete endoscopic ablation, or (3) histologic resolution.[30] However, consensus on this subject is lacking. Similarly, there is no consensus on the definition of resolution of PHG, and it is unlikely for PHG to resolve without correction of underlying portal hypertension (ie, such as after liver transplantation).

Distinguishing GAVE from PHG is extremely important because the treatment of these 2 lesions is fundamentally different. For PHG, although there does not seem to be an ideal treatment approach, the most effective treatment approaches seem to revolve around reduction of elevated portal pressure.[31] Beta-blockers (eg, propranolol, nadolol, and carvedilol) have been widely used to reduce portal pressures and reduce the risk of initial variceal hemorrhage (primary prophylaxis).[32] However, data supporting the use of beta-blockers for primary prophylaxis in PHG are limited. Most experts suggest using beta-blockers in patients with severe PHG but not mild PHG.[15] Several clinical studies suggest that patients with nonbleeding PHG treated with propranolol had better outcomes than patients treated with placebo (bleeding severity and mortality).[33,34] Other studies suggest that TIPS placement and liver transplantation may improve PHG lesions with subsequent reduction in transfusion requirements.[35,36] Other studies have demonstrated significant endoscopic improvement in PHG lesions and transfusion requirements within 2 to 3 months of TIPS and reduction in hepatic venous pressure gradient.[36–38] Liver transplantation also results in amelioration of PHG but is not typically used as a primary treatment modality for PHG.[39]

For acute bleeding due to suspected or possible PHG, management begins as with all GI bleeding—with proper resuscitation.[40] It is important to note that the routine use of nasogastric lavage is not currently recommended in patients with any form of upper GI bleeding.[41] Patients should receive appropriate intravenous fluids as well as packed red blood cell transfusion to maintain hemoglobin levels between 7 and 8 g/dL.[42] Proton pump inhibitors, vasoactive agents, and antibiotics (ie, ceftriaxone) may also be used, although the evidence that they are beneficial is weak.[35,43] Octreotide and terlipressin reduce portal pressure by inducing splanchnic vasoconstriction and thus should be initiated at the time of presentation in all patients with cirrhosis and GI bleeding.[44,45]

ENDOSCOPIC MANAGEMENT

Current guidelines recommend EGD evaluation within 12 or 24 hours in patients with upper GI bleeding in patients with cirrhosis and those without cirrhosis, respectively.[46,47]

Endoscopic management in acute PHG bleeding is often limited as bleeding is typically diffuse. Rather, endoscopic treatment is reserved for situations in which a limited number of lesions are identified. Unlike PHG, GAVE is much less likely to be controlled by reducing portal pressures (eg, through beta blockers, TIPS procedure, or shunt surgery) because it does not seem to be caused by portal hypertension. Nevertheless, GAVE is more amenable to endoscopic measures, specifically thermal ablative methods. Current therapeutic options to treat PHG and GAVE include argon plasma coagulation (APC), hemospray, cryotherapy, endoscopic band ligation (EBL), and laser therapy.[25]

Argon Plasma Coagulation

APC is a noncontact thermal method of hemostasis involving the use of a jet of ionized argon gas (plasma) that is directed through a probe passed through the endoscope, which leads to coagulative necrosis (typically limited to superficial layers).[48] APC has been used for both GAVE and PHG. It is the primary mode of therapy for these lesions because it is more likely to effectively target large bleeding surface areas, which are often involved in these disorders.

A. Portal hypertensive gastropathy

In one study evaluating the efficacy of APC in management of PHG, it was found that APC rapidly and effectively controlled PHG-induced bleeding.[49] In patients admitted to the hospital with UGIB secondary to PHG, APC induced hemostasis in 81% of the patients.[49]

B. Gastric antral vascular ectasia

APC is currently the most commonly used modality to treat GAVE, with a success rate of 40% to 100%.[50] Compared with neodymium-yttrium-aluminum garnet (NAG) laser, APC is relatively easier to use, less expensive, and has less severe side effects.[51–53] Nevertheless, most of the available data are from case series, and there are no available randomized control trials comparing APC to NAG laser. A controversial issue is recurrence of GAVE after APC ablation,[52] which has ranged from 15% to 79%.[54–57] It has been hypothesized that recurrent bleeding following APC ablation is related to the limited depth of penetration of APC (which is typically limited to the mucosal layer), whereas GAVE usually extends to the submucosa.[2,57,58] Similar to NAG laser, APC ablation has been associated with development of hyperplastic polyps.[58] Additionally, Mallory–Weiss syndrome can be observed after APC.[59]

Endoscopic Band Ligation

EBL has evolved as an effective endoscopic mode of therapy for several lesions, including angiodysplasia, Dieulafoy's lesions, GAVE, and others.[60] EBL leads to mechanical strangulation of lesions through the placement of elastic bands, resulting in thrombosis, necrosis, and a subsequent fibrotic wound healing response of the mucosa and submucosa.[61,62] For treatment of GAVE, the estimated success rate of EBL ranges from 78% to 100%.[50] In a recent prospective study evaluating EBL for GAVE, there was a significant improvement in the mean hemoglobin level and a significant decrease in blood transfusion requirements.[63] Further, a recently published systematic review comparing EBL to APC for the treatment of GAVE concluded that EBL was superior to APC in the treatment of GAVE in terms of endoscopic eradication rates, recurrence of bleeding, and transfusion requirements.[64–67] It should be noted that GAVE has been reported to recur following EBL (an estimated rate of up to nearly 50%).[50]

Radiofrequency Ablation

Because of the ability to provide widespread ablation coverage, radiofrequency ablation (RFA) has been proposed as an alternative to other modalities in patients with refractory GAVE.[50] RFA applies a high-energy coaptive coagulation destroying the superficial mucosal capillary ectasia in a uniformed and deeper pattern with the subsequent regeneration of a normal tissue.[30] The endoscopic success rate of RFA has been reported to be 90% to 100% with a recurrence rate from 21% to 33%.[50] A prospective open-label case series of patients with GAVE undergoing RFA found that 83% of the patients were no longer dependent on blood transfusion.[68] Several clinical trials evaluating the role of RFA in GAVE demonstrated a decrease in the need for subsequent blood transfusions, with few procedure-related complications (eg, such as RFA-related bleeding ulcers).[69,70] Collectively, growing evidence suggests that RFA is a feasible and safe method to ablate GAVE lesions.[30] It should also be noted that a multimodal approach (ie, APC ± RFA ± EBL) may be effective, particularly in nodular GAVE.[71]

Cryotherapy

Cryotherapy causes mucosal thermal injury, necrosis, and a wound healing response and thus induces hemostasis. A pilot study evaluated the role of cryotherapy in 26 patients presenting with UGIB (of whom 7 patients had GAVE).[72] Hemostasis was achieved with cryotherapy in 5 out of 7 patients with GAVE (71%). Cryotherapy may also be effective for patients with APC refractory GAVE.[73,74] Adverse events from cryotherapy most commonly include chest pain, esophageal strictures, bleeding, and gastric perforation, so caution is required and it should probably be reserved for refractory cases.[74,75]

Tranexamic Acid

Tranexamic acid (TXA) is an antifibrinolytic agent (through plasmin inhibition) that has been studied in various forms of upper GI bleeding.[76] It was also demonstrated to be effective in controlling GAVE-related bleeding.[77,78] However, it was also noted that TXA increases the risk of thromboembolism (eg, central venous stasis retinopathy or pulmonary embolism).[79]

Neodymium-yttrium-aluminum Garnet Laser Coagulation

NAG laser provides thermal energy that causes an indirect (contactless) tissue destruction. Abundant literature (primarily case series) had discussed the role of NAG laser therapy in GAVE, reporting it as useful and effective method to control the bleeding.[80–82] Nevertheless, because NAG therapy is costly and is associated with significant complications (gastric narrowing, perforations, hyperplastic polyps, and neoplasia), its use has declined.[83]

Thalidomide

Thalidomide, an antiangiogenic agent, has been used in angiodysplasia bleeding[84] and several case reports have suggested its potential role in controlling PHG and GAVE-related bleeding, with subsequent improvement in hemoglobin levels and transfusion requirements.[85–88] Given potential complications of thalidomide including its teratogenicity, it has been used sparingly.

ORTHOTOPIC LIVER TRANSPLANTATION

There is a growing body of evidence that indicates that PHG can be reversed after orthotopic liver transplantation (OLT). Because liver transplantation eliminates portal hypertension, this is not surprising.[15] In one study, PHG (and portal hypertensive enteropathy-related GI bleeding) resolved after liver transplantation.[89] For GAVE, one study demonstrated that 60% (6 out of 10 patients) of patients had complete resolution of GAVE after OLT.[90] Despite these promising data, the authors of this study recommended further studies be performed.

SUMMARY

Although PHG and GAVE may have a similar presentation with chronic GI bleeding and IDA, or acute GI bleeding, they are different entities. However, they often have overlapping endoscopic findings. It is also important to recognize that treatment of GAVE and PHG differ. Therefore, it remains critical to distinguish these 2 diseases. Despite advances in diagnosis and treatment, the optimal medical and/or endoscopic management of PHG and GAVE are not entirely clear. Furthermore, to date, there is no consensus on the definition of treatment success, lesion eradication, recurrence, or clinical response among the available studies. Large high-quality randomized trials evaluating medical and endoscopic therapies are needed.

CLINIC CARE POINTS

- GAVE and PHG are 2 distinct gastrointestinal disorders, yet they often have a similar clinical presentation.
- The exact cause of GAVE is not fully understood but it is often associated with underlying conditions such as cirrhosis, autoimmune diseases, and chronic renal failure. However, PHG is only found in patients with portal hypertension, caused by cirrhosis (most commonly), congestive heart failure, and/or portal vein thrombosis.
- Endoscopically, GAVE is characterized by a typical striped "watermelon" pattern most prominent in the distal stomach, whereas PHG is characterized by the diffuse changes in the gastric mucosa due to increased portal venous pressure, most prominent in the proximal stomach.
- Management of GAVE and PHG requires a multifaceted approach. GAVE can often be treated via endoscopic therapies, whereas PHG management typically depends on addressing underlying portal hypertension.

ACKNOWLEDGMENTS

Ali Khalifa: Review concept and design; acquisition of data; analysis and interpretation of data; drafting of the review article; critical revision of the article for important intellectual content. Email: khalifa@musc.edu.

Don Rockey: Review concept and design; acquisition of data; analysis and interpretation of data; drafting of the review article; critical revision of the article for important intellectual content; supervisory efforts. E-mail: rockey@musc.edu.

CONFLICT OF INTEREST STATEMENT

The authors have no competing interests to disclose.

DISCLOSURE

Grant Support: This project was supported, in part, by the National Institutes of Health, United States—the National Institute of Diabetes and Digestive and Kidney Disease (grant number P30 DK123704—the clinical component), the National Institute of General Medical Sciences, United States (grant number P20 GM 130457—support to D.C. Rockey).

REFERENCES

1. Burak KW, Lee SS, Beck PL. Portal hypertensive gastropathy and gastric antral vascular ectasia (GAVE) syndrome. Gut 2001;49(6):866–72.
2. Patwardhan VR, Cardenas A. Review article: the management of portal hypertensive gastropathy and gastric antral vascular ectasia in cirrhosis. Aliment Pharmacol Ther 2014;40(4):354–62.
3. Dulai GS, Jensen DM, Kovacs TO, et al. Endoscopic treatment outcomes in watermelon stomach patients with and without portal hypertension. Endoscopy 2004;36(1):68–72.
4. Bosch J, Iwakiri Y. The portal hypertension syndrome: etiology, classification, relevance, and animal models. Hepatol Int 2018;12(Suppl 1):1–10.
5. Gjeorgjievski M, Cappell MS. Portal hypertensive gastropathy: A systematic review of the pathophysiology, clinical presentation, natural history and therapy. World J Hepatol 2016;8(4):231–62.
6. Rockey DC, Altayar O, Falck-Ytter Y, et al. AGA technical review on gastrointestinal evaluation of iron deficiency anemia. Gastroenterology 2020;159(3):1097–119.
7. Urrunaga NH, Rockey DC. Portal hypertensive gastropathy and colopathy. Clin Liver Dis 2014;18(2):389–406.
8. Paternostro R, Kapzan L, Mandorfer M, et al. Anemia and iron deficiency in compensated and decompensated cirrhosis: Prevalence and impact on clinical outcomes. J Gastroenterol Hepatol 2020;35(9):1619–27.
9. de Franchis R. Revising consensus in portal hypertension: report of the Baveno V consensus workshop on methodology of diagnosis and therapy in portal hypertension. J Hepatol 2010;53(4):762–8.
10. Lyles T, Elliott A, Rockey DC. A risk scoring system to predict in-hospital mortality in patients with cirrhosis presenting with upper gastrointestinal bleeding. J Clin Gastroenterol 2014;48(8):712–20.
11. Merli M, Nicolini G, Angeloni S, et al. The natural history of portal hypertensive gastropathy in patients with liver cirrhosis and mild portal hypertension. Am J Gastroenterol 2004;99(10):1959–65.
12. Selinger CP, Ang YS. Gastric antral vascular ectasia (GAVE): an update on clinical presentation, pathophysiology and treatment. Digestion 2008;77(2):131–7.
13. Kichloo A, Solanki D, Singh J, et al. Gastric antral vascular ectasia: trends of hospitalizations, biodemographic characteristics, and outcomes with watermelon stomach. Gastroenterology Res 2021;14(2):104–11.
14. Kwon HJ, Lee SH, Cho JH. Influences of etiology and endoscopic appearance on the long-term outcomes of gastric antral vascular ectasia. World J Clin Cases 2022;10(18):6050–9.
15. Rockey DC. An update: portal hypertensive gastropathy and colopathy. Clin Liver Dis 2019;23(4):643–58.
16. de Franchis R. Portal hypertension II. Paper presented at: Proceedings of the second Baveno international consensus workshop on definitions, methodology and therapeutic strategies. Oxford: Blackwell Science; 1996.
17. de Macedo GF, Ferreira FG, Ribeiro MA, et al. Reliability in endoscopic diagnosis of portal hypertensive gastropathy. World J Gastrointest Endosc 2013;5(7):323–31.

18. Rajabnia M, Hatami B, Ketabi Moghadam P, et al. Comparison of portal hypertensive gastropathy and gastric antral vascular ectasia: an update. Gastroenterol Hepatol Bed Bench 2022;15(3):204–18.
19. Aryan M, Jariwala R, Alkurdi B, et al. The misclassification of gastric antral vascular ectasia. J Clin Transl Res 2022;8(3):218–23.
20. Chang D, Levine MS, Ginsberg GG, et al. Portal hypertensive gastropathy: radiographic findings in eight patients. AJR Am J Roentgenol 2000;175(6):1609–12.
21. de Franchis R, Eisen GM, Laine L, et al. Esophageal capsule endoscopy for screening and surveillance of esophageal varices in patients with portal hypertension. Hepatology 2008;47(5):1595–603.
22. Aoyama T, Oka S, Aikata H, et al. Small bowel abnormalities in patients with compensated liver cirrhosis. Dig Dis Sci 2013;58(5):1390–6.
23. Urban BA, Jones B, Fishman EK, et al. Gastric antral vascular ectasia ("watermelon stomach"): radiologic findings. Radiology 1991;178(2):517–8.
24. Barnard GF, Colby JM, Saltzman JR, et al. Endoscopic ultrasound appearance of watermelon stomach. Abdom Imaging 1995;20(1):26–8.
25. Ripoll C, Garcia-Tsao G. The management of portal hypertensive gastropathy and gastric antral vascular ectasia. Dig Liver Dis 2011;43(5):345–51.
26. Chandanwale S, Gupta N, Sheth J, et al. Histopathological study of portal hypertensive gastropathy using gastric biopsy. Medical Journal of Dr DY Patil University 2017;10(6):562–7.
27. Ibrişim D, Cevikbaş U, Akyüz F, et al. Intestinal metaplasia in portal hypertensive gastropathy: a frequent pathology. Eur J Gastroenterol Hepatol 2008;20(9):874–80.
28. Thomas A, Koch D, Marsteller W, et al. An analysis of the clinical, laboratory, and histological features of striped, punctate, and nodular gastric antral vascular ectasia. Dig Dis Sci 2018;63(4):966–73.
29. Al-Taee AM, Cubillan MP, Hinton A, et al. Accuracy of virtual chromoendoscopy in differentiating gastric antral vascular ectasia from portal hypertensive gastropathy: A proof of concept study. World J Hepatol 2021;13(12):2168–78.
30. Peter S, Wilcox CM. Radiofrequency ablation therapy - the grave for GAVE (gastric antral vascular ectasia)? Endosc Int Open 2015;3(2):E128–9.
31. Marrache MK, Bou Daher H, Rockey DC. The relationship between portal hypertension and portal hypertensive gastropathy. Scand J Gastroenterol 2022;57(3):340–4.
32. Rockey DC, Cello JP. Evaluation of the gastrointestinal tract in patients with iron-deficiency anemia. N Engl J Med 1993;329(23):1691–5.
33. Hosking SW, Kennedy HJ, Seddon I, et al. The role of propranolol in congestive gastropathy of portal hypertension. Hepatology 1987;7(3):437–41.
34. Pérez-Ayuso RM, Piqué JM, Bosch J, et al. Propranolol in prevention of recurrent bleeding from severe portal hypertensive gastropathy in cirrhosis. Lancet 1991;337(8755):1431–4.
35. Garcia-Tsao G, Abraldes JG, Berzigotti A, et al. Portal hypertensive bleeding in cirrhosis: Risk stratification, diagnosis, and management: 2016 practice guidance by the American Association for the study of liver diseases. Hepatology 2017;65(1):310–35.
36. Tripathi D, Stanley AJ, Hayes PC, et al. Transjugular intrahepatic portosystemic stent-shunt in the management of portal hypertension. Gut 2020;69(7):1173–92. https://doi.org/10.1136/gutjnl-2019-320221.

37. Urata J, Yamashita Y, Tsuchigame T, et al. The effects of transjugular intrahepatic portosystemic shunt on portal hypertensive gastropathy. J Gastroenterol Hepatol 1998;13(10):1061–7.
38. Mezawa S, Homma H, Ohta H, et al. Effect of transjugular intrahepatic portosystemic shunt formation on portal hypertensive gastropathy and gastric circulation. Am J Gastroenterol 2001;96(4):1155–9.
39. DeWeert TM, Gostout CJ, Wiesner RH. Congestive gastropathy and other upper endoscopic findings in 81 consecutive patients undergoing orthotopic liver transplantation. Am J Gastroenterol 1990;85(5):573–6.
40. Laine L, Laursen SB, Zakko L, et al. Severity and Outcomes of Upper Gastrointestinal Bleeding With Bloody Vs. Coffee-Grounds Hematemesis. Am J Gastroenterol 2018;113(3):358–66.
41. Rockey DC, Ahn C, de Melo SW Jr. Randomized pragmatic trial of nasogastric tube placement in patients with upper gastrointestinal tract bleeding. J Investig Med 2017;65(4):759–64.
42. Stanley AJ, Laine L. Management of acute upper gastrointestinal bleeding. BMJ 2019;364:l536.
43. Fernández J, Ruiz del Arbol L, Gómez C, et al. Norfloxacin vs ceftriaxone in the prophylaxis of infections in patients with advanced cirrhosis and hemorrhage. Gastroenterology 2006;131(4):1049–56 ; quiz 1285.
44. Gralnek IM, Camus Duboc M, Garcia-Pagan JC, et al. Endoscopic diagnosis and management of esophagogastric variceal hemorrhage: European Society of Gastrointestinal Endoscopy (ESGE) Guideline. Endoscopy 2022;54(11):1094–120.
45. Ioannou G, Doust J, Rockey DC. Terlipressin for acute esophageal variceal hemorrhage. Cochrane Database Syst Rev 2003;1:Cd002147.
46. Kumar NL, Cohen AJ, Nayor J, et al. Timing of upper endoscopy influences outcomes in patients with acute nonvariceal upper GI bleeding. Gastrointest Endosc 2017;85(5):945–52.e941.
47. Guo CLT, Wong SH, Lau LHS, et al. Timing of endoscopy for acute upper gastrointestinal bleeding: a territory-wide cohort study. Gut 2022;71(8):1544–50.
48. Zippi M, Traversa G, Cocco A, et al. [Use of argon plasma coagulation in digestive endoscopy: a concise review]. Clin Ter 2012;163(6):e435–40.
49. Hanafy AS, El Hawary AT. Efficacy of argon plasma coagulation in the management of portal hypertensive gastropathy. Endosc Int Open 2016;4(10):E1057–62.
50. Peng M, Guo X, Yi F, et al. Endoscopic treatment for gastric antral vascular ectasia. Ther Adv Chronic Dis 2021;12. 20406223211039696.
51. Kwan V, Bourke MJ, Williams SJ, et al. Argon plasma coagulation in the management of symptomatic gastrointestinal vascular lesions: experience in 100 consecutive patients with long-term follow-up. Am J Gastroenterol 2006;101(1):58–63.
52. Pavey DA, Craig PI. Endoscopic therapy for upper-GI vascular ectasias. Gastrointest Endosc 2004;59(2):233–8.
53. Sebastian S, McLoughlin R, Qasim A, et al. Endoscopic argon plasma coagulation for the treatment of gastric antral vascular ectasia (watermelon stomach): long-term results. Dig Liver Dis 2004;36(3):212–7.
54. Chaves DM, Sakai P, Oliveira CV, et al. Watermelon stomach: clinical aspects and treatment with argon plasma coagulation. Arq Gastroenterol 2006;43(3):191–5.
55. Yusoff I, Brennan F, Ormonde D, et al. Argon plasma coagulation for treatment of watermelon stomach. Endoscopy 2002;34(5):407–10.
56. Chiu YC, Lu LS, Wu KL, et al. Comparison of argon plasma coagulation in management of upper gastrointestinal angiodysplasia and gastric antral vascular ectasia hemorrhage. BMC Gastroenterol 2012;12:67.

57. Boltin D, Gingold-Belfer R, Lichtenstein L, et al. Long-term treatment outcome of patients with gastric vascular ectasia treated with argon plasma coagulation. Eur J Gastroenterol Hepatol 2014;26(6):588–93.

58. Fuccio L, Zagari RM, Serrani M, et al. Endoscopic argon plasma coagulation for the treatment of gastric antral vascular ectasia-related bleeding in patients with liver cirrhosis. Digestion 2009;79(3):143–50.

59. Fábián A, Bor R, Szabó E, et al. Endoscopic treatment of gastric antral vascular ectasia in real-life settings: Argon plasma coagulation or endoscopic band ligation? J Dig Dis 2021;22(1):23–30.

60. Marzano C, Zippi M, Traversa G. Endoscopic band ligation for gastric antral vascular ectasia: time for a new indication? Endoscopy 2016;48(2):196.

61. Eccles J, Falk V, Montano-Loza AJ, et al. Long-term follow-up in patients with gastric antral vascular ectasia (GAVE) after treatment with endoscopic band ligation (EBL). Endosc Int Open 2019;7(12):E1624–9.

62. Wells CD, Harrison ME, Gurudu SR, et al. Treatment of gastric antral vascular ectasia (watermelon stomach) with endoscopic band ligation. Gastrointest Endosc 2008;68(2):231–6.

63. Zepeda-Gómez S, Sultanian R, Teshima C, et al. Gastric antral vascular ectasia: a prospective study of treatment with endoscopic band ligation. Endoscopy 2015; 47(6):538–40.

64. Hirsch BS, Ribeiro IB, Funari MP, et al. Endoscopic Band Ligation Versus Argon Plasma Coagulation in the Treatment of Gastric Antral Vascular Ectasia: A Systematic Review and Meta-Analysis of Randomized Controlled Trials. Clin Endosc 2021;54(5):669–77.

65. McCarty TR, Hathorn KE, Chan WW, et al. Endoscopic band ligation in the treatment of gastric antral vascular ectasia: a systematic review and meta-analysis. Endosc Int Open 2021;9(7):E1145–57.

66. Elhendawy M, Mosaad S, Alkhalawany W, et al. Randomized controlled study of endoscopic band ligation and argon plasma coagulation in the treatment of gastric antral and fundal vascular ectasia. United European Gastroenterol J 2016;4(3):423–8.

67. O'Morain NR, O'Donovan H, Conlon C, et al. Is Endoscopic Band Ligation a Superior Treatment Modality for Gastric Antral Vascular Ectasia Compared to Argon Plasma Coagulation? Clin Endosc 2021;54(4):548–54.

68. Gross SA, Al-Haddad M, Gill KR, et al. Endoscopic mucosal ablation for the treatment of gastric antral vascular ectasia with the HALO90 system: a pilot study. Gastrointest Endosc 2008;67(2):324–7.

69. Dray X, Repici A, Gonzalez P, et al. Radiofrequency ablation for the treatment of gastric antral vascular ectasia. Endoscopy 2014;46(11):963–9.

70. McGorisk T, Krishnan K, Keefer L, et al. Radiofrequency ablation for refractory gastric antral vascular ectasia (with video). Gastrointest Endosc 2013;78(4):584–8.

71. Matin T, Naseemuddin M, Shoreibah M, et al. Case series on multimodal endoscopic therapy for gastric antral vascular ectasia, a tertiary center experience. World J Gastrointest Endosc 2018;10(1):30–6.

72. Kantsevoy SV, Cruz-Correa MR, Vaughn CA, et al. Endoscopic cryotherapy for the treatment of bleeding mucosal vascular lesions of the GI tract: a pilot study. Gastrointest Endosc 2003;57(3):403–6.

73. Cho S, Zanati S, Yong E, et al. Endoscopic cryotherapy for the management of gastric antral vascular ectasia. Gastrointest Endosc 2008;68(5):895–902.

74. Patel AA, Trindade AJ, Diehl DL, et al. Nitrous oxide cryotherapy ablation for refractory gastric antral vascular ectasia. United European Gastroenterol J 2018; 6(8):1155–60.

75. Dhaliwal A, Saghir SM, Mashiana HS, et al. Endoscopic cryotherapy: Indications, techniques, and outcomes involving the gastrointestinal tract. World J Gastrointest Endosc 2022;14(1):17–28.

76. Bennett C, Klingenberg SL, Langholz E, et al. Tranexamic acid for upper gastrointestinal bleeding. Cochrane Database Syst Rev 2014;2014(11):Cd006640.

77. McCormick PA, Ooi H, Crosbie O. Tranexamic acid for severe bleeding gastric antral vascular ectasia in cirrhosis. Gut 1998;42(5):750–2.

78. Khan S, Vaishnavi A. Pharmacotherapy for gastric antral vascular ectasia: dramatic response to tranexamic acid. Gastrointest Endosc 2009;70(1):191 [author reply: 191-192].

79. Manno D, Ker K, Roberts I. How effective is tranexamic acid for acute gastrointestinal bleeding? Bmj 2014;348:g1421.

80. Gostout CJ, Viggiano TR, Ahlquist DA, et al. The clinical and endoscopic spectrum of the watermelon stomach. J Clin Gastroenterol 1992;15(3):256–63.

81. Sargeant IR, Loizou LA, Rampton D, et al. Laser ablation of upper gastrointestinal vascular ectasias: long term results. Gut 1993;34(4):470–5.

82. Potamiano S, Carter CR, Anderson JR. Endoscopic laser treatment of diffuse gastric antral vascular ectasia. Gut 1994;35(4):461–3.

83. Geller A, Gostout CJ, Balm RK. Development of hyperplastic polyps following laser therapy for watermelon stomach. Gastrointest Endosc 1996;43(1):54–6.

84. Ge ZZ, Chen HM, Gao YJ, et al. Efficacy of thalidomide for refractory gastrointestinal bleeding from vascular malformation. Gastroenterology 2011;141(5): 1629–37.e1621, 1624.

85. Karajeh MA, Hurlstone DP, Stephenson TJ, et al. Refractory bleeding from portal hypertensive gastropathy: a further novel role for thalidomide therapy? Eur J Gastroenterol Hepatol 2006;18(5):545–8.

86. Garg H, Gupta S, Anand AC, et al. Portal hypertensive gastropathy and gastric antral vascular ectasia. Indian J Gastroenterol 2015;34(5):351–8.

87. Moser S, Tischer A, Karpi A, et al. Evidence that thalidomide is effective in recurrent bleeding from watermelon stomach associated with liver cirrhosis. Endoscopy 2014;46(Suppl 1 UCTN):E384.

88. Dunne KA, Hill J, Dillon JF. Treatment of chronic transfusion-dependent gastric antral vascular ectasia (watermelon stomach) with thalidomide. Eur J Gastroenterol Hepatol 2006;18(4):455–6.

89. Marupudi S, Tyberg A, Bodin R. Reversal of portal hypertensive enteropathy after liver transplant: 1155. Official journal of the American College of Gastroenterology | ACG 2013;108:S341–2.

90. Ali SE, Benrajab KM, Cruz ACD. Outcome of gastric antral vascular ectasia and related anemia after orthotopic liver transplantation. World J Hepatol 2020;12(11): 1067–75.

Variceal and Nonvariceal Upper Gastrointestinal Bleeding Refractory to Endoscopic Management

Indications and Role of Interventional Radiology

Ece Meram, MD, Elliott Russell, MD, Orhan Ozkan, MD, Mark Kleedehn, MD*

KEYWORDS

- Upper GI bleeding • Interventional radiology • Embolization • Empirical embolization
- Prophylactic embolization • Hemobilia • Hemosuccus pancreaticus
- Variceal bleeding

KEY POINTS

- A recent meta-analysis concluded that empirical embolization after negative angiogram for upper GI bleeding seems to be as effective as targeted embolization after a positive angiogram in preventing rebleeding and mortality.
- The decision to use one embolic agent versus the other for upper GI arterial bleeding is impacted by proximal versus distal location, end versus redundant arterial supply, permanent versus temporary embolic requirements, and desired degree of reduced blood flow impact.
- For patients admitted for acute variceal bleeding with Child–Pugh B disease with active bleeding or Child-Pugh C disease, the early use of transjugular intrahepatic portosystemic shunt (TIPS) (ie, within <72 hours of index endoscopy) with a covered stent is associated with significant reductions in the failure to control bleeding, in rebleeding, and in mortality, with no increase in the risk of hepatic encephalopathy.
- Balloon-occluded retrograde transvenous obliteration and its variants including plug- or coil-assisted retrograde transvenous obliteration are established treatments for management of gastric varices.
- Occlusive ectopic varices are usually managed with recanalization initially, whereas oncotic types benefit from variceal embolization and/or TIPS.

University of Wisconsin School of Medicine and Public Health, University of Wisconsin Hospitals and Clinics, 600 Highland Avenue, Madison, WI 53792, USA
* Corresponding author.
E-mail address: mkleedehn@uwhealth.org

Gastrointest Endoscopy Clin N Am 34 (2024) 275–299
https://doi.org/10.1016/j.giec.2023.09.014
1052-5157/24/© 2023 Elsevier Inc. All rights reserved.

PREPROCEDURE IMAGING

To aid in procedure planning and to help stratify patients in whom catheter-based intervention would be successful, there are several radiologic studies that can be performed to aid in diagnosis and potential treatment planning.[1,2] These radiologic studies include computer tomography angiography (CTA), technetium-99m-labeled red blood cell scintigraphy, and computed tomography enterography.[2,3]

Computer Tomography Angiography

Recent American College of Radiology (ACR) appropriateness criteria list CTA as the most appropriate noninvasive imaging modality for identification of etiology and location in four specific patient variants who present with gastrointestinal bleeding.[4] These include (1) endoscopy revealing a nonvariceal upper gastrointestinal arterial bleeding source, (2) endoscopy confirming nonvariceal upper gastrointestinal bleeding without a clear source, (3) nonvariceal upper gastrointestinal bleeding with negative endoscopy, and (4) postsurgical and traumatic causes of nonvariceal upper gastrointestinal bleeding (when endoscopy is contraindicated).

CTA is performed without oral contrast and as a three-phase examination.[2,3] The noncontrast phase is helpful for identifying any intrinsically hyperattenuating material within the body. which could confound findings. Next, a late arterial phase is obtained, which should show contrast throughout the visceral arteries and early contrast opacification of the portal vein. This is useful for two distinct reasons. First, any new, nonvascular hyperattenuating foci (when compared with the non-contrast phase) are suspicious for areas of bleeding. Second, if intervention is indicated, this phase offers the best evaluation of visceral and systemic arteries for the purpose of pre-procedural planning. Finally, a delayed phase (typically 2-minute delay or portal venous phase is obtained). This phase provides a few additional data points. First, if new hyperattenuating foci are identified on the arterial phase, any evolution of the shape or margin of these foci suggests the presence of extravasated contrast and is consistent with active bleeding. Second, routine pathology in the abdomen and pelvis are often best evaluated on portal venous phase and underlying clinical manifestations of certain diseases and processes, such as cirrhosis, portal hypertension, postsurgical anatomy, and bowel ischemia can be evaluated.[3] Historically, the generally accepted threshold of CTA to detect bleeding has been reported to be rates of bleeding as low as 0.3 mL/min[2,3,5]; however, improvements in CT technique have likely lowered this threshold to as low as 0.1 mL/min[6]. Disadvantages of CTA include disadvantages inherent to all contrast-enhanced CT studies, including radiation dose and iodinated contrast side effects and possible risks.

Scintigraphy

The use of radiotracer-labeled red blood cells to detect gastrointestinal bleeding was first introduced in 1979.[2] The technique involves labeling red blood cells with technetium-99m and injecting them intravenously. Dynamic and then delayed images are acquired using standard planar imaging equipment. Aggregation of extravasated radiolabeled red blood cells within the GI lumen produces characteristic findings. Reported diagnostic criteria suggesting active GI bleeding include (1) a new focus of radiotracer activity identified, (2) demonstrating an increasing size over time, (3) with movement of radiotracer activity suggesting peristalsis, and (4) general intraluminal appearance matching shape and location of bowel.[2] The advantages of this technique include no use of iodinated contrast, no required gastrointestinal tract preparation, and relatively low threshold to detect bleeding, reported as low as 0.05 to 0.1 mL/min.[2,5,7] The disadvantages of this technique are well established and have informed ACR appropriateness criteria to delegate this technique to "may be appropriate" and "usually not appropriate" for the clinical variants described above.[3,4] These disadvantages include lack of information on bleeding etiology, no pre-procedural vascular evaluation, and possible false positives including splenosis and non-enteric bleeding.

Computer Tomography Enterography

Computer tomography enterography is a similar technique to CTA with the principal difference of administration of a large volume of neutral enteric contrast.[2,3] This technique is often used in chronic, occult GI bleeds in patients who are stable and have failed multiple endoscopic evaluations.

PROGNOSTIC FACTORS FOR A POSITIVE ARTERIOGRAM

Although pre-intervention imaging may show evidence of bleeding, this does not definitively predict that active bleeding will be seen on invasive angiography (positive angiogram) as GI bleeding can be intermittent and have decreased conspicuity on invasive angiography if below the threshold bleeding rate (0.5–1 mL/min).[7,8] With the hope of differentiating which patients will demonstrate active bleeding on angiogram, several attempts have been made to identify prognostic factors for a positive arteriogram. In 1997, it was demonstrated that a positive tagged red blood cell (RBC) scan did not increase the probability of a positive angiogram and did not identify any clinical factors that would predict positive angiogram.[8] However, several subsequent studies have since identified that red blood cell transfusion requirements in the preceding 24 hours are positively correlated to probability of a positive angiogram.[9–11] Time to invasive angiography has also been evaluated, and the studies demonstrate mixed results. Choi and colleagues demonstrated that the only significant predictor for a positive angiographic study was the time from clinical presentation to invasive angiogram[12]; however, Akshaar and colleagues demonstrated that time to invasive angiography after diagnostic identification of bleeding (on endoscopy, CTA, or tagged RBC scan) did not affect the rate of positive angiogram.[10] Because few individual clinical factors have been identified to accurately predict positive angiogram, a few more comprehensive clinical decision scores have been developed to help prognosticate patients with GI bleeding. Although the Rockall score and Glasgow-Blatchford scores have been previously evaluated,[13,14] the utility of the shock index (heart rate divided by systolic blood pressure) has been less well studied in gastrointestinal bleeding. Nakasone and colleagues demonstrated that shock index and patient's age could be used in a logarithmic equation to fairly accurately predict a subsequently positive angiogram.[15] In 2015, The National Confidential Enquiry into Patient Outcome and Death (NCEPOD) report on GI bleeding discussed the utility of the shock index stating that increasing shock index was associated with higher mortality.[16] However, more recently in a small retrospective and a large prospective study shock index has proven inferior to other pre-endoscopy scores and has not been found to correlate with clinically significant outcomes in upper GI bleeding.[17,18] Overall, these mixed data suggest that further research is required to successfully identify prognostic factors for angiography in patients with upper GI bleeding.

TECHNIQUES OF TRANSCATHETER ARTERIAL INTERVENTION

When a patient has failed endoscopic and/or conservative treatment options of GI bleeding, catheter angiography can be performed. Invasive angiography is less sensitive for detecting active bleeding than scintigraphy or CTA, with reported threshold bleeding rates of 0.5 to 1.0 mL/min[5,7]; however, several treatment techniques have been developed, which can be performed immediately after and based on angiographic findings. To perform catheter-directed angiography, femoral or radial arterial access is obtained. Commonly, a 21-gauge micro-puncture system is initially used to gain arterial access, followed by system upsizing with placement of a 4 to 6 French vascular sheath over a 0.035 inch guidewire. Next, if a bleeding artery has been identified, selective catheterization of that vessel is performed. In upper gastrointestinal bleeding, most commonly the source of bleeding will arise from the celiac artery; thus, this is a common artery to initially catheterize. Digital subtraction angiography is performed looking for active extravasation of contrast. If identified, superselective catheterization of the culprit artery is performed. A microcatheter system (<3 French microcatheter) is introduced into the parent vessel and with a wire (≤0.018 inch guidewire), the microcatheter is advanced as close to the site of bleeding as possible. At this point, with a microcatheter system in place, a few treatment options exist.[5,7] The most commonly used treatment is transcatheter arterial embolization. Several different embolic agent options exist. These include temporary gelatin sponge, spherical particulates, microcoils, plugs, and liquid embolic agents. Numerous factors including proximal versus distal location, end versus redundant arterial supply, permanent versus temporary embolic requirements, and desired degree of reduced blood flow impact the decision to use one embolic agent versus the other. Given the robust collateral supply in the upper GI tract, it is usually required to perform "sandwich" embolization of the afferent and efferent artery across the site of bleeding and to carefully evaluate for additional collateral supply to the site of bleeding. For example, in the setting of a duodenal ulcer bleed, the superior mesenteric artery which feeds the inferior pancreaticoduodenal artery should usually be interrogated after gastroduodenal artery embolization (**Figs. 1** and **2**). A rarely used treatment option in the setting of GI bleeding is selective infusion of vasoactive medications in an attempt to decrease perfusion pressure and promote clot formation at the location of bleeding.[1,5,7] Vasopressin, a vasoactive peptide synthesized in the hypothalamus, is most commonly used. Intra-arterial infusion of vasopressin for treatment of GI bleeding was more commonly performed before the invention of microcatheters which allow for superselective embolization. Further, vasopressin infusion technique is typically reserved for bleeding in the lower GI tract where there is not dual blood supply and where culprit vessels tend to me smaller in caliber in the setting of diffuse mucosal bleeding.

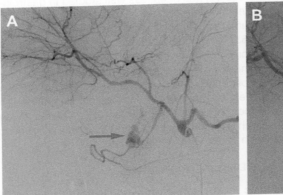
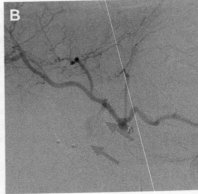

Fig. 1. (*A*) Digital subtraction celiac arteriogram showing brisk duodenal ulcer bleeding from the gastroduodenal artery (*red arrow*). (*B*) Digital subtraction celiac arteriogram following "sandwich" coil embolization (*red arrows*) across the bleeding gastroduodenal artery.

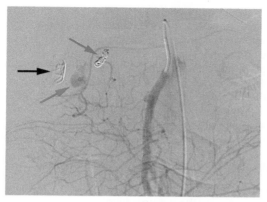

Fig. 2. Digital subtraction superior mesenteric arteriogram following coil embolization of the gastroduodenal artery (*blue arrow*) with persistent duodenal ulcer bleeding (*red arrow*) at the site of endoscopic clamp placement (*black arrow*).

SUCCESS RATES AND COMPLICATIONS AFTER EMBOLIZATION

Transcatheter arterial embolization has been demonstrated to be an effective treatment strategy, with high technical success rates ranging from 93% to 100%.[19–22] In a large meta-analysis that analyzed 15 studies, clinical success rate was reported as 67%.[19] Rebleeding is a known occurrence after embolization, with rates ranging from 27% to 37%.[19,21,22] Risk factors that are known to increase the risk of rebleeding include coagulopathy and large blood transfusion requirements.[19,20] Other factors that have been described but are less well established include coil only embolization, greater than 2 comorbidities, and renal failure.[19–21] With any invasive procedure, there is always risk for adverse outcomes. Complications related to arterial access not specific to embolization include access site hematoma, pseudoaneurysm, and arteriovenous fistula and have been reported in up to 6% of all arterial accesses.[23] Complications related to iodinated contrast administration are also not specific to embolization and include allergic contrast reaction.[19] Contrast-induced nephropathy has recently become a debated and controversial topic with multiple studies not showing a difference in the risk of acute kidney injury between patients who underwent procedures with intravenous administration of iodinated contrast and those who underwent procedures without it.[24] Embolization-related complications are rare, however, include post-embolization ischemia and/or infarction, although this is felt to be lower risk as the stomach and duodenum have rich collateral pathways. However, prior anatomy-altering surgery significantly raises the risk of ischemia, as collateral pathways are often disrupted.[19] An additional distinct risk to embolization is nontarget embolization, defined as inadvertent delivery of embolization material to nontarget tissues.[19] One of the most common sites of nontarget embolization is the liver, as reflux of embolic material can occur during embolization of the gastroduodenal artery.[19] This can manifest as a broad spectrum of clinical entities, from mild elevation of liver enzymes or post-embolization syndrome (fever, pain, nausea/vomiting) to fulminant liver failure, depending on the degree of embolization.

EMPIRICAL EMBOLIZATION IN ANGIOGRAPHICALLY NEGATIVE STUDIES

Without robust predictors for a positive angiogram, operators encountering a negative invasive angiogram arise frequently. This can be seen in a few different clinical scenarios, including cessation of bleeding or slow bleeding below the angiographic threshold of detection. Although intrinsic cessation of bleeding usually correlates with initial patient improvement, this leaves the patient at a high risk of rebleeding, as the underlying lesion remains untreated.[25] Thus, substantial effort has been given toward determining if empirical embolization in the area of highest clinical or radiographic concern will improve outcomes. A recent meta-analysis concluded that empirical embolization after negative angiogram seems to be as effective compared with targeted embolization after positive angiogram in preventing rebleeding and mortality.[26] Empirical gastroduodenal coil embolization is frequently performed in the setting of bleeding duodenal ulcers that cannot be controlled endoscopically.

PROPHYLACTIC EMBOLIZATION AFTER ENDOSCOPIC TREATMENT

Transcatheter arterial embolization may play an additional role in the subacute setting of gastrointestinal bleeding. In the subpopulation of patients who present with high-risk (defined by Rockall score, Forrest classification, or endoscopic evaluation) bleeding peptic ulcers who undergo successful endoscopic treatment with control of bleeding, further prophylactic embolization of the gastroduodenal and/or left gastric arteries to prevent rebleeding has been described.[27,28] Meta-analyses have shown hemodynamic instability at admission, active bleeding at endoscopy, and ulcer size and location to be the most consistent prognostic variables for rebleeding in patients who received endoscopic treatment.[29] A large meta-analysis has evaluated differences in outcomes in patients who underwent endoscopic treatment with prophylactic embolization versus endoscopic treatment alone.[30] There was statistically significant improvement in 30-day rebleeding rate and 30-day mortality rates in patients who underwent embolization. There was no significant difference in reintervention rates or length of hospital stay, and there was a relatively low (0.18%) reported rate of complication associated with embolization.

HEMOBILIA AND HEMOSUCCUS PANCREATICUS

Hemobilia is defined as bleeding into the biliary tract. Clinically, this usually presents as either melena or bright red blood per rectum, with large volume hematemesis encountered less often as rapid bleeding is rare.[31] Etiologies of hemobilia are numerous and include iatrogenic (biopsy, endoscopy, surgery), traumatic, vasculitides, neoplastic, and infectious.[32] Given the inherent difficulties with endoscopic management of hemobilia, transcatheter arterial embolization has been used as definitive treatment. Described as early as 1976[32,33] in case reports, gelfoam embolization has been successful in stopping clinically significant hemobilia. Larger retrospective series have described relative success achieving hemostasis, with clinical success reported between 75% and 92%.[31,34,35] Patients who did not respond to embolization required surgery for definitive bleeding control. Ischemic adverse outcomes are rare, owing to the dual blood supply to the liver. Of the larger case series, only one adverse outcome was reported, which was infarction of the gallbladder and was incidentally noted during surgery and resulted in cholecystectomy.[31] No significant hepatic infarctions were reported.[31,34,35] In conclusion, transcatheter arterial embolization for clinically significant hemobilia is a safe and effective treatment and frequently avoids the need for operative intervention.

Hemosuccus pancreaticus (**Fig. 3**) is defined as bleeding from a pancreatic or peripancreatic vessel into the pancreatic ducts.[36] Although rare, bleeding may be substantial and life-threatening.[37] As in the case of hemobilia, clinical presentation is often of melena, bright red blood per rectum, or hematemesis.[37] Etiology of hemosuccus

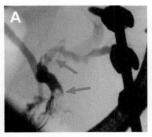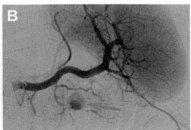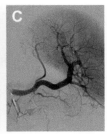

Fig. 3. (A) Endoscopic retrograde cholangiopancreaticography (ERCP) image showing clots as filling defects (*red arrows*) in the pancreatic duct. (B) Splenic arteriogram showing a pancreatica magna pseudoaneurysm (*red arrow*). (C) Splenic arteriogram showing successful coil embolization (*red arrow*) across the pancreatica magna pseudoaneurysm.

pancreaticus is most often from pancreatitis and subsequent development of pseudoaneurysm; however, tumors, vascular malformations, and iatrogenic causes have been identified.[38,39] More rare etiologies such as pancreatolithiasis, ectopic pancreatic tissue, and segmental arterial mediolysis have also been described.[40–42] Given the low incidence of this entity, the literature is limited to case reports and small case series; however, successful treatment with arterial embolization has been described in numerous cases.[37–39,42] In the largest review to date looking at all case reports of hemosuccus pancreaticus between 1976 and 2011, initial clinical success rates were reported between 79% and 100%.[43] In cases of endovascular treatment failure, surgical intervention to excise the pseudoaneurysm is attempted before pancreatic resection.[44]

ESOPHAGEAL BLEED

Nonvariceal arterial bleeding from the esophagus is a major cause of morbidity and mortality. Upper endoscopy is the gold standard for evaluation and treatment of esophageal bleeding. However, transarterial catheter embolization remains an option in the treatment of these patients.

Although originally described in 1980 at a similar time to other gastrointestinal embolization techniques, esophageal angiography and embolization has been less well evaluated and established in the literature.[45] Few case reports over the proceeding years have reported success, but no large series has been performed.[46,47] In one of the largest and most recent studies, Arashidi and colleagues describe their single-center experience with nine patients and reported a clinical success rate of 77.8%.[48]

The technique of esophageal angiography and embolization is inherently difficult, as arterial anatomy is not as simple or consistent when compared with the gastroduodenal vascular supply. Most commonly, the proximal esophagus is supplied by branches of the inferior thyroid artery, the mid-esophagus is supplied by branches of the highly variable bronchial arteries and esophageal arteries arising directly from the aorta (**Fig. 4**), and the distal esophagus is supplied by branches of the left gastric, splenic, or left inferior phrenic arteries.[45,49] Commonly, these arteries are only a few millimeters in diameter, making angiographic detection and catheter selection more difficult.

If esophageal angiography and detection of active bleeding is successful, embolization can be performed similar to elsewhere in the gastrointestinal tract, using coil, liquid, or gelatin sponge embolic agents. One of the dreaded complications of embolization in the thoracolumbar region is spinal cord ischemia and infarct. This has been specifically reported as a complication of bronchial artery embolization,[50–52] abdominal aortic

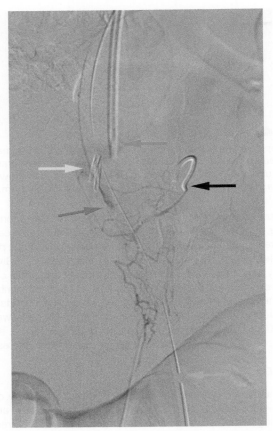

Fig. 4. A digital subtraction image shows a reverse curve catheter (*black arrow*) has accessed a direct esophageal branch of the aorta and active bleeding is seen (*red arrow*) from the site of endoscopically placed clips (*yellow arrow*). A central line (*blue arrow*) and nasogastric tube are noted (*orange arrow*).

interventions,[53] and post-traumatic intercostal and lumbar artery embolization.[54] Additional anatomy relevant to esophageal embolization is the artery of Adamkiewicz.[55] This artery is the most prominent anterior radiculomedullary artery, usually arises on the left side between the T8 and L2 level, and makes a characteristic hairpin turn. Thus, whenever performing nonvisceral angiography in the thoracolumbar region, attention should be made to identify any possible area of spinal cord perfusion and proceed with extreme caution if embolization is required.

VARICEAL BLEEDING BACKGROUND

Variceal bleeding is a sequela of portal hypertension, which is defined as absolute portal venous pressure greater than 10 mm Hg or elevated portosystemic pressure gradient greater than 5 mm Hg.[56] Portal hypertension can affect isolated segments or entirety of portal venous system resulting in venous congestion with or without reversal of blood flow (ie, hepatofugal) and ultimately venous remodeling with formation of extrahepatic venous collaterals decompressing into systemic circulation.[56] Porta hypertension can be diagnosed indirectly with identification of its clinical sequelae such as ascites, variceal hemorrhage, and encephalopathy. The supporting imaging sequelae include cirrhotic liver morphology with splenomegaly, portosystemic collaterals (eg, varices and shunts), or hepatofugal flow on Doppler US.[56] Further confirmatory testing can be done via catheter-based measurement of hepatic sinusoidal pressures to determine hepatic vein pressure gradient (indicate of portal hypertension if > 5 mm Hg).[57] This is an indirect method but reflects the direct portal venous pressure and is more practical to measure. It should be noted, however, it may fail to diagnose portal hypertension with prehepatic or posthepatic etiology as an increased hepatic venous pressure gradient (HVPG) would not be observed in these cases given lack of sinusoidal involvement.[56,57] More invasive, transhepatic or transjugular access of portal vein can be performed to obtain absolute portal vein pressure if indicated.[56]

The etiology of portal hypertension is important to differentiate and can be prehepatic, intrahepatic, or posthepatic. Prehepatic causes included arterioportal fistulas and portal or splenic vein thrombosis.[56] Intrahepatic causes are further divided into pre-sinusoidal, sinusoidal, and post-sinusoidal.[56] Pre-sinusoidal intrahepatic portal hypertension can be caused by sarcoidosis, toxins, schistosomiasis, Wilson disease, and so forth.[56] Sinusoidal intrahepatic portal hypertension is caused by alcohol abuse, primary sclerosing cholangitis, or Gaucher disease.[56] Post-sinusoidal portal hypertension is caused by veno-occlusive disease or Budd-Chiari syndrome.[56] Finally, posthepatic causes include inferior vena cava obstruction, right heart failure, constrictive pericarditis, or mitral valve disease.[56] Regardless of the etiology, a portosystemic gradient of greater than 12 mm Hg has been associated with an increased risk of variceal bleeding.[57] Particularly, gastroesophageal variceal bleeding is a dire sequela of portal hypertension, resulting in GI bleeding in 60% to 90% of patients with cirrhosis and portal hypertension with a yearly bleeding rate or 5% to 15%, a mortality rate of 20% at 6 weeks, and rebleeding rate of 70% if untreated.[56,58–60] In contrast to bleeding from submucosal varices and/or intraperitoneal gastro-renal shunts, which can be life-threatening, bleeding from retroperitoneal shunts is less worrisome as it is usually contained in the retroperitoneal space.[61]

TRANSJUGULAR INTRAHEPATIC PORTOSYSTEMIC SHUNT INDICATIONS AND PATIENT SELECTION

Although the etiology of portal hypertension may not be reversible, the portal hypertension itself can be addressed by decreasing the portosystemic gradient.[56] When initial treatment with medical therapy or endoscopic management of varices and gastropathy is not adequate and liver transplant is not an option, a transjugular intrahepatic portosystemic shunt (TIPS) can be created to lower the splanchnic congestion by the way of shunting the portal inflow to systemic hepatic outflow bypassing the liver.[62,63] TIPS is indicated for acute or recurrent variceal hemorrhage unresponsive to medical therapy, refractory ascites/hydrothorax, or Budd-Chiari syndrome with established evidence.[62–66] Newer evidence suggests promising results for portal hypertensive gastropathy, hepatorenal syndrome, and early TIPS for ascites or first variceal hemorrhage.[59,62,63,66–69] However, not everyone is a TIPS candidate with absolute contraindications including severe hepatic failure, sepsis, heart failure, and significant pulmonary hypertension.[56,63,69,70] There are several criteria to determine who can and should undergo TIPS. A patient's nutritional status and coagulation parameters should be interrogated, and the correction of any coagulopathy should be based on thromboelastography due to unreliable International Normalized Ratio (INR) in the setting of liver disease.[66] The patency of portal and hepatic vein should be interrogated with Doppler ultrasound or contrast-enhanced CT or MR.[56,66,71] The use of cross-sectional imaging is preferred to demonstrate the portal and hepatic vein anatomy in addition to their patency as well as to determine the presence of any liver malignancy or biliary obstruction that may alter procedural plan.[56,66,71] Large-volume ascites should also be evacuated to minimize displacement of liver from its normal anatomic position.[56,71] Given projected increase in central venous pressures and cardiac index after TIPS creation, the evaluation of cardiac function such as with transthoracic echocardiography is important to ensure patients can tolerate hemodynamic changes as a result of the shunt creation.[56,66,71,72] Model for end stage liver disease (MELD) score, which was developed to predict risk and survival for patient undergoing TIPS creation, is an invaluable indicator of liver function[73,74] as well as predictor of other comorbidities, length of hospital stay, and mortality.[75] With regard to TIPS outcomes, MELD score has been shown to be equal or superior to MELD-Na score and should be preferred for patient selection.[76,77] It has been shown that TIPS mortality is higher in patients with MELD score greater than 18 with potential for worsening in liver failure.[74] In more recent years, different MELD cutoffs have been suggested in elective versus emergency settings. For example, Montgomery and colleagues found that early death rate was highest in patient with pre-TIPS MELD of greater than 24 and recommended avoiding elective TIPS in this patient population.[78] Casadaban and colleagues reported an optimal MELD cutoff of greater than 20 for considering TIPS in emergency setting with median survival less than 3 month in patients with MELD score greater than 14 and less than 1 month in patients with MELD score greater than 18.[79] Nevertheless, despite the associated higher mortality rates for patients with higher MELD scores, it is difficult to evaluate hepatic reserve in acute period and TIPS can be performed as an emergency salvage treatment for acute variceal GI bleeding when refractory to medical or endoscopic treatment and/or nothing else can be offered.[79,80] Of note, salvage TIPS is not recommended in patients with Child-Pugh score greater than 13.[66]

TRANSJUGULAR INTRAHEPATIC PORTOSYSTEMIC SHUNT TECHNICAL CONSIDERATIONS

Several technical considerations have been studied with impact on early and long-term procedural outcomes. For example, incorporation of intravascular ultrasound guidance into TIPS procedures has been shown to decrease number of needle passes, procedure time, and radiation dose and improve technical outcomes with decreased morbidity and mortality (**Fig. 5**).[81–85]

Late TIPS dysfunction can be seen with shunt stenosis resulting in absent or elevated TIPS velocities greater than 190 to 200 cm/s on Doppler ultrasound and/or recurrent symptoms.[56,69,70,86] Unassisted TIPS patency has been shown to be superior with stent grafts (80%–90% at 1 year; 76% at 2 year) compared with bare metal stents (25%–66% at 1 year; 36% at 2 year).[56,87] Covered stents also offer improved survival at 3 month, 1 year, and 2 year with survival rate of 93%, 88%, and 76% for the covered stent group compared with 83%, 73%, and 62% for bare stent group.[88] Meta-analyses also confirmed significantly higher overall survival and shunt patency for covered stents compared with bare stents as well as a lower risk of hepatic encephalopathy.[89,90] Of note, nearly all stenoses that occur in stent grafts are at the hepatic vein end related to short length of the stent graft, which should be slightly extended into the inferior vena cava (IVC).[56]

The ideal diameter for TIPS has recently been studied and debated. The use of 8-mm compared with 10-mm stent grafts has been shown to reduce hepatic encephalopathy

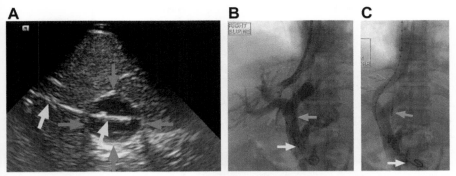

Fig. 5. (A) Side-firing intravascular ultrasound image showing a TIPS needle (*yellow arrows*) accessing the right portal vein (*red arrows*). (B) Portal venogram injection with a marking pigtail catheter (*yellow arrow*) following transjugular transhepatic access from a hepatic vein (*blue arrow*) into the right portal vein (*red arrow*) under side-firing intravascular ultrasound guidance (*green arrow*). (C) Portal venogram with a marking pigtail flush catheter (*yellow arrow*) showing a widely patent TIPS (*red arrows*). Note again made of intravascular ultrasound (US) probe (*green arrow*).

with similar effectiveness in the setting of secondary prevention of variceal bleeding.[91] However, a randomized study was interrupted early because it showed that 8-mm diameter stent grafts were associated with higher recurrent of ascites and the same rate of hepatic encephalopathy when compared with 10-mm stent grafts.[92] A National Data Registry in Germany found patients who received 8-mm stents survived significantly longer than patient who received 10-mm stents, regardless of whether they were fully dilated or underdilated.[93] Recently, Viatorr Controlled Expansion stent grafts (W.L. Gore and Associates, Phoenix, AZ, USA) that have a nominal diameter of 10 mm but that can be underdilated to 8 or 9 mm in diameter have been developed. These have been shown to maintain their underdilated caliber with reported lower rates of readmission for hepatic encephalopathy, uncontrolled ascites and heart failure, and improved 1-year survival.[94]

Although the shunt connection can be made from portal vein into the hepatic vein, direct intrahepatic portosystemic shunt can also be performed with direct access from inferior vena cava into the main portal vein with puncture through the caudate lobe.[81,95] This method can be preferred in patients with hepatic parenchymal lesions or difficult anatomies including small liver, unfavorable portal or hepatic vein relationship, or occlusion.[56,81,95]

TIPS reduction can be considered in cases of refractory hepatic encephalopathy, heart failure, and liver dysfunction following TIPS placement. Methods of TIPS reduction include parallel placement of a balloon-expandable bare metal stent and a new stent graft in the originally placed TIPS (**Fig. 6**), placement of a constrained self-expandable or incompletely dilated balloon-expandable stent graft within the TIPS, or placement of a tapered stent graft within the TIPS. Studies having reported TIPS reduction in improving or resolving hepatic encephalopathy in 63% to 92% of cases.[96]

TRANSJUGULAR INTRAHEPATIC PORTOSYSTEMIC SHUNT OUTCOMES

The outcomes and clinical success rate depend on patient selection, indication for performing TIPS, and the initial MELD scores.[56,63,74] For recurrent variceal bleeding, the clinical success rate of TIPS ranges between 97% and 100%, although

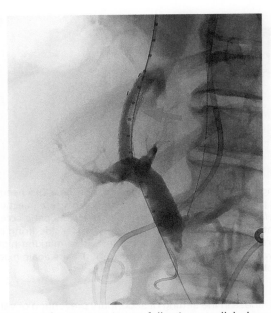

Fig. 6. TIPS reduction portal venogram image following parallel placement of a balloon-expandable bare metal stent (*red arrow*) and a new stent graft in the originally placed TIPS with a subsequent reduction in the caliber of the TIPS and corresponding increase in the pressure gradient across it.

lower rates (60%–70%) have been reported for refractory ascites indication.[56,58,59] In a meta-analysis, TIPS has been found superior for lower variceal bleeding rates compared with medical and endoscopic therapy together (OR 0.24) though at a cost of increased rate of HE (OR 2.07).[64] A more recent meta-analysis, however, failed to show any conclusive superiority between the two methods for overall survival or rebleeding rate.[97] Regardless, guidelines recommend TIPS creation in patients with gastroesophageal bleeding refractory to medical and endoscopic treatment.[60,66] More recently, in patients admitted for acute variceal bleeding with Child–Pugh B disease with active bleeding or Child-Pugh C disease, the early use of TIPS (ie, within <72 hours of index endoscopy) with a covered stent was associated with significant reductions in the failure to control bleeding, in rebleeding, and in mortality, with no increase in the risk of hepatic encephalopathy.[67,98] Again, compared with conventional medical and endoscopic treatment regardless of active bleeding or stage of liver disease, early TIPS was shown to have a better transplant-free survival at 6 weeks and 1 year (HR 0.50, 95% CI 0.25–0.98; $P = .04$) and improved control of bleeding (HR 0.26 (95% CI 0.12–0.55; $P<0 \cdot 0001$).[68] Unfortunately, hepatic encephalopathy risk increases after TIPS in 30% to 50% of patients, which is more prevalent in patients being treated for refractory ascites due to lower target gradients.[56,62,63] Increased age, history of hepatic encephalopathy before TIPS, hypoalbuminemia, and nonalcoholic cirrhosis are considered risk factors for post-TIPS encephalopathy.[56,62,63,99] Most patients respond to medical treatment with lactulose and/or rifaximin with less than 10% experiencing persistent hepatic encephalopathy or can be treated prophylactically after TIPS creation.[99] In these patients, TIPS reduction or occlusion can be considered as well as liver transplantation if applicable.[56,62,63,69] Other complications include liver laceration from wedged-hepatic venography, biliary puncture and fistula formation with hemobilia or cholangitis, biliary obstruction, shunt malposition or migration, vascular injury, liver ischemia, infarction or liver failure, TIPS occlusion, and radiation injury.[69,70]

GASTRIC VARICES

Although the most common etiology of variceal bleeding related to portal hypertension is due to esophageal varices with up to 50% of cirrhotic patients having esophageal varices at initial endoscopy,[56,58] another important cause of portal hypertension-related GI bleeding is gastric varices. Gastric varices have a lower rate of bleeding (10%–36%) but are associated with higher transfusion rates and mortality (14%–45%) compared with esophageal varices.[100] Gastric varices can be formed from several gastric veins and drain into single or multiple veins (**Figs. 7** and **8**). Most gastric varices are formed by the left gastric or posterior gastric veins and the majority of the varices at the lesser curvature and fundus drain into the paraesophageal or inferior phrenic veins with a gastro-renal shunt.[100] Different classifications exist based on location of the varices or number of afferent or efferent veins, and the Sarin classification has been widely adapted (**Fig. 9**).[100,101] Type 1 gastroesophageal varices seen at the lesser curvature represent 70% of all gastric varices, whereas type 1 isolated gastric varices at the gastric fundus have the highest rate of bleeding.[101] TIPS has been shown to have decreased rebleeding rate in management of gastric varices compared with endoscopic sclerotherapy though with similar survival and increased rate of hepatic encephalopathy.[102] Related to their complexity and distance to the portal system, gastric varices can persist and bleed at lower portal pressures compared with esophageal varices.[101,103] Therefore, TIPS with adjunctive embolotherapy has been preferred over TIPS alone given lower rebleeding rates.[104–106] Alternatively, embolotherapy alone with antegrade or retrograde transvenous obliteration can be used in the treatment of gastric varices, especially in patients with isolated gastric varices, poor hepatic reserve, or higher risk of hepatic encephalopathy.[107] Balloon-occluded retrograde transvenous obliteration (BRTO) method and its variants including plug- or coil-assisted retrograde transvenous obliteration (PARTO or CARTO, respectively) became established treatments for management of gastric varices by occlusion of portosystemic shunt using balloon, plug, or coils followed by injection of a sclerosing agent directly into the varix endovascularly (**Fig. 10**).[107] Modified techniques were also shown to be effective in treatment of gastric varices with improved procedural times and decreased complication rates related to nontarget embolization, hemolysis, or renal failure.[107] Although

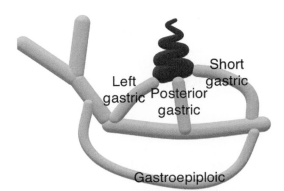

Fig. 7. Potential afferent veins that feed gastric varices are shown.

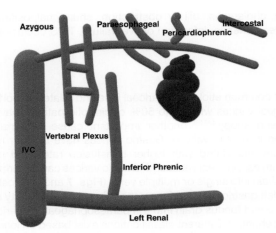

Fig. 8. Potential efferent veins that drain gastric varices are shown.

PARTO is mostly preferred due to convenience and shorter procedure times, CARTO can be considered when the shunt angles are too large for available plugs or not compatible with placement of any vascular plug.[107] If no gastrorenal shunt for retrograde approach or TIPS is being planned or present, an antegrade approach (BATO) can be used for sclerotherapy, which can help minimize overspill of sclerosant and nontarget embolization.[56,107] These methods also have been associated with worsening esophageal varices, as such, they should be used with care in patients with known esophageal varices or concurrent TIPS should be considered.[56,103,107]

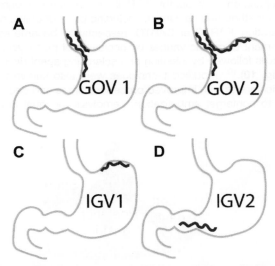

Fig. 9. (A) Type 1 gastroesophageal varices with extension along the lesser curvature of the stomach. (B) Type 2 gastroesophageal varices with extension along the greater curvature of the stomach. (C) Type 1 isolated gastric varices are in the fundus of the stomach only. (D) Type 2 isolated gastric varices can appear anywhere in the stomach including in the body, antrum, or pylorus.

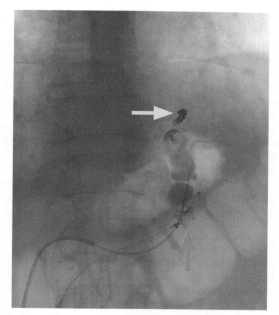

Fig. 10. Fluoroscopic image from a plug-assisted retrograde transvenous obliteration of a gastric varix showing plugs occluding the inferior phrenic outflow, coils in a small embolized systemic outflow vein, and sclerosant filling the gastric varix (*red arrow*).

Portal Hypertensive Gastropathy and Gastric Antral Vascular Ectasia

TIPS creation for portal hypertensive gastropathy with congestion of gastric mucosal capillaries and associated iron deficiency has weaker evidence with mostly small case series. Improved endoscopic outcomes were reported after TIPS creation for patients with portal gastropathy,[66,108] but it remains a less frequent indication for TIPS though still may be considered in patients with portal hypertensive gastropathy and iron deficiency refractory to beta-blockers and iron supplementation.[66] Gastric antral vascular ectasia can have overlapping findings with portal gastropathy, but it is important to differentiate the two as TIPS does not have a role in the management of bleeding solely from gastric antral vascular ectasia.[66]

ECTOPIC VARICES

Ectopic varices, including duodenal, jejunal, ileal, colonic, rectal, or stomal, can also be seen in the setting of portal hypertension, composing 2% to 5% of gastrointestinal variceal bleeds with a fourfold bleeding rate compared with esophageal varices.[66,109,110] Hemodynamic classification of ectopic varices divides them into type a if nonocclusive related to osmotic pressures and type b if related to occlusion of porto-mesenteric vessels including splenic vein.[110] In addition, they are categorized as types 1, 2, or 3 depending on the presence of pure porto-portal, predominantly porto-portal, or predominantly porto-systemic collaterals, respectively.[110] Occlusive types are usually managed with recanalization initially, whereas oncotic types benefit from variceal embolization and/or TIPS.[110] TIPS creation addresses the underlying etiology of portal hypertension and has been shown to be a feasible option for those who are TIPS candidates.[109,111–114] However, rebleeding rates of 18% to 42% have been reported with

TIPS despite a patent shunt.[66] Therefore, embolization of ectopic varices has been recommended at the time of TIPS creation to minimize rebleeding risk.[112] For those who are not safe to undergo TIPS such as poor cardiac function, variceal embolization only can still help manage acute GI bleeding.

As a type of extraperitoneal ectopic varix, stomal varices are particularly associated with an obstructive mechanism either as extrinsic compression or venous occlusion, resulting in localization of varix in the parastomal region.[115] This is mostly in addition to underlying portal hypertension but can be seen with isolated mesenteric occlusion as well.[115] Bleeding from stomal varices can present as focal bleeding, which usually responds to manual compression, but if diffuse oozing, requires TIPS and/or variceal embolization.[115] When TIPS is not indicated or feasible, variceal embolization techniques including BATO can be considered from a percutaneous or transhepatic variceal access (**Fig. 11**).[116,117] These methods, however, do not address the elevated portosystemic gradients and repeat treatments may be necessary due to higher rates of recurrent bleeding compared with TIPS with or without variceal embolization.[112]

SINISTRAL PORTAL HYPERTENSION

Although most of the portal hypertension cases are related to hepatic etiology, sinistral (left-sided) portal hypertension can be seen in isolation related to splenic vein thrombosis usually in the setting of acute or chronic pancreatitis.[118,119] Most common clinical manifestations are splenomegaly and isolated gastric varices with relatively preserved liver function and absence of other sequelae of portal hypertension.[118,119] Splenic vein recanalization and stenting can maintain patency of splenic outflow and decrease venous congestion and flow diversion into gastric collaterals with improved bleeding rates compared with splenic artery embolization (**Fig. 12**).[120] If this cannot be achieved, partial splenic embolization can be performed to decrease inflow to the spleen and in turn splenic outflow while preserving some splenic function.[121] It is particularly important to identify the splenic outflow whether it is partly

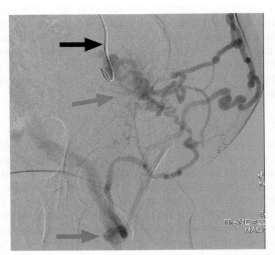

Fig. 11. Digital subtraction venogram with percutaneous access into afferent superior mesenteric branch (*black arrow*) feeding end ileostomy varices (*red arrow*) with dominant drainage to the iliofemoral junction (*blue arrow*). Obliteration was then be performed with injection of sclerosant and manual compression of the systemic draining veins.

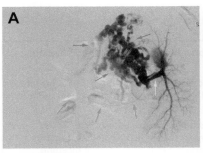 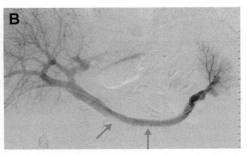

Fig. 12. (A) Splenic digital subtraction venogram after transhepatic portal access was obtained and an occluded splenic vein was crossed (*blue arrows*) with the catheter positioned in the splenic hilum (*yellow arrow*). There is robust filling of gastric varices (*red arrows*). (B) Splenic digital subtraction venogram after splenic stent placement showing the gastric varices are no longer filling.

or entirely drained via the gastric varices. If the gastric variceal complex includes a nonvariceal splenorenal shunt, then its preservation is important to help with decompression of the portal system.[122] In patients with drainage of entire or majority of splenic outflow via gastric varices as well as with splenomegaly and associated thrombocytopenia, partial splenic embolization is preferred.[121,122] In the presence of acute gastric variceal bleeding, transvenous obliteration of gastric varices is recommended in addition to splenic vein recanalization or partial splenic embolization.[56,60,106,122,123] Hybrid procedures can also be considered with endoscopy-guided cyanoacrylate injection to gastric varices during transvenous retrograde balloon-occlusion for treatment of only high-risk varices related to complexity of variceal system and feasibility and/or safety of the BRTO technique.[122]

ARTERIAL CLINICS CARE POINTS

- Recent ACR appropriateness criteria list computer tomography angiography as the most appropriate noninvasive imaging modality for identification of etiology and location in four specific patient variants who present with gastrointestinal bleeding. These include (1) endoscopy revealing a nonvariceal upper gastrointestinal arterial bleeding source, (2) endoscopy confirming nonvariceal upper gastrointestinal bleeding without a clear source, (3) nonvariceal upper gastrointestinal bleeding with negative endoscopy, and (4) postsurgical and traumatic causes of nonvariceal upper gastrointestinal bleeding (when endoscopy is contraindicated).

- Although pre-intervention imaging may show evidence of bleeding, this does not definitively predict that active bleeding will be seen on invasive angiography (positive angiogram) as GI bleeding can be intermittent and have decreased conspicuity on invasive angiography if below the threshold bleeding rate (0.5–1 mL/min).

- A recent meta-analysis concluded that empirical embolization after negative angiogram seems to be as effective compared with targeted embolization after positive angiogram in preventing rebleeding and mortality.

- A large meta-analysis has evaluated differences in outcomes in patients who underwent endoscopic treatment with prophylactic embolization versus endoscopic treatment alone. There was statistically significant improvement in 30-day rebleeding rate and 30-day mortality rates in patients who underwent embolization. There was no significant difference in reinvention rates or length of hospital stay, and there was a relatively low (0.18%) reported rate of complication associated with embolization.

VENOUS CLINICS CARE POINTS

- Portal hypertension etiologies can be categorized as prehepatic, intrahepatic, or posthepatic.
- It has been shown that transjugular intrahepatic portosystemic shunt (TIPS) mortality is higher in patients with MELD score greater than 18 to 24 with potential for worsening in liver failure.
- The ideal diameter for TIPS has recently been studied and debated. The use of 8-mm compared with 10-mm stent grafts has been shown to reduce hepatic encephalopathy with similar effectiveness in the setting of secondary prevention of variceal bleeding.
- In patients admitted for acute variceal bleeding with Child–Pugh B disease with active bleeding or Child-Pugh C disease, the early use of TIPS (ie, within <72 hours of index endoscopy) with a covered stent was associated with significant reductions in the failure to control bleeding, in rebleeding, and in mortality, with no increase in the risk of hepatic encephalopathy.
- Gastric varices have a lower rate of bleeding (10%–36%), but are associated with higher transfusion rates and mortality (14%–45%) compared with esophageal varices.
- Balloon-occluded retrograde transvenous obliteration method and its variants including plug- or coil-assisted retrograde transvenous obliteration became established treatments for management of gastric varices by occlusion of portosystemic shunt using balloon, plug, or coils followed by injection of a sclerosing agent directly into the varix endovascularly.
- Ectopic varices, including duodenal, jejunal, ileal, colonic, rectal, or stomal, can also be seen in the setting of portal hypertension, composing 2% to 5% of gastrointestinal variceal bleeds with a fourfold bleeding rate compared with esophageal varices. Hemodynamic classification of ectopic varices divides them into type a if nonocclusive related to osmotic pressures and type b if related to occlusion of porto-mesenteric vessels including splenic vein.
- Although most of the portal hypertension cases are related to hepatic etiology, sinistral (left-sided) portal hypertension can be seen in isolation related to splenic vein thrombosis usually in the setting of acute or chronic pancreatitis. Splenic vein recanalization and stenting can maintain patency of splenic outflow and decrease venous congestion and flow diversion into gastric collaterals with improved bleeding rates compared with splenic artery embolization. If this cannot be achieved, partial splenic embolization can be performed to decrease inflow to the spleen and in turn splenic outflow while preserving some splenic function.

DISCLOSURE

The authors have nothing to disclose.

REFERENCES

1. Baum S. Role of Angiography in the Diagnosis and Treatment of Gastrointestinal Bleeding: Historical Perspective. J Vasc Intervent Radiol 2018;29(6):905–7.
2. Carney BW, Khatri G, Shenoy-Bhangle AS. The role of imaging in gastrointestinal bleed. Cardiovasc Diagn Ther 2019;9:S88–96.
3. Wells ML, Hansel SL, Bruining DH, et al. CT for evaluation of acute gastrointestinal bleeding. Radiographics 2018;38(4):1089–107.
4. Singh-Bhinder N, Kim DH, Holly BP, et al. ACR Appropriateness Criteria ® Nonvariceal Upper Gastrointestinal Bleeding. J Am Coll Radiol 2017;14(5S):S177–88.
5. Ramaswamy RS, Won Choi H, Mouser H, et al. Role of interventional radiology in the management of acute gastrointestinal bleeding. World J Radiol 2014; 6(4):82.

6. Tse JR, Shen J, Shah R, et al. Extravasation Volume at Computed Tomography Angiography Correlates with Bleeding Rate and Prognosis in Patients with Overt Gastrointestinal Bleeding. Invest Radiol 2021;56(6):394–400.
7. Walker G, Salazar GM, Waltman AC. Angiographic evaluation and management of acute gastrointestinal hemorrhage. World J Gastroenterol 2012;18(11):1191–201.
8. Pennoyer WP, Vignati PV, Cohen JL. Mesenteric Angiography for Lower Gastrointestinal Hemorrhage Are There Predictors for a Positive Study? Disease of the Colon and Rectum 1997;40(9). http://journals.lww.com/dcrjournal.
9. Abbas SM, Bissett IP, Holden A, et al. Clinical variables associated with positive angiographic localization of lower gastrointestinal bleeding. ANZ J Surg 2005; 75(11):953–7.
10. Brahmbhatt A, Rao P, Cantos A, et al. Time to catheter angiography for gastrointestinal bleeding after prior positive investigation does not affect bleed identification. J Clin Imaging Sci 2020;10(1). https://doi.org/10.25259/JCIS_132_2019.
11. Lee L, Iqbal S, Najmeh S, et al. Mesenteric angiography for acute gastrointestinal bleed: Predictors of active extravasation and outcomes. Can J Surg 2012; 55(6):382–8.
12. Choi C, Lim H, Kim MJ, et al. Relationship between angiography timing and angiographic visualization of extravasation in patients with acute non-variceal gastrointestinal bleeding. BMC Gastroenterol 2020;20(1). https://doi.org/10.1186/s12876-020-01570-y.
13. Bryant RV, Kuo P, Williamson K, et al. Performance of the Glasgow-Blatchford score in predicting clinical outcomes and intervention in hospitalized patients with upper GI bleeding. Gastrointest Endosc 2013;78(4):576–83.
14. Rockall TA, Logan FA, Devlin B, Northfield TC. Risk Assessment after Acute Upper Gastrointestinal Haemorrhage. Vol 38.; 1996.
15. Nakasone Y, Ikeda O, Yamashita Y, et al. Shock index correlates with extravasation on angiographs of gastrointestinal hemorrhage: A logistics regression analysis. Cardiovasc Intervent Radiol 2007;30(5):861–5.
16. McPherson SJ, Sinclair MT, Smith NCE, Kelly K, Eliis D, Mason M. Time to Get Control? A Review of the Care Received by Patients Who a Severe Gastrointestinal Haemorrhage.; 2015.
17. Jawad N, Horlick S, Robbins A, Seward E. PTH-037 The Shock Index: A Novel and Useful Predictor of Mortality and Morbidity in Upper Gastrointestinal Bleeds? Gut 2016;65(Suppl 1). https://doi.org/10.1136/gutjnl-2016-312388.442.
18. Saffouri E, Blackwell C, Laursen SB, et al. The Shock Index is not accurate at predicting outcomes in patients with upper gastrointestinal bleeding. Aliment Pharmacol Ther 2020;51(2):253–60.
19. Loffroy R, Favelier S, Pottecher P, et al. Transcatheter arterial embolization for acute nonvariceal upper gastrointestinal bleeding: Indications, techniques and outcomes. Diagn Interv Imaging 2015;96(7–8):731–44.
20. Aina R, Oliva VL, Therasse É, et al. Arterial Embolotherapy for Upper Gastrointestinal Hemorrhage: Outcome Assessment. Vol 12.; 2001.
21. Lee S, Kim T, Han SC, et al. Transcatheter arterial embolization for gastrointestinal bleeding: Clinical outcomes and prognostic factors predicting mortality. Medicine (United States) 2022;101(31):E29342.
22. Širvinskas A, Smolskas E, Mikelis K, et al. Transcatheter arterial embolization for upper gastrointestinal tract bleeding. Wideochirurgia Inne Tech Malo Inwazyjne 2017;12(4):385–93.

23. Hetrodt J, Engelbertz C, Reinecke H, et al. Access site related vascular complications following percutaneous cardiovascular procedures. J Cardiovasc Dev Dis 2021;8(11). https://doi.org/10.3390/jcdd8110136.
24. Mehran R, Dangas GD, Weisbord SD. Contrast-Associated Acute Kidney Injury. N Engl J Med 2019;380(22):2146–55.
25. Lang EV, Picus D, Marx MV, et al. Massive upper gastrointestinal hemorrhage with normal findings on arteriography: Value of prophylactic embolization of the left gastric artery. AJR Am J Roentgenol 1992;158(3). https://doi.org/10.2214/ajr. 158.3.1738991.
26. Yu Q, Funaki B, Navuluri R, et al. Empiric transcatheter embolization for acute arterial upper gastrointestinal bleeding: A meta-analysis. Am J Roentgenol 2021;216(4):880–93.
27. Mille M, Huber J, Wlasak R, et al. Prophylactic Transcatheter Arterial Embolization After Successful Endoscopic Hemostasis in the Management of Bleeding Duodenal Ulcer. J Clin Gastroenterol 2014;49(9):738–45. Available at: www. jcge.com.
28. Kuyumcu G, Latich I, Hardman RL, et al. Gastrodoudenal embolization: Indications, technical pearls, and outcomes. J Clin Med 2018;7(5). https://doi.org/10. 3390/jcm7050101.
29. García-Iglesias P, Villoria A, Suarez D, et al. Meta-analysis: Predictors of rebleeding after endoscopic treatment for bleeding peptic ulcer. Aliment Pharmacol Ther 2011;34(8):888–900.
30. Chang JHE, TJY Lye, Zhu HZ, et al. Systematic Review and Meta-Analysis of Prophylactic Transarterial Embolization for High-Risk Bleeding Peptic Ulcer Disease. J Vasc Intervent Radiol 2021;32(4):576–84.e5.
31. Srivastava DN, Sharma S, Pal S, et al. Transcatheter arterial embolization in the management of hemobilia. Abdom Imaging 2006;31(4):439–48.
32. Perlberger R. Control of Hemobilia by Angiographic Embolization. Am J Roentgenol 1977;128:672–3.
33. Walter JF, Paaso BT, Cannon3 WB. Successful Transcatheter Embolic Control of Massive Hematobilia Secondary to Liver Biopsy. Am J Roentgenol 1976;127: 847–9. www.ajronline.org.
34. Hidalgo F, Narváez JA, Reñé M, et al. Treatment of Hemobilia with Selective Hepatic Artery Embolization. J Vasc Intervent Radiol 1995;6(5):793–8.
35. Shi Y, Chen L, Zhao B, et al. Transcatheter arterial embolization for massive hemobilia with N-butyl cyanoacrylate (NBCA) Glubran 2. Acta Radiol 2022;63(3): 360–7.
36. Sandblom P. Gastrointestinal Hemorrhage Through the Pancreatic Duct. Ann Surg 1970;171(1):61–6.
37. Tarar ZI, Khan HA, Inayat F, et al. Hemosuccus Pancreaticus: A Comprehensive Review of Presentation Patterns, Diagnostic Approaches, Therapeutic Strategies, and Clinical Outcomes. J Investig Med High Impact Case Rep 2022;10 https://doi.org/10.1177/23247096211070388.
38. Sul HR, Lee HW, Kim JW, et al. Endovascular management of hemosuccus pancreaticus, a rare case report of gastrointestinal bleeding. BMC Gastroentero 2016;16(1). https://doi.org/10.1186/s12876-016-0418-3.
39. Ekezie C, Gill KG, Pfau PR, et al. Hemosuccus Pancreaticus Following Acute Pancreatitis in a 12-years-old Boy Secondary to Pancreatic Pseudoaneurysm Treated With Endovascular Coil Embolization. JPGN Rep 2021;2(4):e125.
40. Meneu JA, Fernandez-Cebrian JM, Alvarez-Baleriola I, et al. Hemosuccus pancreaticus in a Heterotopic jejunal Pancreas. Vol 46.; 1999.

41. Jakobs R, Riemann JF. Haemosuccus pancreaticus (haemoductal pancreatitis) due to a pressure ulcer in pancreolithiasis. DMW (Dtsch Med Wochenschr) 1992;117(51–52):1956–61.
42. Obara H, Matsubara K, Inoue M, et al. Successful endovascular treatment of hemosuccus pancreaticus due to splenic artery aneurysm associated with segmental arterial mediolysis. J Vasc Surg 2011;54(5):1488–91.
43. Han B, Song ZF, Sun B. Hemosuccus pancreaticus: A rare cause of gastrointestinal bleeding. Hepatobiliary Pancreat Dis Int 2012;11(5):479–88.
44. Yu P, Gong J. Hemosuccus pancreaticus: A mini-review. Annals of Medicine and Surgery 2018;28:45–8.
45. Michal JA, Brody WR, Walter J, Wexier L. Transcatheter Embohization of an Esophageal Artery for Treatment of a Bleeding Esophageal Ulcer1.; 1980.
46. Ji HP, Kim HC, Jin WC, et al. Transcatheter arterial embolization of arterial esophageal bleeding with the use of N-butyl cyanoacrylate. Korean J Radiol 2009;10(4):361–5.
47. Vogten JM, Overtoom TTC, Lely RJ, et al. Superselective Coil Embolization of Arterial Esophageal Hemorrhage. J Vasc Intervent Radiol 2007;18(6):771–3.
48. Alrashidi I, Kim TH, Shin JH, et al. Efficacy and safety of transcatheter arterial embolization for active arterial esophageal bleeding: a single-center experience. Diagn Interventional Radiol 2021;27(4):519–23.
49. Swigart L, Siekert R. The esophageal arteries; an anatomic study of 150 specimens. Surgery, Gynecology, Obstetrics 1950;90(2).
50. Brown AC, Ray CE. Anterior spinal cord infarction following bronchial artery embolization. Semin Intervent Radiol 2012;29(3):241–4.
51. Ishikawa H, Ohbe H, Omachi N, et al. Spinal cord infarction after bronchial artery embolization for hemoptysis: A nationwide observational study in Japan. Radiology 2021;298(3):673–9.
52. Balasubramanian S, Thind G, Krishnan S. Anterior spinal cord infarction complicating bronchial artery embolization in a patient with massive hemoptysis. Chest 2019;156(4):A1925.
53. Picone AL, Green RM, Ricotta JR, et al. Spinal cord ischemia following operations on the abdominal aorta. J Vasc Surg 1986;3(1):94–103.
54. Ozoilo K, Stein M. Paraplegia complicating embolization for bleeding intercostal artery in penetrating trauma. Inj Extra 2013;44(8):70–3.
55. Boll DT, Bulow H, Blackham KA, et al. MDCT angiography of the spinal vasculature and the artery of Adamkiewicz. Am J Roentgenol 2006;187(4):1054–60.
56. Kaufman JA, Fsir MS. Chapter 14 - portal and hepatic veins. Elsevier Inc.; 2017. Accessed March 22, 2023. Available at: https://doi.org/10.1016/B978-0-323-04584-1.00011-5.
57. Merkel C, Montagnese S. Hepatic venous pressure gradient measurement in clinical hepatology. Dig Liver Dis 2011;43(10):762–7.
58. Opio CK, Garcia-Tsao G. Managing varices: drugs, bands, and shunts. Gastroenterol Clin North Am 2011;40(3):561–79.
59. Diaz-Soto MP, Garcia-Tsao G. Management of varices and variceal hemorrhage in liver cirrhosis: a recent update. Therap Adv Gastroenterol 2022;15. https://doi.org/10.1177/17562848221101712.
60. Jakab SS, Garcia-Tsao G. Evaluation and Management of Esophageal and Gastric Varices in Patients with Cirrhosis. Clin Liver Dis 2020;24(3):335–50.
61. Saad WE, Nicholson DB. Optimizing logistics for balloon-occluded retrograde transvenous obliteration (BRTO) of gastric varices by doing away with the

indwelling balloon: concept and techniques. Tech Vasc Interv Radiol 2013; 16(2):152–7.

62. Boyer TD, Haskal ZJ. The role of transjugular intrahepatic portosystemic shunt in the management of portal hypertension. Hepatology 2005;41(2):386–400.

63. Boyer TD, Haskal ZJ. The Role of Transjugular Intrahepatic Portosystemic Shunt (TIPS) in the management of portal hypertension: Update 2009. Hepatology 2010;51(1):306.

64. Khan S, Tudur Smith C, Williamson P, et al. Portosystemic shunts versus endoscopic therapy for variceal rebleeding in patients with cirrhosis. Cochrane Database Syst Rev 2006;2006(4). https://doi.org/10.1002/14651858.CD000553. PUB2.

65. Fagiuoli S, Bruno R, Debernardi Venon W, et al. Consensus conference on TIPS management: Techniques, indications, contraindications. Dig Liver Dis 2017; 49(2):121–37.

66. Tripathi D, Stanley AJ, Hayes PC, et al. Transjugular intrahepatic portosystemic stent-shunt in the management of portal hypertension. Gut 2020;69(7):1173–92.

67. Nicoară-Farcău O, Han G, Rudler M, et al. Effects of Early Placement of Transjugular Portosystemic Shunts in Patients With High-Risk Acute Variceal Bleeding: a Meta-analysis of Individual Patient Data. Gastroenterology 2021; 160(1):193–205.e10.

68. Lv Y, Yang Z, Liu L, et al. Early TIPS with covered stents versus standard treatment for acute variceal bleeding in patients with advanced cirrhosis: a randomised controlled trial. Lancet Gastroenterol Hepatol 2019;4(8):587–98.

69. Dariushnia SR, Haskal ZJ, Midia M, et al. Quality Improvement Guidelines for Transjugular Intrahepatic Portosystemic Shunts. J Vasc Interv Radiol 2016; 27(1):1–7.

70. Gaba RC, Khiatani VL, Knuttinen MG, et al. Comprehensive review of TIPS technical complications and how to avoid them. AJR Am J Roentgenol 2011;196(3): 675–85.

71. Clark TWI. Stepwise Placement of a Transjugular Intrahepatic Portosystemic Shunt Endograft. Tech Vasc Interv Radiol 2008;11(4):208–11.

72. Saugel B, Phillip V, Gaa J, et al. Advanced hemodynamic monitoring before and after transjugular intrahepatic portosystemic shunt: implications for selection of patients–a prospective study. Radiology 2012;262(1):343–52.

73. Kamath PS, Wiesner RH, Malinchoc M, et al. A model to predict survival in patients with end-stage liver disease. Hepatology 2001;33(2):464–70.

74. Malinchoc M, Kamath PS, Gordon FD, et al. A model to predict poor survival in patients undergoing transjugular intrahepatic portosystemic shunts. Hepatology 2000;31(4):864–71.

75. Roth JA, Chrobak C, Schädelin S, et al. MELD score as a predictor of mortality, length of hospital stay, and disease burden: A single-center retrospective study in 39,323 inpatients. Medicine (United States) 2017;96(24). https://doi.org/10. 1097/MD.0000000000007155.

76. Lee BT, Yang AH, Urban S, et al. Applying the original model for end-stage liver disease score rather than the model for end-stage liver disease-Na score for risk stratification prior to transjugular intrahepatic portosystemic shunt procedures. Eur J Gastroenterol Hepatol 2021;33(4):541–6.

77. Young S, Rostambeigi N, Golzarian J, et al. MELD or Sodium MELD: A Comparison of the Ability of Two Scoring Systems to Predict Outcomes After Transjugular Intrahepatic Portosystemic Shunt Placement. AJR Am J Roentgenol 2020; 215(1):215–22.

78. Montgomery A, Ferral H, Vasan R, et al. MELD score as a predictor of early death in patients undergoing elective transjugular intrahepatic portosystemic shunt (TIPS) procedures. Cardiovasc Intervent Radiol 2005;28(3):307–12.

79. Casadaban LC, Parvinian A, Zivin SP, et al. MELD score for prediction of survival after emergent TIPS for acute variceal hemorrhage: derivation and validation in a 101-patient cohort. Ann Hepatol 2015;14(3):380–8.

80. Bosch J. Salvage transjugular intrahepatic portosystemic shunt for uncontrolled variceal bleeding in patients with decompensated cirrhosis. J Hepatol 2001; 35(5):590–7.

81. Hong R, Dhanani RS, Louie JD, et al. Intravascular ultrasound-guided mesocaval shunt creation in patients with portal or mesenteric venous occlusion. J Vasc Interv Radiol 2012;23(1):136–41.

82. Gipson MG, Smith MT, Durham JD, et al. Intravascular US–Guided Portal Vein Access: Improved Procedural Metrics during TIPS Creation. J Vasc Intervent Radiol 2016;27(8):1140–7.

83. Kao SD, Morshedi MM, Narsinh KH, et al. Intravascular Ultrasound in the Creation of Transhepatic Portosystemic Shunts Reduces Needle Passes, Radiation Dose, and Procedure Time: A Retrospective Study of a Single-Institution Experience. J Vasc Intervent Radiol 2016;27(8):1148–53.

84. Dastmalchian S, Aryafar H, Tavri S. Intravascular Ultrasound Guidance for TIPS Procedures: A Review. Am J Roentgenol 2022;219(4):634–46.

85. Farsad K, Fuss C, Kolbeck KJ, et al. Transjugular intrahepatic portosystemic shunt creation using intravascular ultrasound guidance. J Vasc Interv Radiol 2012;23(12):1594–602.

86. Clark TWI. Management of Shunt Dysfunction in the Era of TIPS Endografts. Tech Vasc Interv Radiol 2008;11(4):212–6.

87. Bureau C, Pagan JCG, Layrargues GP, et al. Patency of stents covered with polytetrafluoroethylene in patients treated by transjugular intrahepatic portosystemic shunts: long-term results of a randomized multicentre study. Liver Int 2007;27(6):742–7.

88. Angermayr B, Cejna M, Koenig F, et al. Survival in patients undergoing transjugular intrahepatic portosystemic shunt: ePTFE-covered stentgrafts versus bare stents. Hepatology 2003;38(4):1043–50.

89. Qi X, Tian Y, Zhang W, et al. Covered versus bare stents for transjugular intrahepatic portosystemic shunt: an updated meta-analysis of randomized controlled trials. Therap Adv Gastroenterol 2017;10(1):32–41.

90. Triantafyllou T, Aggarwal P, Gupta E, et al. Polytetrafluoroethylene-covered stent graft versus bare stent in transjugular intrahepatic portosystemic shunt: Systematic review and meta-analysis. J Laparoendosc Adv Surg Tech 2018;28(7): 867–79.

91. Wang Q, Lv Y, Bai M, et al. Eight millimetre covered TIPS does not compromise shunt function but reduces hepatic encephalopathy in preventing variceal rebleeding. J Hepatol 2017. https://doi.org/10.1016/j.jhep.2017.05.006.

92. Riggio O, Ridola L, Angeloni S, et al. Clinical efficacy of transjugular intrahepatic portosystemic shunt created with covered stents with different diameters: Results of a randomized controlled trial. J Hepatol 2010. https://doi.org/10.1016/j.jhep.2010.02.033.

93. Trebicka J, Bastgen D, Byrtus J, et al. Smaller-Diameter Covered Transjugular Intrahepatic Portosystemic Shunt Stents Are Associated With Increased Survival. Clin Gastroenterol Hepatol 2019;17(13):2793–9.e1.

94. Praktiknjo M, Abu-Omar J, Chang J, et al. Controlled underdilation using novel VIATORR® controlled expansion stents improves survival after transjugular intrahepatic portosystemic shunt implantation. JHEP Rep 2021;3(3):100264.

95. Petersen BD, Clark TWI. Direct intrahepatic portocaval shunt. Tech Vasc Interv Radiol 2008;11(4):230–4.

96. Sarwar A, Esparaz AM, Chakrala N, et al. Efficacy of TIPS reduction for refractory hepatic encephalopathy, right heart failure, and liver dysfunction. Am J Roentgenol 2021;216(5). https://doi.org/10.2214/AJR.19.22497.

97. Simonetti RG, Perricone G, Robbins HL, et al. Portosystemic shunts versus endoscopic intervention with or without medical treatment for prevention of rebleeding in people with cirrhosis. Cochrane Database Syst Rev 2020; 2020(10). https://doi.org/10.1002/14651858.CD000553.pub3.

98. García-Pagán JC, Caca K, Bureau C, et al. Early Use of TIPS in Patients with Cirrhosis and Variceal Bleeding. N Engl J Med 2010;362(25):2370–9.

99. De Wit K, Schaapman JJ, Nevens F, et al. Prevention of hepatic encephalopathy by administration of rifaximin and lactulose in patients with liver cirrhosis undergoing placement of a transjugular intrahepatic portosystemic shunt (TIPS): a multicentre randomised, double blind, placebo controlled trial (PEARL trial). BMJ Open Gastroenterol 2020;7(1):e000531.

100. Kiyosue H, Mori H, Matsumoto S, et al. Transcatheter obliteration of gastric varices. Part 1. Anatomic classification. Radiographics 2003;23(4):911–20.

101. Philips CA, Ahamed R, Rajesh S, et al. Beyond the scope and the glue: update on evaluation and management of gastric varices. BMC Gastroenterol 2020; 20(1):1–14.

102. Bai M, Qi XS, Yang ZP, et al. EVS vs TIPS shunt for gastric variceal bleeding in patients with cirrhosis: a meta-analysis. World J Gastrointest Pharmacol Ther 2014;5(2):97–104.

103. Saad WEA, Darcy MD. Transjugular Intrahepatic portosystemic shunt (TIPS) versus balloon-occluded retrograde transvenous obliteration (BRTO) for the management of gastric varices. Semin Intervent Radiol 2011;28(3):339–49.

104. Giri S, Patel RK, Varghese J, et al. Comparative outcome of transjugular intrahepatic portosystemic shunt with or without variceal obliteration: a systematic review and meta-analysis. Abdominal Radiology 2023. https://doi.org/10.1007/s00261-023-03843-y.

105. Tesdal IK, Filser T, Weiss C, et al. Transjugular intrahepatic portosystemic shunts: adjunctive embolotherapy of gastroesophageal collateral vessels in the prevention of variceal rebleeding. Radiology 2005;236(1):360–7.

106. Kiyosue H, Mori H, Matsumoto S, et al. Transcatheter Obliteration of Gastric Varices: Part 2. Strategy and Techniques Based on Hemodynamic Features. Radiographics 2003;23(4):921–37.

107. Kim DJ, Darcy MD, Mani NB, et al. Modified Balloon-Occluded Retrograde Transvenous Obliteration (BRTO) Techniques for the Treatment of Gastric Varices: Vascular Plug-Assisted Retrograde Transvenous Obliteration (PARTO)/Coil-Assisted Retrograde Transvenous Obliteration (CARTO)/Balloon-Occluded Antegrade Transvenous Obliteration (BATO). Cardiovasc Intervent Radiol 2018; 41(6):835–47.

108. Urata J, Yamashita Y, Tsuchigame T, et al. The effects of transjugular intrahepatic portosystemic shunt on portal hypertensive gastropathy. J Gastroenterol Hepatol 1998;13(10):1061–7.

109. Norton ID, Andrews JC, Kamath PS. Management of ectopic varices. Hepatology 1998;28(4 I):1154–8.

110. Saad WEA, Lippert A, Saad NE, et al. Ectopic Varices: Anatomical Classification, Hemodynamic Classification, and Hemodynamic-Based Management. Tech Vasc Interv Radiol 2013;16(2):108–25.
111. Shibata D, Brophy DP, Gordon FD, et al. Transjugular intrahepatic portosystemic shunt for treatment of bleeding ectopic varices with portal hypertension. Dis Colon Rectum 1999;42(12):1581–5.
112. Vangeli M, Patch D, Terreni N, et al. Bleeding ectopic varices - Treatment with transjugular intrahepatic porto-systemic shunt (TIPS) and embolisation. J Hepatol 2004;41(4):560–6.
113. Vidal V, Joly L, Perreault P, et al. Usefulness of transjugular intrahepatic portosystemic shunt in the management of bleeding ectopic varices in cirrhotic patients. Cardiovasc Intervent Radiol 2006;29(2):216–9.
114. Kochar N, Tripathi D, Mcavoy NC, et al. Bleeding ectopic varices in cirrhosis: the role of transjugular intrahepatic portosystemic stent shunts. Aliment Pharmacol Ther 2008;28(3):294–303.
115. Saad WE, Saad NE, Koizumi J. Stomal varices: management with decompression tips and transvenous obliteration or sclerosis. Tech Vasc Interv Radiol 2013;16(2):126–34.
116. Ozaki M, Jogo A, Yamamoto A, et al. Transcatheter embolization for stomal varices: A report of three patients. Radiol Case Rep 2021;16(4):801–6.
117. Samaraweera RN, Feldman L, Widrich WC, et al. Stomal varices: percutaneous transhepatic embolization. Radiology 1989;170(3 l):779–82.
118. Liu Q, Song Y, Xu X, et al. Management of bleeding gastric varices in patients with sinistral portal hypertension. Dig Dis Sci 2014;59(7):1625–9.
119. Fernandes A, Almeida N, Ferreira AM, et al. Left-Sided Portal Hypertension: A Sinister Entity. GE Port J Gastroenterol 2015;22(6):234–9.
120. Wei B, Zhang L, Tong H, et al. Retrospective Comparison of Clinical Outcomes Following Splenic Vein Stenting and Splenic Arterial Embolization in Sinistral Portal Hypertension-Related Gastrointestinal Bleeding. AJR Am J Roentgenol 2021;216(6):1579–87.
121. Koconis KG, Singh H, Soares G. Partial splenic embolization in the treatment of patients with portal hypertension: a review of the English language literature. J Vasc Interv Radiol 2007;18(4):463–81.
122. Saad WEA, Kitanosono T, Koizumi J, et al. The conventional balloon-occluded retrograde transvenous obliteration procedure: indications, contraindications, and technical applications. Tech Vasc Interv Radiol 2013;16(2):101–51.
123. Akahoshi T, Hashizume M, Tomikawa M, et al. Long-term results of balloon-occluded retrograde transvenous obliteration for gastric variceal bleeding and risky gastric varices: A 10-year experience. J Gastroenterol Hepatol 2008; 23(11):1702–9.

Surgical Management of Upper Gastrointestinal Bleeding

Teresa Soldner, MD, Katherine Bakke, MD, MPH,
Stephanie Savage, MD, MS*

KEYWORDS

- Upper GI bleeding • Portal hypertension • General surgery • Peptic ulcer disease
- Hemostasis • Vagotomy • Portosystemic shunt

KEY POINTS

- Surgical management of upper gastrointestinal (GI) bleeding is increasingly rare given advances in endoscopy and interventional radiology technologies.
- Surgical management of peptic ulcer disease involves denervation of the acid-secreting cells, which also affects stomach drainage and GI motility.
- Portosystemic shunt surgery has largely been replaced by transjugular intrahepatic portosystemic shunt (TIPS) procedures, but the superiority of TIPS over shunt surgery has yet to be definitively demonstrated.
- Surgeries used to treat the underlying causes of upper GI bleeding can have long-term sequelae and syndromes with which both surgeons and gastroenterologists should be familiar.

INTRODUCTION

Endoscopic management for patients with acute upper gastrointestinal (GI) bleeding has been the standard of care since the early 1990s.[1] Advancement in endoscopic technology, instrumentation, and technical skill, as well as the discovery of proton-pump inhibitors (PPI) and Helicobacter pylori infection as the etiology of most peptic ulcers, has made once-common surgeries for GI bleeding a rare event. Today, only 2% to 8% of patients with upper GI bleeding are managed surgically, though open surgical intervention remains common internationally in areas without advanced endoscopy or interventional radiology.[2]

Approximately 80% of all gastrointestinal bleeding originates in the upper GI tract, defined as the esophagus, stomach, and duodenum to the Ligament of Treitz.[2]

Acute Care and Regional General Surgery, University of Wisconsin School of Medicine and Public Health, Clinical Science Center, 600 Highland Avenue, Madison, WI 53792, USA
* Corresponding author.
E-mail address: sasavage2@wisc.edu

Gastrointest Endoscopy Clin N Am 34 (2024) 301–316
https://doi.org/10.1016/j.giec.2023.09.005
1052-5157/24/© 2023 Elsevier Inc. All rights reserved.

Common practice dictates that a patient with an acute upper GI bleed should be resuscitated and undergo an endoscopy with possible intervention within 24 hours of admission.[3] If bleeding recurs, either a repeat endoscopy, angioembolization, or surgery should be considered.[4] Incidence of recurrent bleeding after endoscopy ranges from 11% to 33%.[2,5,6] Incidence of recurrent bleeding after angioembolization is similar, ranging from 10% to 20%.[2] Surgery is rarely needed for management of acute upper GI bleeding. A 2012 study looking at the use of surgery or angioembolization after failed endoscopic management for upper GI bleeding in 4478 patients found that only 533 patients experienced rebleeding (11.9%), with 163 of these patients requiring surgery, 60 angioembolization, and 6 undergoing both interventions.[7] Mortality was equivalent between patients with recurrent GI bleeding undergoing repeat endoscopy (23%), angioembolization (23%) and surgery (29%).[7]

While the majority of patients can be stabilized with endoscopy alone, management of acute upper GI bleed requires a collaborative, multidisciplinary approach between gastroenterologists, radiologists, and surgeons. Although the need for surgical intervention is rare, surgical management of acute upper GI bleed remains an essential skill of the general surgeon. Knowing when to do surgery, and what surgery to do, for both hemostasis and disease treatment, is important. Furthermore, surgery for upper GI bleeding can alter anatomy and lead to unique postoperative syndromes that require long-term management by a surgeon and/or gastroenterologist.

PEPTIC ULCER DISEASE
Gastric Ulcer

Peptic ulcer disease (PUD) is the most common cause of upper GI bleeding, representing 40% of all cases.[2] Before advances in endoscopic and interventional radiology (IR) technology in the early 1990s, surgery was the mainstay of treatment for patients with PUD. Now, only 4.3% of patients with upper GI bleeding due to peptic ulcer disease require surgical management.[8] Surgery should be considered for patients who are hemodynamically unstable secondary to hemorrhage or continue to bleed despite multiple endoscopic and/or IR interventions. Additionally, early surgical consultation should be considered for patients with a high risk of rebleeding based on the Forrest Classification, ulcers greater than 2 cm in size, and ulcers located in the stomach or posterior duodenum; patients with these ulcer characteristics are more likely to require surgery for recurrent or refractory bleeding.[2] Although simultaneous peptic ulcer bleeding and perforation is unusual, this situation also requires surgical intervention.[5] Particularly in elderly and medically frail populations, using endoscopy or interventional radiology approaches and avoiding major abdominal surgery is an advantage.[9]

There are 2 basic methods by which a bleeding peptic ulcer can be managed: oversewing or resection. Oversewing involves making an intentional gastrotomy in the anterior aspect of the stomach in order to visualize the gastric lumen, identifying the bleeding ulcer, and using sutures to ligate vessels and achieve hemostasis. Oversewing is helpful if an ulcer is present in an area of the stomach where resection is difficult. It is essential that the surgeon biopsy a stomach ulcer when oversewing, as 6% of gastric ulcers will be malignant.[2] Oversewing addresses the acute problem—hemorrhage—but does not address the underlying cause of the ulcer. Since medical therapy for peptic ulcer disease has become routine, it is unusual to perform acid-reducing and resection procedures, such as vagotomy and antrectomy (**Table 1**), which were commonly performed in the past.

After oversewing, continued histamine H2-receptor antagonist (H2 blocker) but preferably PPI therapy is necessary in the postoperative period to reduce acid and assist in

Table 1
Types of acid-reducing procedures

	Definition	Advantages	Disadvantages
Truncal Vagotomy	Transection of the right and left vagus nerves at or above the level of the diaphragmatic hiatus. Must send 2 cm of each nerve for pathologic confirmation. Disrupts the acid-secreting parietal cells, and slows stomach emptying.	Decreases acid secretion by 60%–70%.	Drainage procedure required due to denervation of pylorus. Dumping syndrome. Diarrhea.
Highly Selective Vagotomy	Division of the vagus nerve branches 7 cm proximal to the pylorus and 6 cm from the distal esophagus. Goal is disruption of branches that innervate parietal cells only.	Minimize motility and drainage issues that result from a truncal vagotomy.	Highest risk of ulcer recurrence.
Gastric Antrectomy	Resection of the gastric antrum, pylorus, and first portion of duodenum to remove the gastrin-secreting cells, which also stimulate HCl secretion.	When combined with vagotomy, reduces acid secretion up to 85%.	Requires reconstruction to restore foregut continuity.

ulcer healing. Repeat endoscopy should be performed in 8 to 12 weeks after surgery for a bleeding gastric ulcer to document ulcer healing. If biopsies were not performed at the time of surgery, these should be done at interval endoscopy in order to rule out malignancy. If the ulcer is refractory and not healing, risk factor evaluation including smoking, alcohol, non-steroidal anti-inflammatory drug (NSAID) use, gastrinomas, Helicobacter pylori infection, and non-adherence to medications should be investigated.[10]

Surgical resection of a peptic ulcer is more involved, both in terms of surgical decision-making and technical nature of the surgery. Typically, surgeons will build an operative plan by answering the following questions.

1. Does the bleeding peptic ulcer need resection back to healthy tissue (due to perforation or tissue ischemia)?
2. Does the patient need an acid-reducing procedure to prevent future ulcers (see **Table 1**)?
3. How will one drain and reconstruct the foregut following a resection (**Figs. 1** and **2**, **Table 2**)?

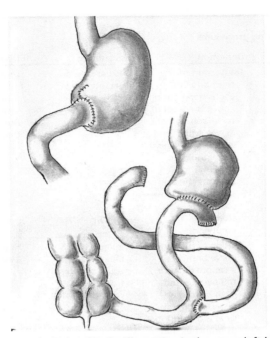

Fig. 1. Billroth I anatomy is depicted in the illustration in the upper left-hand corner. Billroth I reconstruction involves gastric antrectomy and restoration of gastrointestinal (GI) continuity with an anastomosis between the remaining portion of the stomach and the duodenum. Roux-en-Y gastric bypass anatomy is depicted in the illustration in the lower right-hand corner. After antrectomy, GI continuity is restored by creating a gastrojejunostomy (Roux limb or efferent limb). The duodeno-biliopancreatic limb (afferent limb) joins the efferent limb with an anastomosis of small bowel to small bowel. The small intestine distal to this anastomosis is called the common channel.

In the acute setting, surgical resections are more often employed to treat perforation with destruction of the tissues or gastric outlet obstruction secondary to PUD. These surgeries are less likely to be employed to control hemorrhage. In fact, given the high success of medical management, it is atypical to see the use of acid-reducing and drainage procedures unless maximal medical therapy has already been tried and failed.[11]

In addition to addressing upper GI bleeding, acid-reducing and resection procedures can be indicated in the semi-elective setting for patients who have refractory ulcers and cannot modify risk factors such as patients allergic to PPIs, patients with arthritis and require NSAID use for symptom management, and those who have persistent H pylori infections despite treatment. If indicated, the surgeon must determine what kind of acid-reducing and drainage procedure is needed for the patient based on the patient's disease process and desire to avoid chronic side effects. Furthermore, a bleeding ulcer may represent gastric malignancy, so a surgeon must consider what impact resection will have on future oncologic margins and outcomes.

Surgeons who trained in recent decades have limited exposure to acid-reducing and drainage operations. This lack of experience, combined with the fact that the patients nowadays who undergo these procedures have refractory PUD, may very well contribute to poor clinical outcomes despite other advances in general hospital and

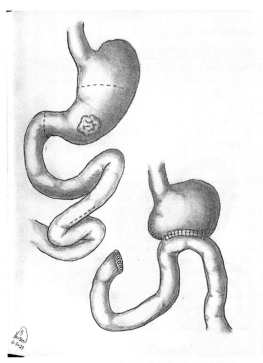

Fig. 2. Illustration depicts a stomach with ulcer pathology and subsequent Billroth II recon-struction after partial gastric resection. The Billroth II differs from the Billroth I in that there is no gastroduodenal anastomosis; a loop of proximal jejunum is instead connected to the remainder of the stomach to restore intestinal continuity.

perioperative care. A recent retrospective review of complications across 2007 to 2015 at a single center showed a high mortality at 20% (highest in the elderly and those presenting with hemorrhage) and noted that readmissions and reoperations are not uncommon.[12]

Duodenal Ulcer

Duodenal ulcers can be treated with oversewing or resection in a similar manner to surgical management of gastric ulcers. Unlike gastric ulcers, duodenal ulcers are rarely malignant, do not require routine endoscopic surveillance for healing, and nearly all are caused by H pylori infection.[13] Unique to duodenal ulcers, however, is the pos-sibility of life-threatening hemorrhage from ulcer erosion of the gastroduodenal artery, located at the posterior aspect of the first portion of duodenum. Posterior location of a duodenal ulcer is a risk factor for failed endoscopy therapy compared to those located anteriorly.[6] Indeed, in a study reviewing the ulcer location of patients requiring emer-gency surgery for upper GI bleed, 72% of the patients had ulcers located in the pos-terior duodenal wall.[6]

Today, with PPI therapy and H pylori treatment, vagotomy and drainage procedure is rarely necessary for duodenal ulcers.[2] Thus, oversewing a bleeding posterior duodenal ulcer is commonly taught and tested surgical knowledge. The retroperito-neal duodenum is mobilized via a "Kocher maneuver" and a generous longitudinal incision along the pylorus and first portion of the duodenum provides access to the

Table 2
Types of drainage/reconstructive procedures

	Surgical Description	Advantages	Disadvantages
Pyloroplasty (Heineke-Mikulicz, Finney, Jaboulay)	Transverse closure of a longitudinal incision along the pylorus.	Widens pylorus to assist in gastric emptying.	Does not include resection of antrum, which may result in additional acid secretion.
Billroth I	Antrectomy + gastro-duodenostomy reconstruction.	Addresses residual acid secretion.	Diarrhea. Dumping syndrome. Alkaline reflux gastritis.
Billroth II	Antrectomy + loop gastrojejunostomy reconstruction.	Addresses residual acid secretion. Lower anastomotic tension.	Diarrhea. Dumping syndrome. Alkaline reflux gastritis. Risk of duodenal stump blowout.
Roux-en-Y	Antrectomy + Roux-en-Y gastrojejunostomy and jejunojejunostomy reconstruction.	Addresses residual acid secretion. Reduces alkaline reflux.	Marginal ulcer. Internal hernia.

posterior wall of the duodenum. Ligation of the gastroduodenal artery is performed by placing a suture at the anterior, posterior, and lateral aspects of the ulcer to ligate the artery and its branches. Care is taken when placing a suture laterally, as the common bile duct is below the duodenum in this region and can be injured with ligation. The incision along the pylorus is closed transversely so as not to narrow the pyloric channel and cause obstruction.

SURGICAL MANAGEMENT OF PORTAL HYPERTENSION AND ACUTE VARICEAL BLEEDING

Though there are several different etiologies of portal hypertension, and therefore varied strategies of optimization, medical management is the ideal approach in order to control the development of gastric and/or esophageal varices (primary prophylaxis). Acute bleeding requires both rapid control of the bleeding source and, frequently, shunting procedures are performed to decrease the degree of portal hypertension and thereby diminish rebleeding risk (secondary prophylaxis). Approaches to shunting include interventional radiology,transjugular intrahepatic portosystemic shunt (TIPS), or portosystemic shunt surgery (PSSS) which has several variations. Just as surgical management of PUD is now rare given advances in medication and endoscopic treatment of PUD, the use of surgical shunts for management of portal hypertension is increasingly rare in high-income countries.

In current practice, gastric varices are commonly managed with endoscopic therapy of bleeding varices, and subsequent maximal medical therapy to decrease portal hypertension which may necessitate portosystemic shunting. The surgical alternative is to perform a gastrotomy and ligate the bleeding varices directly, which should be followed by some form of shunting to decrease underlying portal hypertension.[14] Patients with bleeding esophageal varices who have failed endoscopic intervention, should have a Sengstaken–Blakemore tube placed to tamponade the bleeding for several hours to allow for aggressive resuscitation prior to any surgical or interventional radiology intervention. This converts an emergent surgery into a semi-urgent surgery, which in turn can improve patient outcomes given time for resuscitation.[14] Surgical shunting is relatively well tolerated with 1 study reporting a specific surgical approach (distal splenorenal shunt, described in a table later) resulting in a 6% perioperative mortality (within a literature supported 0%–14% and lower than the TIPS comparison of 7%–45%) and an 85% 1-year survival.[15]

TIPS rapidly replaced surgical shunt procedures due to the ease of placement, avoidance of a major abdominal surgery for the patient, and reduction in cost and length of hospitalization. However, use of TIPS became widespread before data demonstrated its superiority over PSSS.[16] At the beginning of their clinical use, the upfront benefits of TIPS compared to surgery were compromised by the use of bare-metal stents, which had an 80% in-stent thrombosis rate at 2 years and required routine surveillance to monitor for these types of complications.[17] Studies at the time showed perioperative survival to be equivalent between TIPS with bare-metal stents and distal spleno-renal shunt surgery resulting in a practice favoring TIPS due to ease of insertion albeit the need for frequent re-intervention and surveillance.[18] However, introduction of polytetrafluoroethylene (PTFE)-covered stents has resulted in improved stent patency, decreased rates of encephalopathy, and decreased mortality.[17] It is therefore important to note that there is limited literature to compare PSSS to TIPS with PTFE stents, given the ubiquity of TIPS and waning surgical expertise in shunt procedures in high-income countries.

Keeping this in mind while evaluating available literature, our meta-analyses include data from bare-metal and PTFE-stent papers. Multiple Cochrane Reviews on portosystemic surgical shunts (PSSS) suggest the superiority of surgery over TIPS with low-certainty,[19] offered no recommendation on surgery versus endoscopic intervention,[20] and gave no recommendation on shunts versus devascularization procedures.[21] Another Cochrane review has a submitted protocol on selective versus nonselective shunts (discussed later) and including TIPS of varying diameter, which has not been published.[22] In conclusion, there are no strong data for or against one type of intervention to hold sway over the others.

The use of PSSS should be reconsidered despite the ease and ubiquity of TIPS. A 2010 meta-analysis found similar morbidity and mortality at 30-days and 1-year follow-up, but significantly improved 2-year mortality and decreased shunt failure with PSSS over TIPS.[23] A 2009 randomized control trial called into question the current low rate of surgical shunting nationwide, suggesting that surgery is superior to TIPS for permanent bleeding control, transfusion need, and survival at all time intervals and with all Child's classes.[24] These studies indicate that surgical shunting should not be abandoned and may merit updated research and re-evaluation.

Based on consensus guidelines, indications to consider surgical shunts (in centers where expertise exists) are similar to that of TIPS: prevention of recurrent variceal hemorrhage (secondary prophylaxis) and acute variceal bleeding which has failed endoscopic intervention.[25,26] Specifically, under consideration are patients with advanced cirrhosis already complicated by encephalopathy (who are not candidates for TIPS), patients with variceal bleeding and well-compensated cirrhosis not nearing transplant, or patients with portal hypertension due to extra-hepatic veno-occlusive disease, who may be appropriate candidates for surgical shunt procedures.[19,27,28]

There are several surgical options to address the different needs of a patient with portal hypertension which can be grouped into 3 categories based on the patient's needs.

1. Esophagogastric devascularization ± splenectomy ± transection & reanastomosis

Usually used in extreme cases to prevent further variceal rebleeding. Devascularization procedures could also play a role in preventing a primary bleeding in select cases, particularly for patients who reside physically far from medical access points.[14]

2. Porto-systemic surgical shunts (PSSS) (**Figs. 3** and **4**, **Table 3**):

Nonselective shunts, preferred for greater control of variceal bleeding, work by offloading a greater volume of blood through the shunt. Unfortunately, this causes them to also be associated with higher immediate postoperative encephalopathy and greater deterioration of liver function, yet without notable difference in mortality. Interestingly, there is no appreciable difference in long-term survival, encephalopathy, and bleeding between the selective and nonselective types, likely due to a loss of selectivity over time.[29]

3. Orthotopic liver transplantation: As the only curative option to refractory/recurrent variceal bleeding and its associated underlying liver disease, shunting procedures (including TIPS) are often considered a logical "bridge to transplant." Yet, only 3% to 14% of patients with TIPS go on to transplant.[19] If surgical shunting is warranted prior to transplantation, surgeons often prefer H-graft or splenorenal shunt surgery to minimize portal dissection in a future surgical field.[14,15] The complex patient selection and several variations in the surgical techniques in liver transplantation are beyond the scope of this article.

The selection of surgical shunt or devascularization is highly dependent on the etiology of the patient's portal hypertension, vascular anatomy, and transplant prospects in the future. No standardized algorithm exists due to the complex interplay between the afore mentionede considerations, and careful planning is necessary to decrease portal venous pressure without risking encephalopathy by offloading too much volume through the shunt. This anatomy-dependent choice may be aided in the modern age by the assistance of radiologists and advanced imaging.[30]

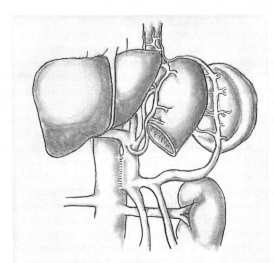

Fig. 3. Illustration of a side-to-side porto-caval shunt. The portal vein is sewn to the inferior vena cava in an attempt to divert portal blood flow into the systemic venous circulation to decrease portal hypertension.

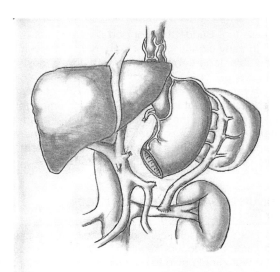

Fig. 4. Illustration of a spleno-renal shunt, where the ligation of the gastric and pancreatic veins lowers portal blood flow and decreases portal hypertension. The splenic vein is attached to the left renal vein to maintain venous outflow into the inferior vena cava.

Ultimately, perioperative morbidity and mortality from shunt procedures are primarily due to the residual hepatic function and resuscitation status of the patient at the time of surgery, and not the type of surgery that is performed. In patients with early/well-compensated cirrhosis not nearing transplant, or patients with

Table 3
Types of portosystemic shunts

	Concept	Illustrated Example	Additional Examples:
Nonselective Shunts	Divert portal and mesenteric blood flow into the IVC. Requires delicate balance of shunting and also maintaining transhepatic pressure gradient, ensuring residual portal venous flow.	Side-to-side portacaval shunt: inferior vena cava (IVC) and portal vein (PV) are isolated and mobilized to create a side-to-side PV-IVC anastomosis.	Mesocaval shunt, Interposition 16 mm H graft, Proximal spleno-renal shunt, Side-to-side splenorenal shunt.
Selective Shunts	Exploit dilated variceal anatomy to divert blood flow to more resistant venous flow, lowering portal venous pressure. Short-term advantages include maintenance of portal venous flow and less liver function derangement.	Distal spleno-renal shunt (DSRS): Ligation of the gastric and pancreatic veins lowers drainage into the portal vein. Distal splenic vein is mobilized to create an end-to-side anastomosis with the left renal vein.	Interposition 8 mm H-graft, Coronary-caval shunt ("coronary" referring to the left gastric vein)

veno-occlusive disease (eg, Budd–Chiari or portal vein thrombosis), surgery still offers benefits.[14,27,28] In early cirrhosis, shunt surgery may prevent rebleeding events while offering a durable long-term patency with lower costs and health care usage.[14,15]

In conclusion, there remains controversy about the role of surgery in the management of portal hypertension, but it is undeniably less common for surgeons to have extensive shunting experience in the modern era of TIPS and advanced endoscopy. Therefore, the surgical options for any patient will be fundamentally influenced by the expertise available at your center of practice. It is important, however, to keep an open mind before relegating PSSS to historical status.

OTHER SOURCES OF UPPER GASTROINTESTINAL BLEED
Mallory–Weiss Tear

A Mallory–Weiss tear is a mucosal laceration, typically at the junction between the esophagus and stomach, that occurs secondary to forceful coughing, vomiting, or retching. While these tears are known to cause upper GI bleeding, they are typically self-limited. Only 10% of patients require intervention and rebleeding after intervention is even more unusual, occurring in 7% of patients.[2] Endoscopic management with clips or epinephrine injection is the first step in management. Recurrent bleeding should be addressed with either repeat endoscopy or angiography.[2] The morbidity of the open thoracotomy needed to access the lower esophagus, and the potential for esophageal leak, makes surgical management unfavorable in all but the most severe of circumstances.

Hemobilia

Hemobilia occurs due to a fistulous connection between the hepatic blood vessels and the bile ducts. It is a rare cause of GI bleeding. Causes of hemobilia include traumatic liver injury, hepatobiliary intervention (such as liver biopsy, endoscopic retrograde cholangiopancreatography (ERCP), or percutaneous transhepatic cholangiography), vascular malformations, inflammatory processes resulting in pseudoaneurysm, and malignancy.[31] While endoscopy can be performed to confirm diagnosis of hemobilia—with blood or clot seen emerging from the ampulla of Vater—it is not a therapeutic modality.[31] Computed tomography (CT) angiography can be used to localize a site of bleeding.

Hemobilia can often be managed with conservative and supportive treatment. If intervention is needed, preferred therapy would be angiography and embolization, vascular stenting, and thrombin injection.[2,31] Surgery is much more invasive, usually requiring resection of the segment or lobe in order to gain control of the vascular pedicle. While surgery carries a 90% success rate for hemorrhage control, it also is burdened by a high mortality rate (10%).[31]

Cameron Ulcer

Cameron ulcers are linear ulcers or erosions resulting from an ischemic insult to the folds of gastric mucosa due to a paraesophageal hernia; they are seen in 3% to 5% of hiatal hernia patients. Patients with Cameron ulcers present with chronic anemia, and up to 80% of Cameron lesions are missed on initial endoscopy. If presenting as an acute gastrointestinal bleed, these are usually controlled with endoscopic means. If Cameron ulcers are implicated in chronic gastrointestinal bleeding, there is strong evidence to suggest the superiority of hiatal hernia repair over medical management.[32]

Dieulafoy Lesions

Dieulafoy lesions are dilated submucosal arteries in the stomach that can erode through the mucosa and cause upper GI bleeding. They are rare sources of bleeding, and endoscopic and IR angio-embolization are the ideal therapy for their success in hemostasis and minimally-invasive technique.[2]

Aortoenteric Fistula

Aortoenteric fistulas can occur after abdominal aortic aneurysm (AAA) repair. Aortoenteric fistula is rare, and can occur in patients who have undergone either an open AAA repair or an endovascular repair (EVAR). The classic presentation is one of a "herald bleed" that is often minor, followed later by massive exsanguination. Frustratingly, these fistulas can form at any time—early in the postoperative period, or years to decades after surgery. Because the fistula typically forms in the third-fourthth portion of the duodenum, endoscopic management is challenging and is not the standard of care. Esophagogastroduodenoscopy (EGD) also has low diagnostic sensitivity, approaching only 50%.[33] Thus, CTangiography (CTA) is recommended for diagnosis in a stable patient. If the CTA is negative for fistula, then EGD and colonoscopy should be performed to seek an alternative source of GI bleed. In an unstable patient with GI bleed and history of AAA, operative exploration in an open fashion or endovascular method is appropriate.[33]

UNIDENTIFIED GASTROINTESTINAL BLEEDING IN THE UNSTABLE PATIENT

Due to the evolution of contrast-enhanced radiography and evolving endoscopy techniques (capsule, double-balloon enteroscopy), intraoperative endoscopy is no longer recommended as first-line treatment for obscure gastrointestinal bleeding. It may still be indicated for adjunctive use during planned surgical intervention, and can be useful for identifying a mass or lesion that cannot otherwise be palpated by the surgeon in the operating room.[34] The surgeon can make a controlled enterotomy and introduce a port or the scope itself, guiding the advancement of the scope whilst the gastroenterologist controls insufflation and deflection. Without any tattoo or serosal findings to guide the surgeon, intraoperative enteroscopy is critical for localization of culprit lesions or confirming the absence of such lesions and avoiding unnecessary resection.[35]

In cases of exsanguinating hemorrhage with negative upper endoscopy and with suspicion for lower GI bleeding, the classic surgical teaching is to perform a total colectomy. This approach has not necessarily incorporated the advances in endoscopy and IR in the recent decades, and also fails to address small bowel sources. Most patients would instead have a multi-disciplinary collaboration to attempt to locate the bleed with intraoperative enteroscopy or on-table angiography during exploratory laparotomy.

In the rare cases of exsanguinating hemorrhage in which the patient is unstable for exclusively endoscopic or radiographic intervention, surgical intervention may be required to gain vascular control and resuscitation before truly identifying the source of bleeding. These events are more likely to occur with aorto-enteric fistula (discussed earlier) or duodenal ulcer erosion into the gastroduodenal artery (GDA) (discussed earlier). In these cases, the surgeon begins an exploratory laparotomy by first gaining control (vascular clamping) of the celiac and superior mesenteric artery (SMA) axes, allowing the anesthesia team to catch up with resuscitation. Once ready, the surgeon can employ endoscopy (upper, lower, or through an enterotomy as discussed earlier) to localize the lesion for resection. Additionally, centers with available IR could attempt on-table angiography to accomplish the same. Without a target, the surgeons cannot necessarily see any evidence to localize and resect a bleeding lesion, as the area of bleeding is often not apparent from the extra-luminal vantage point of the peritoneum. Without any ability to localize, surgeons can intraoperatively isolate segments of the gastrointestinal tract with sequential bowel clamping and controlled enterotomies for intraluminal investigation in order to localize the bleeding source for resection. No data or algorithms currently exist for this method given the rarity of the case and the high mortality of patients in such extremis.

LONG-TERM COMPLICATIONS AFTER MAJOR FOREGUT SURGERY

Any procedure which alters the drainage of the stomach carries long-term sequelae. Given how rare it is nowadays to care for a patient with a history of vagotomy and drainage procedure, the authors thought it worthwhile to review the complications of these surgeries to aid physicians who care for these patients.

Dumping Syndrome

Dumping can occur after vagotomy and drainage procedure. The underlying pathophysiology is not well understood, but the symptoms appear to be related to a food bolus rapidly entering the small intestine, particularly sugars. There are 2 primary forms of dumping syndrome. Early dumping occurs immediately after a meal and includes symptoms of nausea, epigastric discomfort, palpitations, sweating, and rarely, syncope. This is believed to be due to fluid shifts into the small intestine, causing intestinal distention and lower blood volume. Late dumping occurs 1 to 3 hours after a meal and is notable for reactive hypoglycemia in addition to symptoms of early dumping. Dumping syndrome is usually mild, occurs in the early post-operative period, and resolves in the vast majority of patients over time. A small subset of patients experience dumping syndrome beyond their recovery from surgery. Somatostatin analogues, injected prior to a meal, can help alleviate dumping symptoms by decreasing plasma insulin levels and intestinal transit time. For patients with Billroth I or Billroth II anatomy, surgical conversion to Roux-en-Y anatomy can alleviate dumping syndrome.

Diarrhea

Diarrhea can occur after vagotomy, and may be associated with the afore-mentioned dumping syndrome and present as osmotic diarrhea. While the issue has not been studied in depth since the 1970s, studies conducted during this time period demonstrated that cholestyramine, which chelates bile salts, can improve post-vagotomy diarrhea.[36]

Alkaline Reflux

Alkaline reflux is seen in patients with Billroth I and Billroth II anatomy. It can also occur in patients with Roux-en-Y anatomy and a "short" intestinal limb. Alkaline reflux is characterized by postprandial epigastric pain, bile reflux or staining of the stomach seen during endoscopy, and histologic changes of chronic inflammation on gastric biopsy. With significant inflammation, this can also cause gastritis and bleeding. Medical therapy, including PPI, H2 blockers, and bile salt chelators, are usually not beneficial. Persistent symptoms from alkaline reflux can be treated with conversion to a Roux-en-Y gastrojejunostomy, with the intestinal limb measuring 50 to 60 cm to avoid reflux of bile and other intestinal secretions back into the stomach.

Marginal Ulcer

Classically, patients with a gastro-duodenal or gastro-jejunal anastomosis need to be on PPI medication for the rest of their lives. Failure to do so can result in marginal ulcers due to the acidity of the gastric contents eroding the jejunal mucosa. Smoking and NSAID use are also significant risk factors for marginal ulcers. At times, marginal ulcers can become so significant as to result in perforation or bleeding. Depending on the size of perforation and whether it is an uncontained leak, a patient may need surgery and, depending on the quality of the tissue, complete revision of the anastomosis may be necessary.

Internal Hernia

Internal hernia is primarily a complication of postsurgical patients; usually due to Roux-en-Y anatomy or any gastro-jejunal anastomosis. It is often a late complication, and occurs in 0.5% to 9% of patients.[37] There are typically 2 mesenteric windows created in the Roux-en-Y construction through which the small bowel can herniate, causing an acute small bowel obstruction. Symptoms can be pronounced, such as acute abdominal pain, nausea, and vomiting; however, symptoms can also be episodic and associated with vague abdominal discomfort, distension, or even back pain. Acute pain and internal hernia, however, is a surgical emergency as they are typically closed loop morphology and can rapidly progress to intestinal ischemia and necrosis if not reduced. Reduction can often be achieved laparoscopically, with closure of the mesenteric defect and bowel resection if needed.

SUMMARY

Management of acute upper gastrointestinal bleeding demands a multidisciplinary approach when the patient is unstable or initial endoscopic intervention is unsuccessful. Surgery, once common with well-delineated open approaches, is now uncommon in the United States due to access to and advancement of endoscopy and interventional radiology techniques. As with any surgical intervention, outcomes improve with higher volume (several cases per year), and this is now relatively uncommon to encounter in surgical training. It is unclear whether surgical approaches to PUD or portal hypertension will continue to wane, though data from the past 20 years indicate a need for reconsideration of how surgery can be useful in modern treatment algorithms.

CLINICS CARE POINTS

Bleeding Ulcer:
- Oversewing bleeding ulcers is a way to gain rapid hemostasis.
- Vagotomy and drainage procedures are reserved for patients with refractory PUD and may cause long-term management issues.

Portal Hypertension:
- Several different surgical shunting options exist to address portal hypertension, each with advantages and drawbacks.
- Expertise in the area of surgical shunts is limited in the current era of TIPS, but certain patient populations would benefit from surgical consideration and further research.

Unidentified GI Bleeding:
- On-table enteroscopy is particularly useful to use for occult GI bleeding in the small bowel, helping to isolate culprit lesion and avoid unnecessary intestinal resection.

- In cases of exsanguinating hemorrhage, a multidisciplinary approach is critical to localize a lesion for hemorrhage control.

ACKNOWLEDGMENTS

Many thanks to Bryar Hansen, MD for illustrating the figures in this article.

DISCLOSURE

None of the authors have any conflicts of interest or financial disclosures.

REFERENCES

1. Sivak MV. Gastrointestinal endoscopy: past and future. Gut 2006;55(8):1061–4.
2. Nelms DW, Pelaez CA. The acute upper gastrointestinal bleed. Surg Clin 2018; 98(5):1047–57.
3. Barkun AN, Almadi M, Kuipers EJ, et al. Management of nonvariceal upper gastrointestinal bleeding: guideline recommendations from the international consensus group. Ann Intern Med 2019;171(11):805–22.
4. Gralnek IM, Dumonceau JM, Kuipers EJ, et al. Diagnosis and management of nonvariceal upper gastrointestinal hemorrhage: European Society of Gastrointestinal Endoscopy (Esge) Guideline. Endoscopy 2015;47(10):a1–46.
5. Donohoe CL, Rockall TA. Is there still a role for the surgeon in the management of gastrointestinal bleeding. Best Pract Res Clin Gastroenterol 2019;42–3, 101622.
6. Millat B, Fingerhut A, Borie F. Surgical treatment of complicated duodenal ulcers: controlled trials. World J Surg 2000;24(3):299–306.
7. Jairath V, Kahan BC, Logan RF, et al. National audit of the use of surgery and radiological embolization after failed endoscopic haemostasis for non-variceal upper gastrointestinal bleeding. Br J Surg 2012;99(12):1672–80.
8. Quan S, Frolkis A, Milne K, et al. Upper-gastrointestinal bleeding secondary to peptic ulcer disease: incidence and outcomes. World J Gastroenterol 2014; 20(46):17568–77.
9. Beggs AD, Dilworth MP, Powell SL, et al. A systematic review of transarterial embolization versus emergency surgery in treatment of major nonvariceal upper gastrointestinal bleeding. Clin Exp Gastroenterol 2014;7:93–104.
10. Napolitano L. Refractory peptic ulcer disease. Gastroenterol Clin N Am 2009; 38(2):267–88.
11. Lee CW, Sarosi GA. Emergency ulcer surgery. Surg Clin North Am 2011;91(5) 1001–13.
12. Hasadia R, Kopelman Y, Olsha O, et al. Short- and long-term outcomes of surgical management of peptic ulcer complications in the era of proton pump inhibitors. Eur J Trauma Emerg Surg 2018;44(5):795–801.
13. Gurusamy KS, Pallari E. Medical versus surgical treatment for refractory or recurrent peptic ulcer. Cochrane Upper GI and Pancreatic Diseases Group. Cochrane Database of Systematic Reviews 2016;2016(3).
14. Pal S. Current role of surgery in portal hypertension. Indian J Surg 2012;74(1) 55–66.
15. Elwood DR. Distal splenorenal shunt: preferred treatment for recurrent variceal hemorrhage in the patient with well-compensated cirrhosis. Arch Surg 2006 141(4):385.

16. Rosemurgy AS, Molloy DL, Thometz DP, et al. Tips in florida: is its application a result of evidence-based medicine? J Am Coll Surg 2007;204(5):794–801.

17. Bureau C, Pagan JCG, Layrargues GP, et al. Patency of stents covered with poly-tetrafluoroethylene in patients treated by transjugular intrahepatic portosystemic shunts: long-term results of a randomized multicentre study. Liver Int 2007;27(6): 742–7.

18. Henderson JM, Boyer TD, Kutner MH, et al. Distal splenorenal shunt versus trans-jugular intrahepatic portal systematic shunt for variceal bleeding: a randomized trial. Gastroenterology 2006;130:1643–51.

19. Brand M, Prodehl L, Ede CJ. Surgical portosystemic shunts versus transjugular intrahepatic portosystemic shunt for variceal hemorrhage in people with cirrhosis. Cochrane Database Syst Rev 2018;10(10):CD001023.

20. Simonetti RG, Perricone G, Robbins HL, et al. Portosystemic shunts versus endo-scopic intervention with or without medical treatment for prevention of rebleeding in people with cirrhosis. Cochrane Database Syst Rev 2020;10(10):CD000553.

21. Ede CJ, Nikolova D, Brand M. Surgical portosystemic shunts versus devascular-isation procedures for prevention of variceal rebleeding in people with hepatos-plenic schistosomiasis. Cochrane Database Syst Rev 2018;8(8):CD011717.

22. Ede CJ, Ede R, Brand M. Selective versus non-selective shunts for the prevention of variceal rebleeding. Cochrane Hepato-Biliary Group. Cochrane Database Syst Rev 2019. https://doi.org/10.1002/14651858.CD013471.

23. Clark W, Hernandez J, McKeon B, et al. Surgical shunting versus transjugular in-trahepatic portasystemic shunting for bleeding varices resulting from portal hy-pertension and cirrhosis: a meta-analysis. Am Surg 2010;76(8):857–64.

24. Orloff MJ, Isenberg JI, Wheeler HO, et al. Randomized trial of emergency endo-scopic sclerotherapy versus emergency portacaval shunt for acutely bleeding esophageal varices in cirrhosis. J Am Coll Surg 2009;209(1):25–40.

25. Orloff MJ, Vaida F, Haynes KS, et al. Randomized controlled trial of emergency transjugular intrahepatic portosystemic shunt versus emergency portacaval shunt treatment of acute bleeding esophageal varices in cirrhosis. J Gastrointest Surg 2012;16(11):2094–111.

26. Bari K, Garcia-Tsao G. Treatment of portal hypertension. World J Gastroenterol 2012;18(11):1166–75.

27. Gur I, Diggs BS, Orloff SL. Surgical portosystemic shunts in the era of TIPS and liver transplantation are still relevant. HPB (Oxford) 2014;16(5):481–93.

28. Orloff MJ, Isenberg JI, Wheeler HO, et al. Budd–chiari syndrome revisited: 38 years' experience with surgical portal decompression. J Gastrointest Surg 2012;16(2):286–300.

29. Yoshida H, Makino H, Yokoyama T, et al. Surgical treatment: selective shunt sur-gery. In: Obara K, editor. Clinical investigation of portal hypertension. Singapore: Springer; 2019. p. 439–46.

30. Fehrenbach U, Gül-Klein S, de Sousa Mendes M, et al. Portosystemic shunt sur-gery in the era of TIPS: imaging-based planning of the surgical approach. Abdom Radiol 2020;45(9):2726–35.

31. Navuluri R. Hemobilia. Semin Intervent Radiol 2016;33(4):324–31.

32. Verhoeff K, Dang JT, Deprato A, et al. Surgical management of hiatal hernia vs medical therapy to treat bleeding Cameron lesions: a systematic review and meta-analysis. Surg Endosc 2021;35(12):7154–62.

33. Dorosh J, Lin JC. Aortoenterofistula. In: StatPearls. 2022. Available at: https://www.ncbi.nlm.nih.gov/books/NBK567729/#. Accessed May 25, 2023.

34. Bonnet S, Douard R, Malamut G, et al. Intraoperative enteroscopy in the management of obscure gastrointestinal bleeding. Dig Liver Dis 2013;45(4):277–84.
35. Green J, Schlieve CR, Friedrich AK, et al. Approach to the diagnostic workup and management of small bowel lesions at a tertiary care center. J Gastrointest Surg 2018;22(6):1034–42.
36. Duncombe VM, Bolin TD, Davis AE. Double-blind trial of cholestyramine in postvagotomy diarrhoea. Gut 1977;18(7):531–5.
37. Mulholland M, editor. Greenfield's surgery: scientific principles and practice. 6th edition. Philadelphia, PA: Wolters Kluwer Health; 2016.

Diagnosis of Occult and Obscure Gastrointestinal Bleeding

Durga Thakral, MD, PhD, Daniel Joseph Stein, MD, MPH,
John R. Saltzman, MD*

KEYWORDS

- Occult gastrointestinal bleeding • Obscure gastrointestinal bleeding
- Video capsule endoscopy • Deep enteroscopy • CT • Angiography
- Iron deficiency anemia

KEY POINTS

- Occult bleeding has no visible blood but rather presents with a positive fecal occult blood test and/or iron deficiency anemia (IDA). In contrast, overt bleeding has visible evidence of blood in the emesis or stool.
- Obscure bleeding is defined as gastrointestinal (GI) bleeding with a negative complete endoscopic evaluation of the bowel.
- Workup of IDA with no other obvious cause should include bidirectional endoscopy, potential small bowel investigation, and evaluation for iron malabsorption.
- Strategies for evaluating obscure GI bleeding include repeat bidirectional endoscopy, deep enteroscopy, radiologic enterography, tagged red blood cell scan, and Meckel scan.

DEFINITIONS

The definition of obscure gastrointestinal (GI) bleeding has evolved along with endoscopic advances in evaluating the source of GI bleeding. Before the routine use of endoscopy, obscure GI bleeding referred to bleeding whose source remained unknown after standard radiologic investigations such as barium radiography.[1] After upper endoscopy and colonoscopy became widely available, obscure GI bleeding referred to bleeding without a source found on bidirectional endoscopy. After the addition of video capsule endoscopy, the definition of obscure GI bleeding further evolved to GI bleeding without a source seen on pan-endoscopy.[2]

Overt (visible) bleeding is defined as visible bright red blood or altered blood (such as coffee-grounds, melena, or clots) in emesis or stool.[2] Occult bleeding has no visible

Division of Gastroenterology, Hepatology and Endoscopy, Brigham and Women's Hospital and Harvard Medical School, 75 Francis Street, Boston, MA 02115, USA
* Corresponding author.
E-mail address: jsaltzman@bwh.harvard.edu

Gastrointest Endoscopy Clin N Am 34 (2024) 317–329
https://doi.org/10.1016/j.giec.2023.09.006
1052-5157/24/© 2023 Elsevier Inc. All rights reserved.

giendo.theclinics.com

blood in the stool and may present as iron deficiency anemia (IDA) and/or a positive fecal occult blood test (FOBT) with anemia of suspected GI origin. Obscure bleeding includes both occult and overt GI bleeding and is commonly invoked after endoscopic examinations do not demonstrate a source. Overt-obscure bleeding is visible bleeding with negative endoscopic examinations. Occult-obscure bleeding may be due to IDA and/or a positive FOBT with negative endoscopic examinations and a clinical suspicion of a GI source.

Small bowel bleeding is estimated to accounts for 5% to 10% of all cases of GI bleeding and used to be considered obscure bleeding.[2,3] In 2015, the American College of Gastroenterology redefined obscure bleeding to GI bleeding of unknown cause after upper and lower endoscopy along with small bowel evaluation such as with video capsule endoscopy, enteroscopy, or radiographic imaging.[2]

INITIAL EVALUATION WITH CLINICAL HISTORY AND PHYSICAL EXAMINATION

Clinical history can suggest the source of bleeding when localizing symptoms are present. Hematemesis or dysphagia suggests an upper GI source, whereas hemodynamically stable hematochezia suggests a lower GI source.[4] Clinical history in obscure GI bleeding should include an exploration of factors that may cause or exacerbate mucosal GI injury such as the use of nonsteroidal anti-inflammatory drugs (NSAIDs), aspirin, bisphosphonates, and anticoagulants.[1] Earlier history of GI surgery including gastric bypass or gastrectomy may suggest a possible anastomotic or excluded anatomic source of bleeding. A history of cirrhosis or risk factors for liver disease suggests varices, which may occur anywhere in the GI tract, as well as portal hypertensive gastropathy, enteropathy, and colopathy.[2] In addition to personal or family history of bleeding disorders, factors contributing to acquired coagulopathy or thrombocytopenia should be investigated. For example, patients with increased circulatory turbulence from mechanical valves, left ventricular-assist devices, hypertrophic cardiomyopathy, and severe mitral regurgitation are more likely to develop angiodysplasias, as are patients with aortic stenosis with Heyde syndrome and acquired von Willebrand syndrome.[2]

Additional history should explore for other risk factors including travel or unusual exposures to suggest parasitic infections (eg, *Strongyloides stercoralis*) that may cause iron deficiency or GI bleeding in immunocompromised hosts with hyperinfection syndrome.[1] Family history and physical examination may suggest genetic or rare disorders as the source of GI bleeding, listed in **Table 1**.[1] Family history of polyposis syndromes (including Gardner syndrome, Cowden disease, Cronkhite-Canada syndrome, Peutz-Jeghers syndrome, and familial adenomatosis polyposis) and malignancies may cause obscure or occult GI bleeding.[1]

POTENTIAL SOURCES OF BLEEDING

Occult bleeding may be due to GI mucosal lesions with slow or intermittent bleeding. Common causes of obscure GI bleeding are outlined in **Fig. 1**, with additional examination findings as detailed in **Table 1**.[4]

GI polyps and malignancies may be causes of occult or overt obscure GI bleeding. These include polyposis syndromes, leiomyomas, and malignancies including GI stromal tumors, leiomyosarcomas, adenocarcinomas, lymphomas, neuroendocrine tumors including carcinoids, esophageal or anal squamous cell carcinomas, and metastases such as from melanoma, breast cancer, renal cell carcinoma, and lung cancer.[4]

The diagnosis of occult GI bleeding manifested as IDA or a positive FOBT thought to be secondary to bleeding polyps may be presumptive if no other sources are seen

Table 1
Physical examination findings of rare or genetic disorders that can result in gastrointestinal bleeding

Condition	Possible Source of GI Bleeding	Features on Physical Examination
HHT	Stomach or small bowel telangiectasias	Telangiectasias on the upper extremities, lips, and oral mucosa
Plummer-Vinson syndrome	Unknown (consequence of chronic IDA, which may be secondary to GI source)	Atrophic tongue; brittle, spoon-shaped nails
Blue rubber bleb nevus syndrome	Bowel hemangiomas	Cutaneous hemangiomas
AIDS	Kaposi's sarcoma of the GI tract	Cutaneous Kaposi sarcomas
Pseudoxanthoma elasticum	Raised, yellow, plaque-like lesions of the GI tract	Retinal hemorrhage, retinopathy, and angioid streaks; yellow papular lesions; cutaneous laxity
Ehlers-Danlos syndrome	Hernias, prolapse, intestinal diverticula, diaphragmatic eventration, and vascular involvement	Hypermobile joints; lax skin around eyes and face; tissue fragility
Tuberous sclerosis complex	Gastric angiomyolipomas, neuroendocrine tumors, hamartomatous polyps, and stromal tumors of the bowel	Ash leaf spots, facial angiofibromas, and shagreen patches
Neurofibromatosis	Bowel neurofibromas	Axillary freckles, cutaneous neurofibromas, café-au lait macules
Malignant atrophic papulosis	Gastric, small bowel, and colonic ulcers from vasculopathy	Papular skin lesions with central white atrophy and surrounding telangiectatic rim
Amyloidosis	Gastric, small bowel, and colonic ulcers from vasculopathy	Waxy papules of the eyelids, macroglossia, postproctoscopic periorbital purpura
Polyarteritis nodosa	Pseudoaneurysms	Subcutaneous erythematous nodules; cutaneous ulcers and plaques; livedo reticularis; gangrene

Abbreviations: AIDS, acquired immunodeficiency syndrome; IDA, iron-deficiency anemia.

because polyps are rarely bleeding at the time of endoscopy.[1] However, colonic hyperplastic and serrated polyps are unlikely to bleed while adenomatous polyps greater than 1 cm in size are more likely to bleed.[1] It has been estimated that 50% to 60% of colon cancers may bleed but only 11% of adenomas bleed.[1] In contrast, large hyperplastic or inflammatory polyps of the stomach have a greater propensity for bleeding.[5]

DIAGNOSTIC APPROACH
Occult Gastrointestinal Bleeding

In the evaluation of occult GI bleeding, the gold standard for initial evaluation is bidirectional endoscopy with upper endoscopy and colonoscopy. When a culprit lesion is identified, 29% to 56% of lesions are in the upper GI tract compared with 20% to 30% in the lower GI tract.[1] A meta-analysis of 6993 patients who underwent endoscopy for

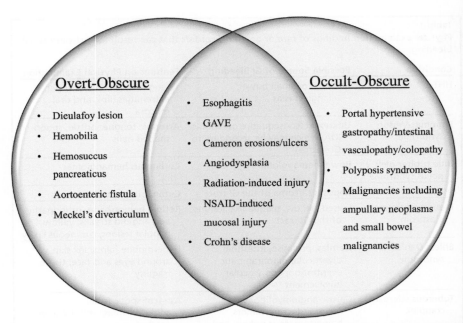

Fig. 1. Common causes of GI bleeding categorized by their general pattern of presentation as overt-obscure bleeding or occult-obscure GI bleeding. GAVE, gastric antral vascular ectasia.

positive FOBT found that the prevalence of upper GI malignancy was 0.8% and that of any GI lesions was 30.4%, whereas the prevalence of colon malignancy was 3.3% and that of any colonic lesions was 31.9%.[6] Of note, even if a lesion is found on upper endoscopy, it may not fully explain occult blood positivity or IDA because additional sources may exist.[1]

Many of the colon cancer-screening studies using FOBT were not consistent in dietary restrictions before FOBT testing, and unlike with fecal immunochemical test (FIT) testing, false-positive and false-negative results may occur after ingestion of high peroxidase-containing foods (such as fruits and raw vegetables), red meat, poultry, fish, vitamin C, and aspirin.[4] In addition, the results may vary with spontaneously passed stools compared with a stool sample obtained from a digital rectal examination (which may cause trauma and a false-positive test).[4] The expanded use of immunochemical testing has improved accuracy when used for colon cancer screening, although FOBT remains in use in some clinic and hospital settings.

Iron Deficiency Anemia

Anemia may be defined as a hemoglobin concentration of less than 13 g/dL in men and less than 12 g/dL in people who menstruate. When anemia is present, a low mean corpuscular volume (MCV) can be suggestive of IDA, whereas a ferritin concentration less than 45 ng/mL is consistent with IDA.[7] In patients with inflammation or chronic kidney disease, ferritin levels may be reactive and elevated despite low total body iron stores, and alternative tests including serum iron concentration or soluble transferrin receptor should be used for diagnosing IDA.[7]

An adequate trial of iron supplementation is a thrice-weekly dose of 35 to 65 mg of elemental iron, and response is a hemoglobin increase by 2 g/dL after 4 weeks of therapy.[4] Studies have demonstrated similar effectiveness in raising hemoglobin and ferritin levels with every other day iron dosing compared with daily dosing with improved compliance due to reduced side effects.[8] Every other day iron dosing should be first used compared with more frequent dosing. After normalization of anemia, iron repletion therapy should be continued for 3 to 6 months to replenish iron stores.[9] If side effects limit tolerance or there is concern for malabsorption, intravenous iron can be administered. Intravenous iron carries a higher risk of adverse reactions including anaphylactic shock and arthralgia-myalgia syndrome.[4]

In patients with IDA, a thorough history and physical examination should be obtained to assess for localizing or GI symptoms. In patients with a negative GI workup, it is important to assess for other causes such as dietary nutrient deficiencies, non-GI blood losses, frequent blood donation, and malabsorption syndromes. Hematology consultation may be warranted.

Workup of Iron Deficiency Anemia

In asymptomatic men and postmenopausal women with IDA and no other obvious cause, bidirectional endoscopy with upper endoscopy and colonoscopy should be performed. An upper GI malignancy can be detected in 2% of patients and lower GI malignancy in 9% of patients.[10] Endoscopic evaluation can visualize findings to suggest other GI causes of chronic blood loss or malabsorption including inflammatory bowel disease, celiac disease, peptic ulcer disease, gastric antral vascular ectasia (also called watermelon stomach), and erosive esophagitis. The management of premenopausal asymptomatic women with IDA and no other obvious cause is less clear; it is reasonable to initiate an empiric trial of iron supplementation and assess response before bidirectional endoscopy.

The American Gastroenterological Association (AGA) does not recommend routine concurrent duodenal biopsies for celiac disease or gastric biopsies for *Helicobacter pylori*/atrophic gastritis during the index endoscopy unless there are gross abnormalities due to cost ineffectiveness.[7] Noninvasive serologic testing for celiac disease is recommended before bidirectional endoscopy, and small bowel biopsies can be obtained if these are positive or there are risk factors for celiac disease based on history such as symptoms, concurrent autoimmune disease, or positive family history. If endoscopic findings suggest celiac disease (mucosal scalloping, effacement of circular folds and villi, and pale or smooth, atrophic-appearing mucosa of the small bowel), duodenal biopsies should be obtained.

Noninvasive testing for *H pylori* (with treatment if positive) is also recommended by the AGA before endoscopy, due to the association of *H pylori* and gastric adenocarcinoma and peptic ulcer disease.[10] In clinical practice, many patients directly referred for endoscopic evaluation of iron deficiency have not had earlier testing for *H pylori* or celiac disease, and it is our practice to routinely obtain biopsies for both in this scenario.

Workup of Occult Gastrointestinal Bleeding

In patients with positive fecal occult blood testing without IDA, a colonoscopy should be performed, with or without upper endoscopy depending on the patient's symptoms. If no symptoms are present, colonoscopy does not reveal a bleeding source, or IDA is also present, the full bidirectional examination with upper endoscopy and colonoscopy should be completed. If no source of bleeding is identified after bidirectional endoscopy and IDA or positivity of FOBT persists, capsule endoscopy should be performed. If video capsule endoscopy cannot be performed or there is high suspicion for small bowel pathologic condition, we may proceed directly to push enteroscopy to allow for possible therapeutic intervention. If there is any suspicion of bleeding from a pancreatic or biliary source, endoscopy demonstrates an unusual appearance of the ampulla, or lesions are identified that cannot be completely assessed with a forward-viewing endoscope, we perform side-viewing or cap-assisted endoscopy.

Obscure Gastrointestinal Bleeding

Initial management of overt-obscure GI bleeding is similar to any GI bleeding and is focused on resuscitation and achievement of hemodynamic stability. Given that overt-obscure bleeding may be intermittent, the highest diagnostic yield is obtained with rapid investigation. This is optimally within the first 2 hours via radiological methods and 10 to 30 hours via endoscopy after adequate resuscitation.[2,11] A general approach is presented in **Fig. 2** with specific investigations and considerations detailed below.

Repeat Bidirectional Endoscopy

If initial bidirectional endoscopy is negative, patients can be considered as having a "potential" small bowel bleed. These patients should then undergo evaluation for a small bowel source.[2] When the initial upper endoscopy and colonoscopy were not performed recently or if there is any question about the quality of the examinations, it is our practice to repeat bidirectional endoscopy to assess for commonly missed lesions (see **Fig. 2**). Evaluation of the upper GI tract should be repeated in patients with melena or hematemesis. We either start with a push enteroscopy or are prepared to

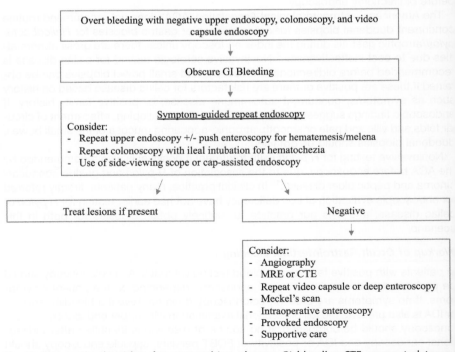

Fig. 2. Diagnostic algorithm for approaching obscure GI bleeding. CTE, computed tomographic enterography; MRE, magnetic resonance enterography.

switch to an enteroscope if the repeat upper endoscopy is unremarkable to assess for commonly missed lesions in the distal duodenum and proximal jejunum, which may be more difficult to visualize with video capsule endoscopy.[2,3]

In a study of 95 patients undergoing push enteroscopy for obscure GI bleeding, a suspected bleeding source was found in 41% of patients, and 64% of the lesions identified were within the reach of standard upper endoscopy.[1] The most common lesions missed on initial endoscopy include Cameron's erosions, arteriovenous malformations of the stomach and proximal duodenum, and peptic ulcer disease, especially with recent NSAID use.[3]

Additional techniques to improve diagnostic yield of repeat upper endoscopy include careful examination of the ampulla and periampullary region to assess for hemobilia and duodenal lesions with side-viewing or cap-assisted endoscopy. Repeat colonoscopy with ileal intubation should be considered if recurrent hematochezia is present and/or if repeat upper endoscopy evaluation is negative.[1]

Video Capsule Endoscopy and Deep Enteroscopy

In both overt and occult GI bleeding, investigation of the small bowel is standard after negative bidirectional endoscopy (see **Fig. 2**). Approximately 5% to 10% of GI bleeding occurs between the Ampulla of Vater and the ileocecal valve with angiodysplasia accounting for 30% to 40% of bleeding lesions.[2,3] Video capsule endoscopy is the first test in most patients to visualize actively or potentially bleeding small bowel lesions.[3] The most common cause of obscure bleeding differs based on age: in patients aged younger than 40 years, the most likely causes are small bowel tumors, Meckel diverticula, angiodysplasia, polyposis syndromes, and Crohn disease. In patients aged older than 40 years, the most likely causes are angiodysplasia, gastric antral vascular ectasias (GAVE), small bowel tumors, Dieulafoy lesions, and drug-induced small bowel injury.[1] In patients with possible small bowel stenoses, including established Crohn disease, earlier small bowel surgery, and earlier radiation, caution is needed due to the risk of capsule retention.[3]

If a source is not clearly visualized on video capsule endoscopy, the presence of blood seen on video capsule endoscopy can help localize the source of bleeding and direct further endoscopic intervention such as push enteroscopy or device-assisted enteroscopy (including single-balloon, double-balloon, and spiral techniques). A meta-analysis of 39 studies of video capsule endoscopy and device-assisted enteroscopy for overt-obscure GI bleeding demonstrated a diagnostic yield of 44% to 100% for device-assisted enteroscopy performed in the first 24 to 48 hours of bleeding or combined video capsule endoscopy and device-assisted enteroscopy during ongoing bleeding.[12] Video capsule endoscopy before deep enteroscopy increases diagnostic yield and directs the approach to be antegrade or retrograde. In massive hemorrhage from the small bowel or when video capsule endoscopy is contraindicated, initial deep enteroscopy may be appropriate, typically starting with an antegrade approach unless bleeding is suspected from the distal third of the small intestine.[2] When no source is identified on a thorough deep enteroscopy examination, we mark the deepest extent of visualization with a clip or tattoo to provide a landmark should we need to repeat enteroscopy from the other direction or proceed with video capsule endoscopy.

Motorized spiral enteroscopy is a new technique that seems to significantly shorten procedure time and have a technical success rate compared with other forms of deep enteroscopy. In addition, motorized enteroscopy is much more likely to allow for total small bowel enteroscopy in one session. The technique of motorized small bowel enteroscopy will likely result in a higher diagnostic and higher therapy yield than other forms of deep enteroscopy.

In patients aged younger than 40 years with obscure GI bleeding, ulceration, or bleeding from a Meckel diverticulum should be considered. This may be assessed with video capsule endoscopy, which may reveal a diverticulum, or "double-lumen sign," and may show active bleeding or colocalization with active bleeding.[13] A Meckel scan may also detect the presence of a Meckel diverticulum (see later discussion).

Computed Tomographic Enterography and Magnetic Resonance Enterography

Computed tomographic or magnetic resonance enterography (CTE/MRE) may help identify a cause of bleeding. We consider CTE/MRE if a small bowel bleed is suspected but capsule endoscopy is negative, particularly if a small bowel space-occupying lesion or metastatic disease is suspected. CTE/MRE can also be used as a noninvasive evaluation when video capsule endoscopy is contraindicated.[2] Both CTE and MRE involve administration of a high volume of oral contrast followed by image acquisition with intravenous contrast in the arterial, enteric, and delayed phases. Both techniques provide high spatial resolution, which may reveal polyps, vascular malformations, or luminal lesion suggestive of neoplasms, strictures, inflammation such as from NSAIDs or inflammatory bowel disease, and ectopic or heterotopic tissue.[14] Angioectasias may show enteric phase enhancement on CTE, due to their thin, tortuous vasculature with an arborizing pattern, which fades on delayed images.[14] Arteriovenous malformations and arteriovenous fistulas may seem as avid enhancement on CTE arterial phase imaging, which becomes undetectable on enteric and delayed phase imaging.[14]

A meta-analysis of 7 studies including 279 patients suggested a diagnostic yield of 34% for CTE compared with 53% for video capsule endoscopy in obscure GI bleeding.[15] Disadvantages of CTE include radiation exposure, iodinated contrast use, and patient need to tolerate oral contrast. MRE, which uses a gadolinium-based IV contrast, is preferable to CTE in cases of iodine contrast allergy, pregnancy before 25 weeks gestation or in younger patients. However, MRE cannot be used in patients with noncompatible metal implants or devices, gadolinium allergy, high risk for nephrogenic systemic fibrosis, or difficulty laying still for longer image acquisition time than CTE.

Angiography

In cases of overt-obscure bleeding in which a source has not been endoscopically identified in which brisk lower GI bleeding is suspected, computed tomography angiography (CTA) is helpful for localization and conventional angiography for potential therapeutic intervention.

Computed tomography angiography

CTA involves initial low-dose noncontrast image acquisition to assess for preexisting hyperdense materials including pills, prior contrast, or retained barium, which could interfere with interpretation.[14] Image acquisition is then done after administration of intravenous iodinated contrast during the arterial phase 8 to 10 seconds after adequate enhancement of the proximal portion of the abdominal aorta, which allows extravasated contrast to accumulate in the lumen of the bowel.[14] A third image acquisition is performed in the portal venous phase about 50 seconds after the arterial phase.[14] Delayed imaging 90 to 120 seconds after injection may also be obtained to assess for lower intensity bleeds.[14]

CTA is considered positive when active extravasation is visualized. This may seem as a "blush" of hyperdense contrast material within the lumen of the bowel, a jet of contrast in the case of a brisk arterial bleed, or a focus of contrast extravasation within the lumen seen on delayed imaging that may be moving distally as the bowel peristalses.[14]

CTA has been shown to detect bleeding rates as low as 0.3 to 0.5 mL/min with a meta-analysis of 672 patients finding a sensitivity of 85% and specificity of 92% for acute GI bleeding in selected patients.[14] It is important to note that CTA only detects acute, active bleeding during the image acquisition, as stigmata of intermittent or earlier bleeding are not visualized. CTA is most helpful in the acutely, briskly bleeding patient including patients who are hemodynamically unstable, especially to aid in localization before directed angiography, which should be performed within 90 minutes of CTA, if feasible. Risks of CTA include radiation exposure and the need for iodinated contrast, which may be contraindicated in renal compromise.

Conventional angiography

Conventional angiography has a lower sensitivity for the detection of active bleeding than CTA, detecting bleeds at rates as low as 0.5 to 1 mL/min.[16] Angiography is typically used for patients who have a GI bleeding source already identified such as on CTA, or have been found to have a nonintervenable lesion or bleed refractory to intervention on endoscopy. It also has a role in select cases with severe, active bleeding that other modalities fail to localize. It is an invasive technique, accessible primarily at large or academic hospitals, and involves administration of iodinated contrast, which may not be possible in patients with significant renal disease or contrast allergy. The primary advantage of angiography is the ability to intervene on identification of a bleeding lesion without the requirement for bowel preparation.[14] It has no role in the management of occult bleeding.

Tagged Red Blood Cell Scan

In cases of overt-obscure GI bleeding, nuclear scintigraphy, or a tagged red blood cell (RBC) scan may be helpful to verify if a GI bleeding source is present. It can detect low-intensity GI bleeds at a rate as low as 0.05 mL/min.[2] RBCs from the patient are radiolabeled with Technetium (Tc) 99m and reinfused before imaging over 90 minutes. If the bleeding rate is in the range of 0.1 to 0.4 mL/min and present during the continuous phase of imaging or an "early blush" is present, a general area of bleeding can be identified to potentially guide angiographic, endoscopic, or surgical therapy.[3] If an initial study is negative but there is concern for rebleeding, the patient can be reimaged with the same-tagged bolus for up to 24 hours.[14] However, sensitivity for GI bleeding is low with up to 85% of GI bleeding sources missed.[3] Furthermore, the utility in localization is limited to a general area in the body rather than an anatomic position in the GI tract to guide further endoscopy and therapy. Surgery should not be performed when the bleeding site is only localized on a tagged RBC scan. Given the poor ability to localize bleeding, CTA has largely supplanted its use, and we no longer routinely obtain tagged RBC scans in our clinical practice.

Meckel Scan

In patients with a suspected bleeding Meckel diverticulum but inconclusive testing including video capsule endoscopy, investigation with 99mTc-pertechnetate scintigraphy (Meckel scan), can detect ectopic gastric mucosa within a Meckel diverticulum.[2] The sensitivity is reported as 85% to 100% in the pediatric population and up to 62% patients in patients aged older than 16 years.[17] False-negative results are possible if the diverticulum contains only ectopic pancreatic tissue and no ectopic gastric tissue (although these types are much less likely to bleed because the acid secreted from the gastric type mucosa causes small bowel ulcerations that bleed) or false positives if other sources of ectopic gastric mucosa (such as duplication cysts, gastrogenic cysts, or enteric duplication cysts) are present.[14] A Meckel scan does not detect GI bleeding, and further workup such as video capsule endoscopy or enteroscopy is necessary to assess if a Meckel diverticulum, if detected, is the bleeding source.

Provoked Angiography and Endoscopy

Provoked endoscopy refers to the administration of antiplatelet and/or anticoagulant agents to provoke bleeding and thereby elucidate bleeding sources during endoscopy or angiography. This strategy can be considered in obscure GI bleeding after other methods of radiographic or endoscopic identification of bleeding have not been successful, especially if bleeding may be due to vascular lesions such as angioectasias and Dieulafoy lesions that may not be visible unless actively bleeding. It is recommended that provoked endoscopy only be performed in centers where there are ample ancillary resources, including intensive care units, angiography, and surgery. In addition, this should be limited to centers capable of performing device-assisted enteroscopy to ensure the entire GI tract may be accessed given the risk for uncontrolled severe bleeding and death. All potential sources (especially variceal) must be appropriately managed before proceeding with provocation, and same-admission panendoscopy should be negative. Additionally, careful attention should be provided to potentially provoking non-GI bleeding, especially at vascular access sites and in the brain.

Provocation agents include antiplatelet agents, anticoagulants, vasodilators, and fibrinolytics. Heparin is most commonly used. Antiplatelet agents such as clopidogrel may be especially helpful for patients in whom bleeding is thought to be worsened by platelet dysfunction such as those with Heyde syndrome with acquired von Willebrand factor deficiency or in patients with left-ventricular assist devices. One study used a bolus of 5000 units of heparin 12 hours before endoscopy, infused to a target partial thromboplastin time (PTT) between 79 and 118 seconds, and held 6 hours before endoscopy.[18] The glycoprotein IIb/IIIa inhibitor abciximab may be a more conservative option due to its short half-life and easy reversibility with platelet administration.[18] Dabigatran is another option, suggested at a dose of 150 mg, which peaks in 2 hours and its reversibility with the administration of idarucizumab.[18] Vasodilators such as tolazoline and nitroglycerine as well as fibrinolytics such as urokinase and streptokinase have also been used.[3] There is no data on the use of newer short-term agents such as bivalirudin. A recent study of 27 patients with obscure GI bleeding who underwent a total of 38 provoked endoscopies demonstrated a diagnostic yield of 27% to 71%. Although this study noted no adverse events, the patients ranged in transfusion requirements from 3 to 67 units of packed RBCs with the average transfusion requirement of 13 units per patient. Others have demonstrated limited benefits and questionable cost-effectiveness and safety.[3]

Intraoperative Enteroscopy

Intraoperative enteroscopy involves endoscopic evaluation during laparotomy. This may be achieved by the introduction of an endoscope through an enterostomy created during the operation or through an oral or anal route with assistance of the surgeon in guiding the instrument through the bowel. Intraoperative enteroscopy may be indicated if a lesion has been identified, which cannot be treated by any other measures or if a significant bleeding lesion remains obscure after extensive earlier investigations have not elucidated a source and overt rapid bleeding is present.[3] Tattoos placed during prior endoscopic examinations may be helpful in guiding intraoperative enteroscopy.[2] Intraoperative enteroscopy can allow for complete evaluation of the small bowel in 57% to 100% of cases with identification of a bleeding source in up to 80% of cases.[19] However, 13% to 52% of patients experience recurrent bleeding, and overall reported mortality is 5% and morbidity is 17%.[19] Given the significant operative morbidity and mortality, the technical difficulties to avoid overdistension and laceration of the mesentery, the extensive time that may be needed, and the required coordination of providers (endoscopists and surgeons), intraoperative enteroscopy is a last-resort diagnostic option primarily in patients with ongoing transfusion dependence with refractory, severe, and active GI bleeding.

SUPPORTIVE CARE

Maintenance of hemodynamic stability is imperative in the management of all GI bleeding. All patients should be resuscitated with intravenous fluids and RBC transfusions to support cardiac output. Thresholds for erythrocyte transfusion are dependent on the clinical scenario because patients with active cardiovascular disease or end-stage renal disease have higher target hemoglobin levels. Erythropoietin administration may be administered to stimulate erythrocyte production in the presence of chronic renal disease in patients with slow occult-obscure GI bleeding. In patients with GI bleeding on medications that are associated with bleeding, such as anticoagulants, P2Y12 inhibitors, aspirin, and NSAIDs, these should be discontinued if no longer indicated. An interdisciplinary risk-benefit discussion that considers the thromboembolic risk versus the bleeding risk may be needed. Comprehensive efforts should be made to control the bleeding source before discontinuing medications with an ongoing indication. It is critical to get patients back on their antithrombotic medications as soon as possible if given for secondary prevention.

Medical therapy includes iron replacement in IDA. In patients with IDA and initial negative upper endoscopy and colonoscopy, empiric iron replacement may result in the resolution of anemia in up to 83% of patients.[10]

Patients with significant aortic stenosis and Heyde syndrome are recommended to have aortic valve replacement.[2] In patients with obscure GI bleeding secondary to angiodysplasias, especially in patients with hereditary hemorrhagic telangiectasia (HHT), additional options for medical therapy include octreotide, thalidomide, and hormonal therapy. Octreotide, a synthetic mimic of somatostatin, can inhibit the release of cholecystokinin, secretin, and vasoactive peptide, which in turn reduces splanchnic blood flow and thus may help to improve GI bleeding.[4]

Thalidomide downregulates vascular endothelial growth factor thus inhibiting angiogenesis and may improve bleeding from angiodysplasia, obscure GI bleeding, HHT, and Crohn disease.[2] Nevertheless, thalidomide must be used with caution and only in select patients due to toxicities including birth defects, neuropathy, rash, constipation, and somnolence.[2] Finally, some studies suggest a possible benefit with hormonal therapy, such as combined estrogen and progesterone therapy, in angiodysplasia, occult GI bleeding, and HHT patients with concurrent renal disease.[2,4]

SUMMARY

The diagnostic approach to occult and obscure GI bleeding continues to evolve because advances in the practice of gastroenterology and endoscopy improve diagnostic and therapeutic abilities. Video capsule endoscopy has allowed noninvasive endoscopic exploration of the entire small bowel and is routine in the investigation of occult and obscure GI bleeding. We provide contemporary definitions of occult and obscure GI bleeding and discuss an approach to the history, physical examination, diagnostic testing, and management. The current recommendations for the diagnostic evaluation of occult and obscure GI bleeding are summarized, and we provide additional perspective from our clinical experience. The management of occult and obscure GI bleeding remains challenging; however, both diagnosis and therapy are improving with advances in endoscopy including motorized small bowel enteroscopy.

CLINICS CARE POINTS

- Overt GI bleeding is bleeding evidenced by visible bright red or altered blood in emesis or stool, and initial management should focus on resuscitation before endoscopic evaluation. In contrast, occult GI bleeding is defined by a positive FOBT and/or IDA with no other obvious cause.
- Occult GI bleeding warrants workup with symptom-guided or bidirectional endoscopy, small bowel investigation, and/or evaluation for iron malabsorption.
- Obscure GI bleeding is defined as GI bleeding without a source after complete endoscopic examinations, including small bowel investigation.
- Evaluation of obscure GI bleeding may be challenging, and strategies include repeat bidirectional endoscopy, deep enteroscopy, radiologic enterography including angiography, tagged RBC scan, Meckel scan, and provoked endoscopy.
- When obscure GI bleeding persists despite a thorough negative workup, management should focus on supportive care and potential pharmacologic management of bleeding.

DISCLOSURE

J.R. Saltzman receives royalties from UpToDate. The other authors have no relevant conflicts of interest.

REFERENCES

1. Zuckerman GR, Prakash C, Askin MP, et al. AGA technical review on the evaluation and management of occult and obscure GI bleeding. Gastroenterology 2000;118:201–21.
2. Gerson LB, Fidler JL, Cave DR, et al. ACG clinical guideline: diagnosis and management of small bowel bleeding. Am J Gastroenterol 2015;110(9):1265–87.
3. Leighton JA, Goldstein J, Hirota W, et al. Obscure GI bleeding. Gastrointest Endosc 2003;58(5):650–5.
4. Concha R, Amaro R, Barkin JS. Obscure GI bleeding: diagnostic and therapeutic approach. J Clin Gastroenterol 2007;41(3):242–51.
5. Yacoub H, Bibani N, Sabbah M, et al. Gastric polyps: a 10-year analysis of 18,496 upper endoscopies. BMC Gastroenterol 2022;22(1):70.
6. Shah A, Eqbal A, Moy N, et al. Upper GI endoscopy in subjects with positive fecal occult blood test undergoing colonoscopy: systematic review and meta-analysis. Gastrointest Endosc 2023;97(6):1005–15.e30.
7. Ko CW, Siddique SM, Patel A, et al. AGA clinical practice guidelines on the GI evaluation of iron deficiency anemia. Gastroenterology 2020;159(3):1085–94.
8. Düzen Oflas N, Demircioğlu S, Yıldırım Doğan N, et al. Comparison of the effects of oral iron treatment every day and every other day in female patients with iron deficiency anaemia. Intern Med J 2020;50(7):854–8.

9. Snook J, Bhala N, Beales ILP, et al. British Society of Gastroenterology guidelines for the management of iron deficiency anaemia in adults. Gut 2021;70(11): 2030–51.

10. Rockey DC, Altayar O, Falck-Ytter Y, et al. AGA technical review on GI evaluation of iron deficiency anemia. Gastroenterology 2020;159(3):1097–119.

11. Uchida G, Nakamura M, Yamamura T, et al. Systematic review and meta-analysis of the diagnostic and therapeutic yield of small bowel endoscopy in patients with overt small bowel bleeding. Dig Endosc 2021;33(1):66–82.

12. Estevinho MM, Pinho R, Fernandes C, et al. Diagnostic and therapeutic yields of early capsule endoscopy and device-assisted enteroscopy in the setting of overt GI bleeding: a systematic review with meta-analysis. Gastrointest Endosc 2022; 95(4):610–25.e9.

13. Wu J, Huang Z, Wu H, et al. The diagnostic value of video capsule endoscopy for Meckel's diverticulum in children. Rev Esp Enferm Dig 2020;112.

14. Kim G, Soto JA, Morrison T. Radiologic assessment of GI bleeding. Gastroenterol Clin N Am 2018;47(3):501–14.

15. Wang Z, Jun qiang C, Liu JL, et al. CT enterography in obscure gastrointestinal bleeding: A systematic review and meta-analysis: CT enterography for OGIB. Journal of Medical Imaging and Radiation Oncology 2013;57(3):263–73.

16. Carney BW, Khatri G, Shenoy-Bhangle AS. The role of imaging in gastrointestinal bleed. Cardiovasc Diagn Ther 2019;9(Suppl 1):S88–96.

17. Irvine I, Doherty A, Hayes R. Bleeding Meckel's diverticulum: A study of the accuracy of pertechnetate scintigraphy as a diagnostic tool. Eur J Radiol 2017; 96:27–30.

18. Raines DL, Jex KT, Nicaud MJ, et al. Pharmacologic provocation combined with endoscopy in refractory cases of GI bleeding. Gastrointest Endosc 2017;85(1): 112–20.

19. Bonnet S, Douard R, Malamut G, et al. Intraoperative enteroscopy in the management of obscure GI bleeding. Dig Liver Dis 2013;45(4):277–84.

Endoscopic Treatment of Small Bowel Bleeding

Sofi Damjanovska, MD[a], Gerard Isenberg, MD, MBA[b],*

KEYWORDS

- Small bowel bleeding • Endoscopic therapy • Small bowel capsule endoscopy
- Push enteroscopy • Device-assisted enteroscopy • Angioectasias
- Dieulafoy lesions

KEY POINTS

- Small bowel capsule endoscopy is the primary method used to investigate the origin of a suspected small bowel bleeding.
- Small bowel endoscopists should review capsule videos before proceeding with endoscopic treatment to not only clarify the diagnosis of the lesion present but to also determine the best endoscopic equipment and insertion route for treatment.
- The most common cause of small bowel bleeding are angioectasias, which preferably are treated with argon plasma coagulation.
- Marking the adjacent area of bleeding can facilitate future repeat endoscopy procedures, interventional radiology angioembolization, and/or surgery, if needed.
- Recurrence rates of small bowel bleeding are high depending on the lesion found, and in many patients, alternatives to endoscopic treatment are needed.

INTRODUCTION

Small bowel bleeding is bleeding of unknown origin that persists or recurs after a negative initial bidirectional endoscopy evaluation.[1,2] Small bowel bleeding originates between the ligament of Treitz and the ileocecal valve. Small bowel bleeding can be challenging to localize and treat. Approximately 5% of all gastrointestinal (GI) bleeding (GIB) in patients originates from the small bowel.[3] The American College of Gastroenterology in 2015 and the American Society for Gastrointestinal Endoscopy published guidelines on the evaluation and management of small bowel bleeding.[3,4] Guidelines published in Europe and Japan are similar.[5–7] This article provides current evidence and a discussion on endoscopic treatment of small bowel bleeding consistent with these guidelines.

[a] Department of Medicine, University Hospitals Cleveland Medical Center/Case Western Reserve University, 11100 Euclid Avenue, Cleveland, OH 44106, USA; [b] Division of Gastroenterology and Liver Disease, University Hospitals Cleveland Medical Center/Case Western Reserve University, 11100 Euclid Avenue, Cleveland, OH 44106, USA
* Corresponding author.
E-mail address: Gerard.Isenberg@uhhospitals.org

Gastrointest Endoscopy Clin N Am 34 (2024) 331–343
https://doi.org/10.1016/j.giec.2023.09.007
1052-5157/24/© 2023 Elsevier Inc. All rights reserved.

ETIOLOGY

Although there are many causes of small bowel bleeding, angioectasias are the most common and account for up to 30% to 40% of cases and are often endoscopically treated.[8] Additional etiologies include other vascular lesions (Dieulafoy lesions, which can be managed endoscopically, and small bowel varices), medications including non-steroidal anti-inflammatory drug (NSAID)-induced erosions and ulcers, ulcers in the setting of Crohn's disease (which can sometimes be managed endoscopically if a bleeding site is visualized), and less commonly, benign and malignant lesions (gastrointestinal stromal tumors, carcinoid tumors, lymphomas, and adenocarcinomas), Meckel's diverticulum–related ulceration, radiation enteropathy, and aortoenteric fistulas, all of which often require surgical management.[9–19] A thorough history and consideration of the patient's age, comorbidities, and medications are important when trying to determine the etiology of a suspected small bowel bleeding as well as subsequent therapeutic options.[1]

EVALUATION

The evaluation of small bowel bleeding should start with a thorough history, physical examination, and review of results of previous evaluations. Once initial bidirectional endoscopy is negative, the first step in evaluating a suspected small bowel bleeding is small bowel capsule endoscopy (SBCE). Additional tests may be indicated and can include push enteroscopy (PE), device-assisted enteroscopy (DAE) such as single-ballon or double-balloon enteroscopy, computed tomographic enterography (CTE), computed tomographic angiography (CTA), magnetic resonance enterography, and intraoperative enteroscopy depending on the clinical situation.

Small Bowel Capsule Endoscopy

SBCE is a minimally invasive, well-tolerated diagnostic tool that allows visualization of the entire GI tract, especially the small bowel in its entirety, without exposing the patient to additional risks, such as sedation.[20,21] Contraindications to SBCE include partial or intermittent small bowel obstruction and pregnancy. For patients unable to swallow due to dysphagia, the capsule can be placed endoscopically. Even though there is a US Food and Drug Administration (FDA) boxed warning that capsule endoscopy is contraindicated in patients with pacemakers and implantable defibrillators, studies have not found evidence that the devices interfere with each other.[22,23] However, in patients with left ventricular assist devices (LVADs), there may be some loss of images with the video recording. Nevertheless, SBCEs are used in these patients as well. SBCE increases the yield of DAE and can be helpful when deciding the optimal DAE approach—anterograde versus retrograde.[24] Evidence suggests that shorter intervals between a bleeding episode and SBCE (including when done as an inpatient) increase the yield and positively influence management and outcomes.[25] Another consideration of SBCE is pre-procedure bowel preparation. Currently, there is no universal guidance on the timing or method of pre-procedure bowel preparation if even needed. Data regarding the timing of pre-procedure bowel preparation are mixed with studies evaluating pre-procedure bowel preparation administration 4 to 12 hours before SBCE.[26,27] There are data to support both pre-procedure bowel preparation and the lack of one. Two randomized controlled trials (RCTs) and a meta-analysis suggest that there is no difference in mucosa visualization when comparing a clear liquid diet to purgative administration before SBCE.[28–30] On the other hand, a recent multi-center RCT showed better mucosal visualization when 1 L of polyethylene glycol was administered before SBCE when compared to fasting alone.[26] Other pre-SBCE interventions have been looked into including antifoaming agents, prokinetics, and combination of purgative and antifoaming agent without any significant clinical impact. The analysis and results of those separate studies are outside of the scope of this review.

Enteroscopy

"Enteroscopy" as a general term refers to the passage of an adult or pediatric colonoscope or dedicated enteroscope beyond the ligament of Treitz. In patients with ongoing bleeding after negative SBCE and CTE, enteroscopy is the next step in the evaluation of small bowel bleeding. There are several different enteroscopy methods. The most significant advantage of enteroscopy over SBCE is the ability to perform therapeutic interventions. Depending on the equipment and techniques used, it is estimated that 25 to 80 cm of the jejunum distal to the ligament of Treitz can be evaluated with PE.[31] In selected patients, such as those with lesions in the distal duodenum or proximal jejunum, PE should be performed after SBCE.

Another enteroscopy method is DAE which can include double-balloon enteroscopy, single-balloon enteroscopy, and spiral enteroscopy (a motorized version of this device which is not available in the United States).[32] Each technique is based on different overtube designs to minimize small bowel looping. With DAE, it is estimated that 240 to 360 cm beyond the pylorus can be evaluated in the anterograde approach and 100 to 140 cm beyond the ileocecal valve with the retrograde approach. The accessibility of DAE is limited by both endoscopist training and equipment availability and may require referral to a center of expertise. Lastly, intraoperative enteroscopy is performed by inserting an enteroscope through an enterotomy site, orally, or rectally during surgery.[33,34] In general, intraoperative enteroscopy is avoided and is considered the last endoscopic resource for persistent bleeding after failure of less invasive methods of evaluation.

ENDOSCOPIC TREATMENT

In this review article, the authors propose an algorithm for endoscopic treatment of small bowel bleeding (**Fig. 1**). In patients that present with GIB, an upper and lower source of bleeding should be ruled out with an esophagogastroduodenoscopy and colonoscopy ("bidirectional endoscopy") before starting an evaluation for small bowel bleeding. The evaluation for small bowel bleeding should start with SBCE as this modality has highest sensitivity in detecting bleeding lesions.[3] If culprit lesions are detected on SBCE, the appropriate endoscopic modality should be chosen based on the location of the lesion. PE should be used for proximal small bowel lesions (distal duodenum and proximal jejunum) and DAE for more distal small bowel lesions (more distal than proximal jejunum), as well as for further diagnostic evaluation of possible small bowel bleeding in the setting of negative SBCE. If PE or DAE are negative, and the patient is hemodynamically stable with reassuring laboratory indices of anemia (eg, stable hemoglobin and hematocrit), observation and supportive treatment (eg, iron supplementation, discontinuation of antiplatelets and/or anticoagulation if clinically appropriate, and periodic blood transfusions) are suggested. If PE or DAE are negative, and the patient has ongoing symptomatic bleeding, CTA with subsequent interventional radiology and/or surgical referrals should take place. Occasionally, tagged *red blood* cells (RBC) scans are done but these are not clinically useful as localization of bleeding is challenging. Meckel's scans are only useful if a Meckel's diverticulum has gastric mucosa; those that do not will have false-negative scans. An

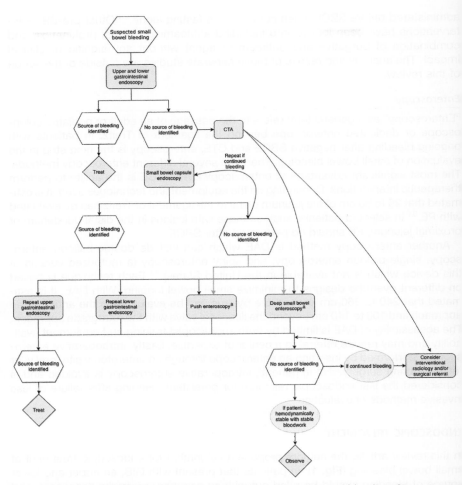

Fig. 1. Proposed algorithm for endoscopic treatment of small bowel bleeding. [a]Enteroscopy method should be chosen based on lesion location in the small bowel, possible contraindications to the procedure, and local availability and expertise.

important rule of thumb is that every patient needs to be assessed individually (eg, age, functionality, comorbidities, medications, life expectancy, and goals) in order to weigh the benefits and risks of the invasive evaluation methods and therapeutics in shared decision-making.

Enteroscopy is the most useful intervention in small bowel bleeding because it facilitates all therapeutic modalities, including hemostatic treatments (by argon plasma coagulation [APC], injection therapy, and hemoclip placement).[7,35–45]

Given that angioectasias are the most common etiology of small bowel bleeding, the endoscopic treatment of small bowel bleeding is largely focused on treating these vascular lesions. Unfortunately, high quality data are unavailable when it comes to the effectiveness of different endoscopic treatment modalities of angioectasias, and small bowel bleeding in general. Additionally, the data available show only modest reduction in blood loss and transfusion requirement.[3,46,47]

Angioectasias

Angioectasias represent a diagnostic and therapeutic challenge. Most small bowel angioectasias are not bleeding at the time of detection during endoscopy, including on SBCE. In addition, bleeding from angioectasias can cease spontaneously. It remains unclear if treating some or all angioectasias seen results in improved patient outcomes related to number of endoscopic procedures, subsequent radiologic studies, hospitalizations, surgical interventions, or mortality. Data suggest that endoscopic treatment can stabilize the hemoglobin level and reduce the need for blood transfusions.[48] However, up to 50% of patients with angioectasias found, that are not treated, do not have bleeding again over several years of follow-up.[2]

Since numerous angioectasias throughout the small bowel can be found in up to 63% of patients,[49] determining a suitable insertion route (anterograde or oral, vs retrograde or rectal) is needed by calculating the burden of angioectasias that are accessible with each potential route. Data suggest that an anterograde or oral route usually represents the highest yield for treatment of angioectasias. Some studies have suggested that using bowel transit time on SBCE may be helpful in determining which insertion route to use.[50] These studies suggest that a lesion found in the first 67% of small bowel transit time is likely to be accessible by the anterograde route. However, a caveat with calculating small bowel transit time in this fashion is that transit delays through the small bowel by the capsule device may impact the percentage of time calculated. For example, a prolonged transit delay in the duodenum could artificially increase the calculated time for the distal small bowel leading to an incorrect decision to pursue a retrograde approach rather than a correct anterograde approach.

Small bowel endoscopists should review capsule videos before proceeding with endoscopic treatment to not only clarify the diagnosis of the lesion present (eg, if a lesion is truly an angioectasia or actually an area of non-specific erythema which would not require endoscopic treatment) but to also determine the best insertion route for treatment (refer to Isenberg G. ASGE Video Tips: Top 10 Tips for Obscure GI Bleeding: Four Part Series. 2023: learn.asge.org). The decision to proceed with endoscopic therapy also depends on the number, size, and distribution of angioectasias as well as the severity of bleeding. For example, a single or few small angioectasias noted on small bowel capsule endoscopy in a patient with mild iron deficiency anemia is not likely to benefit from deep small bowel enteroscopy treatment. In addition, on the other end of the spectrum, an older patient with multiple co-morbidities (including cardiopulmonary and renal diseases) who has intermittent bleeding from angioectasias is unlikely to benefit from repeated deep small bowel enteroscopy therapy as angioectasias in this patient population often recur despite endoscopic treatment.[48] In such patients, periodic iron therapy or intermittent blood transfusions may be a preferable treatment strategy.

The endoscopic techniques and tools used to treat angioectasias have been extrapolated from their use to treat vascular lesions in the upper GI tract, with APC being the most commonly used modality. APC involves the use of a jet of ionized argon gas that is directed through a probe that passes through the endoscope, allowing the transmission of the gas to target the lesion without direct contact with the mucosa.[51] Due to its efficacy and low incidence of complications, APC has become the most widely used method for treating small bowel angioectasias.[52] Another thermal therapy which is less commonly used is bipolar cautery.

Mechanical hemostasis can also be achieved using hemoclips. Hemoclips can be attempted for the management of large angioectasias or arterial lesions such as Dieulafoy lesions and larger arteriovenous malformations (AVMs).[53] Hemoclips can be used in combination with APC and/or epinephrine injection for high-risk lesions as well. Additionally, there are data to suggest that combination therapy when treating large AVMs in LVAD patients has a higher success rate when compared to APC alone.[54] Though less common than APC and mechanical hemostasis, sclerotherapy may be used and has demonstrated moderate success.[55]

Dieulafoy Lesions

Bleeding from small bowel Dieulafoy lesions also represents a diagnostic and therapeutic challenge. These lesions typically present with severe overt GIB requiring transfusion of multiple units of blood. In a study using double-balloon enteroscopy, Dieulafoy lesions were identified as a source for overt GIB in 3.5% of all patients, with most of these lesions located in the jejunum.[16] Dieulafoy lesions are difficult to find and treat as they intermittently bleed and on many occasions are not seen during endoscopic evaluations when they do stop bleeding. Multiple endoscopic and radiologic examinations are sometimes required to ultimately identify these lesions.

The optimal endoscopic therapy for bleeding Dieulafoy lesions is unknown as there are no large clinical trials evaluating endoscopic intervention. Nevertheless, endoscopic intervention is often recommended as a first-line therapy. Because Dieulafoy lesions are arterial in nature, hemostasis with either hemoclip(s) placement or combination treatment using cautery (such as bipolar or APC), epinephrine injection, and hemoclips is recommended.[16,56]

Ulcers

Another source of small bowel bleeding which is identifiable with SBCE and enteroscopy are ulcers, which can be medication related (eg, NSAID), infectious (eg, tuberculosis), or inflammatory (eg, Crohn's disease). Bleeding from ulcers can be treated using similar endoscopic techniques mentioned earlier, including combinations of mechanical hemostasis, coagulation, and/or injection therapy. If ulcers are identified and suspected to be medication-related, the offending agent should be discontinued if possible. If ulcers are identified and thought to be due to infectious etiology, the underlying infection should be treated. In both scenarios, repeat SBCE can be considered in 6 to 8 months to confirm ulcer resolution. If the ulcers are still present on repeat SBCE, PE or DAE can be considered for biopsies. If ulcers are identified on SBCE and suspected to be due to Crohn's disease, the authors suggest either empiric treatment for Crohn's disease with consideration of repeat SBCE in 6 to 8 months to assess for mucosal healing (with an antecedent patency capsule sometimes needed if stricturing Crohn's disease is suspected clinically), or depending on the location of the ulcers, PE or DAE for endoscopic evaluation and biopsy (if doing so would change patient management).[57]

Fig. 2 outlines a proposed algorithm that can be of aid when deciding on the endoscopic treatment modality of commonly encountered small bowel bleeding lesions.

The complication rate of therapeutic enteroscopy is as high as 8%.[35,52,58] There is a risk of pancreatitis (0.3%) associated with anterograde DAE. The mechanism of DAE-related acute pancreatitis is thought to be related to traumatic or ischemic injury to the pancreas during push-and-pull maneuvers.[59–63] The risk of DAE-related acute pancreatitis may be reduced by a careful, atraumatic technique designed to minimize mechanical stress and avoiding balloon inflation in the proximal duodenum.[52]

WHEN ENDOSCOPIC TREATMENT FAILS OR IS NOT FEASIBLE

Patients who present with brisk bleeding suspected to originate from the small bowel and are hemodynamically unstable might not be suitable for endoscopy. In this

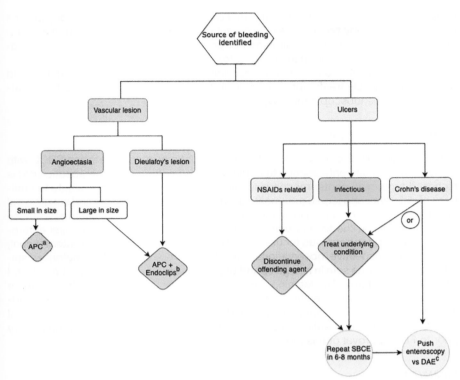

Fig. 2. Proposed algorithm for different endoscopic treatment modalities for most common small bowel bleeding lesions. [a]Argon plasma coagulation is preferred but bipolar therapy and hemoclips can be used. [b]Dieulafoy lesions should be treated with combined therapy that can include epinephrine injection. [c]If the ulcers are still present, depending on the location, push enteroscopy versus device-assisted enteroscopy can be considered for biopsies.

setting, as well as in the case of prior and recently failed endoscopic hemostasis, CTA should be considered with angiography and subsequent embolization, although it should be recognized that interventional radiology is not available in every hospital setting. Surgical treatment of midgut bleeding is generally performed when interventional radiology is unavailable or not feasible. Intraoperative enteroscopy may be performed during laparotomy or laparoscopy through an enterotomy or via peroral or rectal route. This technique is associated with a considerable risk of complications, including prolonged ileus, wound infections, adhesive intestinal obstruction, and mortality.[34,64] SBCE, tattooing and/or hemoclip placement performed during DAE, and/or angiographic techniques are useful to guide surgery.[65,66] In these cases, intraoperative enteroscopy should be available to allow identification of the source of bleeding and allow for both endoscopic and surgical hemostasis.[67]

In the case of angioectasias, unfortunately for many patients, a single endoscopic procedure to treat angioectasias does not result in a durable response. A recent meta-analysis revealed that the pooled re-bleeding rate after treatment of angioectasias was as high as 43%.[68] At 5 years, the incidence of recurrent bleeding from angioectasias increases to 63% despite endoscopic therapy.[69] Recurrence of angioectasias is likely driven by persistent underlying comorbidities (including cardiopulmonary and renal disease as well as the use of antiplatelets and anticoagulants which can increase bleeding risk). In addition, angioectasias missed or beyond the reach of enteroscopy procedures may contribute to recurrent bleeding. In these situations, alternative conservative (iron and/or periodic blood transfusions) and/or medical therapy (such as thalidomide or somatostatin analogs) may be indicated.

Thus, patients with complicated comorbidities would benefit from evaluation and planning of available treatment options, including conservative and/or medical treatments, beyond endoscopic therapy.

FUTURE CONSIDERATIONS

Future research is also needed to determine the optimal interval between SBCE with positive findings and enteroscopy to determine when enteroscopy therapeutic yield is highest. Large multi-center randomized clinical trials are needed to evaluate the efficacy of different endoscopic treatments of small bowel angioectasias and small bowel bleeding lesions in general. However, the relative rarity of these lesions makes these studies difficult. At the time of writing of this review article, motorized spiral enteroscopy has not been approved for use in the United States by the FDA. An international, multicenter, prospective, observational study from Europe showed that motorized spiral enteroscopy was safe in a large cohort of patients, some of them post-surgical and with altered anatomy. The learning curve was short for the endoscopists, and there was no increase in adverse effects when patients had altered anatomy.[70] These findings are promising, but future larger studies and comparison of motorized spiral enteroscopy with other enteroscopic modalities are needed, and may be necessary prior to FDA approval of this modality in the United States.

SUMMARY

Endoscopic therapy of small bowel bleeding should only be undertaken after consideration of the different options, and the risks, benefits, and alternatives of each option. For example, in an older patient with numerous comorbidities who has angioectasias of the small bowel, it may be more prudent to consider periodic iron infusions and blood transfusions with possible medical therapy then to pursue an aggressive and repeated endoscopic treatment approach.

Endoscopic therapy options for small bowel bleeding are like those treatments used for other forms of bleeding in the upper and lower gastrointestinal tract. However, hemostatic powder spray agents, over-the-scope clips, and neodymium:yttrium-aluminium-garnet (Nd:YAG) laser do not have catheters long enough for most of the device-assisted enteroscopes used in practice currently. Typically, injection sclerotherapy with diluted (1:10,000) epinephrine, APC, and hemoclips are used to treat small bowel bleeding. Due to the thin wall of the small bowel, endoscopic therapy should be carefully employed to avoid risk for perforation.

The choice of which method to use is often dependent on the type of bleeding lesion encountered. For example, angioectasias or other vascular malformations are treated with APC or sometimes hemoclips. On occasion, a larger angioectasia requires epinephrine injection for treatment to risk for perforation related to prolonged duration of coagulation. An ulcer or a Dieulafoy lesion is often treated with epinephrine injection and/or hemoclips.

Marking the adjacent area of bleeding with either a submucosal injection of carbon black tattoo (after initial submucosal pillow formation with saline to avoid injecting ink into the peritoneum or mesentery) and/or a hemoclip can facilitate future repeat endoscopic and/or surgical intervention (using the tattoo) and/or interventional radiology angioembolization. The tattoo (endoscopy and surgery) or hemoclips (radiology) serve as a guide for localization for additional treatment as needed.

Future research in the best, most effective type of treatment for each type of small bowel bleeding lesion and the ability of endoscopic treatment to impact on patient outcomes depending on patient characteristics is needed. Further advances in technology, including the use of artificial intelligence in identifying the optimal strategy for endoscopic management of small bowel bleeding, will likely yield improvement in the care of these patients.

CLINICS CARE POINTS

- In many situations, clinical management of small bowel bleeding should involve a multi-disciplinary approach.

- Review of SBCE videos, not images, is important in confirming the lesion(s) of interest, and identifying next steps in management, including decision to pursue an anterograde or retrograde approach for deep small bowel enteroscopy (if needed) and accessory equipment needed during enteroscopy, if pursued.

- Endoscopic treatment of small bowel bleeding is dependent on the lesion(s) encountered.

- Recurrent obscure small bowel bleeding often requires an algorithmic approach, including repeat evaluation to localize the source such as repeat SBCE, deep small bowel enteroscopy, and CT angiography, based on various clinical factors.

- Patients with severe comorbidities often benefit from conservative and/or medical approaches, and shared medical decision-making should be utilized for all patients.

REFERENCES

1. Pasha SF, Leighton JA, Das A, et al. Double-balloon enteroscopy and capsule endoscopy have comparable diagnostic yield in small-bowel disease: a meta-analysis. Clin Gastroenterol Hepatol 2008;6(6):671–6.
2. Zuckerman GR, Prakash C, Askin MP, et al. AGA technical review on the evaluation and management of occult and obscure gastrointestinal bleeding. Gastroenterology 2000;118(1):201–21.
3. Gerson LB, Fidler JL, Cave DR, et al. ACG Clinical Guideline: Diagnosis and Management of Small Bowel Bleeding. Am J Gastroenterol 2015;110(9):1265–87 [quiz: 1288].
4. ASoP Committee, Gurudu SR, Bruining DH, et al. The role of endoscopy in the management of suspected small-bowel bleeding. Gastrointest Endosc 2017; 85(1):22–31.
5. Pennazio M, Spada C, Eliakim R, et al. Small-bowel capsule endoscopy and device-assisted enteroscopy for diagnosis and treatment of small-bowel disorders: European Society of Gastrointestinal Endoscopy (ESGE) Clinical Guideline. Endoscopy 2015;47(4):352–76.
6. Pennazio M, Rondonotti E, Despott EJ, et al. Small-bowel capsule endoscopy and device-assisted enteroscopy for diagnosis and treatment of small-bowel disorders: European Society of Gastrointestinal Endoscopy (ESGE) Guideline - Update 2022. Endoscopy 2023;55(1):58–95.
7. Yamamoto H, Ogata H, Matsumoto T, et al. Clinical Practice Guideline for Enteroscopy. Dig Endosc 2017;29(5):519–46.

8. Raju GS, Gerson L, Das A, et al. American Gastroenterological Association (AGA) Institute technical review on obscure gastrointestinal bleeding. Gastroenterology 2007;133(5):1697–717.

9. Cangemi DJ, Patel MK, Gomez V, et al. Small bowel tumors discovered during double-balloon enteroscopy: analysis of a large prospectively collected single-center database. J Clin Gastroenterol 2013;47(9):769–72.

10. Ross A, Mehdizadeh S, Tokar J, et al. Double balloon enteroscopy detects small bowel mass lesions missed by capsule endoscopy. Dig Dis Sci 2008;53(8): 2140–3.

11. Maiden L. Capsule endoscopic diagnosis of nonsteroidal antiinflammatory drug-induced enteropathy. J Gastroenterol 2009;44(Suppl 19):64–71.

12. Hayashi Y, Yamamoto H, Taguchi H, et al. Nonsteroidal anti-inflammatory drug-induced small-bowel lesions identified by double-balloon endoscopy: endo-scopic features of the lesions and endoscopic treatments for diaphragm disease. J Gastroenterol 2009;44(Suppl 19):57–63.

13. Leighton JA, Triester SL, Sharma VK. Capsule endoscopy: a meta-analysis for use with obscure gastrointestinal bleeding and Crohn's disease. Gastrointest Endosc Clin N Am 2006;16(2):229–50.

14. Kiratli PO, Aksoy T, Bozkurt MF, et al. Detection of ectopic gastric mucosa using 99mTc pertechnetate: review of the literature. Ann Nucl Med 2009;23(2):97–105.

15. Nakamura M, Hirooka Y, Watanabe O, et al. Three cases with active bleeding from radiation enteritis that were diagnosed with video capsule endoscopy without retention. Nagoya J Med Sci 2014;76(3–4):369–74.

16. Blecker D, Bansal M, Zimmerman RL, et al. Dieulafoy's lesion of the small bowel causing massive gastrointestinal bleeding: two case reports and literature review. Am J Gastroenterol 2001;96(3):902–5.

17. Dulic-Lakovic E, Dulic M, Hubner D, et al. Bleeding Dieulafoy lesions of the small bowel: a systematic study on the epidemiology and efficacy of enteroscopic treatment. Gastrointest Endosc 2011;74(3):573–80.

18. Traina M, Tarantino I, Barresi L, et al. Variceal bleeding from ileum identified and treated by single balloon enteroscopy. World J Gastroenterol 2009;15(15): 1904–5.

19. Gerard PS, Gerczuk PZ, Idupuganti R, et al. Massive gastrointestinal bleeding due to an aorto-enteric fistula seen by technetium-99m-labeled red blood cell scintigraphy. Clin Nucl Med 2007;32(7):551–2.

20. Cave DR, Hakimian S, Patel K. Current Controversies Concerning Capsule Endoscopy. Dig Dis Sci 2019;64(11):3040–7.

21. Aliment Pharmacol Ther - 2003 - Lewis - The advent of capsule endoscopy a not %E2%80%90so%E2%80%90futuristic approach to obscure.pdf>. doi:10.1046/ j.0269-2813.2003.01556.x.

22. Bandorski D, Keuchel M, Bruck M, et al. Capsule endoscopy in patients with cardiac pacemakers, implantable cardioverter defibrillators, and left heart devices: a review of the current literature. Diagn Ther Endosc 2011;2011:376053.

23. Stanich PP, Kleinman B, Betkerur K, et al. Video capsule endoscopy is successful and effective in outpatients with implantable cardiac devices. Dig Endosc 2014; 26(6):726–30.

24. Delvaux M, Fassler I, Gay G. Clinical usefulness of the endoscopic video capsule as the initial intestinal investigation in patients with obscure digestive bleeding: validation of a diagnostic strategy based on the patient outcome after 12 months. Endoscopy 2004;36(12):1067–73.

25. Pennazio M, Santucci R, Rondonotti E, et al. Outcome of patients with obscure gastrointestinal bleeding after capsule endoscopy: report of 100 consecutive cases. Gastroenterology 2004;126(3):643–53.
26. Wu S, Zhong L, Zheng P, et al. Low-dose and same day use of polyethylene glycol improves image of video capsule endoscopy: A multi-center randomized clinical trial. J Gastroenterol Hepatol 2020;35(4):634–40.
27. Kotwal VS, Attar BM, Gupta S, et al. Should bowel preparation, antifoaming agents, or prokinetics be used before video capsule endoscopy? A systematic review and meta-analysis. Eur J Gastroenterol Hepatol 2014;26(2):137–45.
28. Gkolfakis P, Tziatzios G, Dimitriadis GD, et al. Meta-analysis of randomized controlled trials challenging the usefulness of purgative preparation before small-bowel video capsule endoscopy. Endoscopy 2018;50(7):671–83.
29. Bahar R, Gupta A, Mann SK. Clear Liquids versus Polyethylene Glycol Preparation for Video Capsule Endoscopy of the Small Bowel: A Randomized Controlled Trial. Digestion 2019;99(3):213–8.
30. Hookey L, Louw J, Wiepjes M, et al. Lack of benefit of active preparation compared with a clear fluid-only diet in small-bowel visualization for video capsule endoscopy: results of a randomized, blinded, controlled trial. Gastrointest Endosc 2017;85(1):187–93.
31. Asge Technology C, DiSario JA, Petersen BT, et al. Enteroscopes. Gastrointest Endosc 2007;66(5):872–80.
32. Mans L, Arvanitakis M, Neuhaus H, et al. Motorized Spiral Enteroscopy for Occult Bleeding. Dig Dis 2018;36(4):325–7.
33. Zaman A, Sheppard B, Katon RM. Total peroral intraoperative enteroscopy for obscure GI bleeding using a dedicated push enteroscope: diagnostic yield and patient outcome. Gastrointest Endosc 1999;50(4):506–10.
34. Ress AM, Benacci JC, Sarr MG. Efficacy of intraoperative enteroscopy in diagnosis and prevention of recurrent, occult gastrointestinal bleeding. Am J Surg 1992;163(1):94–8 [discussion: 98-9].
35. Xin L, Liao Z, Jiang YP, et al. Indications, detectability, positive findings, total enteroscopy, and complications of diagnostic double-balloon endoscopy: a systematic review of data over the first decade of use. Gastrointest Endosc 2011; 74(3):563–70.
36. Zhong J, Ma T, Zhang C, et al. A retrospective study of the application on double-balloon enteroscopy in 378 patients with suspected small-bowel diseases. Endoscopy 2007;39(3):208–15.
37. May A, Nachbar L, Pohl J, et al. Endoscopic interventions in the small bowel using double balloon enteroscopy: feasibility and limitations. Am J Gastroenterol 2007;102(3):527–35.
38. Ell C, May A, Nachbar L, et al. Push-and-pull enteroscopy in the small bowel using the double-balloon technique: results of a prospective European multicenter study. Endoscopy 2005;37(7):613–6.
39. Heine GD, Hadithi M, Groenen MJ, et al. Double-balloon enteroscopy: indications, diagnostic yield, and complications in a series of 275 patients with suspected small-bowel disease. Endoscopy 2006;38(1):42–8.
40. Sun B, Rajan E, Cheng S, et al. Diagnostic yield and therapeutic impact of double-balloon enteroscopy in a large cohort of patients with obscure gastrointestinal bleeding. Am J Gastroenterol 2006;101(9):2011–5.
41. Ramchandani M, Reddy DN, Gupta R, et al. Diagnostic yield and therapeutic impact of single-balloon enteroscopy: series of 106 cases. J Gastroenterol Hepatol 2009;24(10):1631–8.

42. Aktas H, de Ridder L, Haringsma J, et al. Complications of single-balloon entero-scopy: a prospective evaluation of 166 procedures. Endoscopy 2010;42(5): 365–8.

43. Frantz DJ, Dellon ES, Grimm IS, et al. Single-balloon enteroscopy: results from an initial experience at a U.S. tertiary-care center. Gastrointest Endosc 2010;72(2): 422–6.

44. Upchurch BR, Sanaka MR, Lopez AR, et al. The clinical utility of single-balloon enteroscopy: a single-center experience of 172 procedures. Gastrointest Endosc 2010;71(7):1218–23.

45. Morgan D, Upchurch B, Draganov P, et al. Spiral enteroscopy: prospective U.S. multicenter study in patients with small-bowel disorders. Gastrointest Endosc 2010;72(5):992–8.

46. Jackson CS, Gerson LB. Management of gastrointestinal angiodysplastic lesions (GIADs): a systematic review and meta-analysis. Am J Gastroenterol 2014; 109(4):474–83 [quiz 484].

47. Standards of Practice C, Faulx AL, Kothari S, et al. The role of endoscopy in sub-epithelial lesions of the GI tract. Gastrointest Endosc 2017;85(6):1117–32.

48. May A, Friesing-Sosnik T, Manner H, et al. Long-term outcome after argon plasma coagulation of small-bowel lesions using double-balloon enteroscopy in patients with mid-gastrointestinal bleeding. Endoscopy 2011;43(9):759–65.

49. Hadithi M, Heine GD, Jacobs MA, et al. A prospective study comparing video capsule endoscopy with double-balloon enteroscopy in patients with obscure gastrointestinal bleeding. Am J Gastroenterol 2006;101(1):52–7.

50. Rondonotti E, Spada C, Adler S, et al. Small-bowel capsule endoscopy and device-assisted enteroscopy for diagnosis and treatment of small-bowel disor-ders: European Society of Gastrointestinal Endoscopy (ESGE) Technical Review. Endoscopy 2018;50(4):423–46.

51. Vargo JJ. Clinical applications of the argon plasma coagulator. Gastrointest En-dosc 2004;59(1):81–8.

52. Moschler O, May AD, Muller MK, et al. Complications in double-balloon-enteroscopy: results of the German DBE register. Z Gastroenterol 2008;46(3): 266–70. Ergebnisse des deutschen Registers fur die Doppelballonenteroskopie.

53. Chung IK, Kim EJ, Lee MS, et al. Bleeding Dieulafoy's lesions and the choice of endoscopic method: comparing the hemostatic efficacy of mechanical and injec-tion methods. Gastrointest Endosc 2000;52(6):721–4.

54. Zikos TA, Namdaran P, Banerjee D, et al. Arteriovenous malformations respond poorly to argon plasma coagulation in patients with continuous flow left ventricu-lar assist devices. Eur J Gastroenterol Hepatol 2019;31(7):792–8.

55. Igawa A, Oka S, Tanaka S, et al. Major predictors and management of small-bowel angioectasia. BMC Gastroenterol 2015;15:108.

56. Lipka S, Rabbanifard R, Kumar A, et al. A single-center United States experience with bleeding Dieulafoy lesions of the small bowel: diagnosis and treatment with single-balloon enteroscopy. Endosc Int Open 2015;3(4):E339–45.

57. Tun GS, Rattehalli D, Sanders DS, et al. Clinical utility of double-balloon entero-scopy in suspected Crohn's disease: a single-centre experience. Eur J Gastroen-terol Hepatol 2016;28(7):820–5.

58. Hirai F, Beppu T, Sou S, et al. Endoscopic balloon dilatation using double-balloon endoscopy is a useful and safe treatment for small intestinal strictures in Crohn's disease. Dig Endosc 2010;22(3):200–4.

59. Moeschler O, Mueller MK. Deep enteroscopy - indications, diagnostic yield and complications. World J Gastroenterol 2015;21(5):1385–93.

60. Teshima CW, Aktas H, Kuipers EJ, et al. Hyperamylasemia and pancreatitis following spiral enteroscopy. Can J Gastroenterol 2012;26(9):603–6.
61. Tsujikawa T, Bamba S, Inatomi O, et al. Factors affecting pancreatic hyperamylasemia in patients undergoing peroral single-balloon enteroscopy. Dig Endosc 2015;27(6):674–8.
62. Kopacova M, Tacheci I, Rejchrt S, et al. Double balloon enteroscopy and acute pancreatitis. World J Gastroenterol 2010;16(19):2331–40.
63. Pata C, Akyuz U, Erzin Y, et al. Post-procedure elevated amylase and lipase levels after double-balloon enteroscopy: relations with the double-balloon technique. Dig Dis Sci 2010;55(7):1982–8.
64. Bonnet S, Douard R, Malamut G, et al. Intraoperative enteroscopy in the management of obscure gastrointestinal bleeding. Dig Liver Dis 2013;45(4):277–84.
65. Hartmann D, Schmidt H, Bolz G, et al. A prospective two-center study comparing wireless capsule endoscopy with intraoperative enteroscopy in patients with obscure GI bleeding. Gastrointest Endosc 2005;61(7):826–32.
66. Jakobs R, Hartmann D, Benz C, et al. Diagnosis of obscure gastrointestinal bleeding by intra-operative enteroscopy in 81 consecutive patients. World J Gastroenterol 2006;12(2):313–6.
67. Dray X, Riccioni ME, Wurm Johansson G, et al. Feasibility and diagnostic yield of small-bowel capsule endoscopy in patients with surgically altered gastric anatomy: the SAGA study. Gastrointest Endosc 2021;94(3):589–597 e1.
68. Romagnuolo J, Brock AS, Ranney N. Is Endoscopic Therapy Effective for Angioectasia in Obscure Gastrointestinal Bleeding?: A Systematic Review of the Literature. J Clin Gastroenterol 2015;49(10):823–30.
69. Pinho R, Ponte A, Rodrigues A, et al. Long-term rebleeding risk following endoscopic therapy of small-bowel vascular lesions with device-assisted enteroscopy. Eur J Gastroenterol Hepatol 2016;28(4):479–85.
70. Beyna T, Moreels T, Arvanitakis M, et al. Motorized spiral enteroscopy: results of an international multicenter prospective observational clinical study in patients with normal and altered gastrointestinal anatomy. Endoscopy 2022;54(12):1147–55.

Endoscopic Diagnosis and Treatment of Colonic Diverticular Bleeding

Dennis M. Jensen, MD

KEYWORDS

- Diverticular hemorrhage • Colonoscopy • Colonoscopy hemostasis
- Diverticular stigmata of hemorrhage • Monitoring diverticular arterial blood flow

KEY POINTS

- Colonoscopy is the most accurate method to diagnose and treat diverticula hemorrhage.
- Risk stratification with diverticular stigmata of hemorrhage and monitoring underlying arterial blood flow facilitate accurate diagnosis and definitive colon hemostasis.
- Clinical outcomes are improved by urgent colonoscopic diagnosis and treatment of definitive diverticular hemorrhage.

INTRODUCTION
Background

In adult patients who present to the hospital with severe hematochezia (eg, red blood or clots per rectum), the most common colon diagnosis reported is diverticular hemorrhage.[1,2] Hematochezia or lower gastrointestinal (LGI) bleeding is reported to have an annual incidence of about 20 cases/100,000 population, but with a much higher rate in the elderly.[3] The majority of the patients with severe hematochezia from colon sources are older than 70 years and present to the hospital with painless bleeding, anemia with a decrease in hemoglobin from baseline, but usually without syncope or major changes in orthostatic pulse or systolic blood pressure.[1,2] The most common colonic diagnoses by urgent colonoscopy among 882 patients with severe LGI bleeding reported in descending order are diverticular (TIC) hemorrhage (32.3%), ischemic colitis (11.2%), internal hemorrhoids (10.4%), post-polypectomy–induced ulcer hemorrhage (9.1%), rectal ulcers (8.2%), and other forms of colitis (7.1%). Refer to Table 1 for further details.[4]

The current endoscopic diagnosis and treatment of documented, acute colon diverticular hemorrhage is the focus of this report. There are several reasons for this

David Geffen School of Medicine at UCLA, UCLA Medical Center, VA Greater Los Angeles Healthcare System, Building 115 Room 318, 11301 Wilshire Boulevard, Los Angeles, CA 90073-1003, USA

E-mail address: djensen@mednet.ucla.edu

Gastrointest Endoscopy Clin N Am 34 (2024) 345–361
https://doi.org/10.1016/j.giec.2023.10.002
1052-5157/24/Published by Elsevier Inc.

giendo.theclinics.com

Table 1 Eight most common colonic sources of severe hematochezia (882 cases) (expressed as percent of colonic sources)	
Diverticulosis (Def/Pres)	32.3%
Ischemia	11.2%
Internal hemorrhoids	10.4%
Post Polypectomy Ulcer	9.1%
Rectal ulcers	8.2%
Colitis (UC, C. dif, Crohn's other)	7.1%
Colon angiomas/XRT	6.8%
Colon CA or Polyps	6.0%

Diverticulosis Def is definitive and Pres is presumptive. UC is ulcerative colitis. C. dif is Clostridium dificile. XRT is radiation telangiectasia. Colon CA is cancer. (Data from Jensen D. Management of patients with severe hematochezia–with all current evidence available. Am J Gastroenterol 2005;100:2403-2406.)

emphasis. The first is because TIC hemorrhage is the most common diagnosis in older adult patients who are hospitalized with an acute severe LGI hemorrhage. The second is that urgent colonoscopy for diagnosis and hemostasis is feasible, safe, and effective when performed by experienced endoscopists in the United States or elsewhere.[1,2,4–6] Clinical outcomes have been improved with this management. Third, in referral hospitals which have colonoscopists with expertise in performing urgent colonoscopy and diagnosing diverticular hemorrhage, this approach has replaced emergency angiography and surgery. That is because it is more often available, diagnostic, and safer and more cost effective than non-endoscopic treatments, especially for elderly patients.[5,6] Part of the reason for this change in usual treatment is that colonoscopic hemostasis itself has improved over the last 3 decades from treatment with less effective injection of epinephrine[7] to use of more effective hemostasis techniques including thermal coagulation, rubber band ligation, through-the-scope hemoclips, combination treatments, and large over-the-scope hemoclips targeted at the bleeding site.[4–16]

The diagnosis of definite diverticular hemorrhage has also improved. Similar to peptic ulcer bleeding (PUB) where stigmata of recent hemorrhage (SRH) have been utilized to risk stratify for rebleeding,[17] active bleeding and other non-bleeding SRH have been applied for diagnosis, risk stratification, and treatment of definitive TIC hemorrhage.[2,4,5,18–21] To improve risk stratification and treatment of definitive TIC hemorrhage beyond utilizing visual SRH alone, Doppler endoscopic probe (DEP) monitoring of arterial blood flow underneath SRH has also been utilized.[18,20,22] DEP has helped define the natural history of definitive diverticular hemorrhage which has led to recognition that all TIC SRH have a high risk for rebleeding. By expanding TIC SRH to include flat spots and blood flow detection by DEP, there is an overall increase in the rate of diagnosis of definitive TIC hemorrhage on urgent colonoscopy.[20] DEP monitoring of arterial blood flow after colonoscopic hemostasis has also resulted in higher rates of definitive hemostasis when there is obliteration of arterial blood flow underneath TIC SRH, similar to reports for non-variceal upper gastrointestinal (UGI) lesions.[22] These technical advances and changes have contributed to an evolution in patient management, colonoscopic diagnosis, and colon hemostasis with subsequent improvements in clinical outcomes. That is when clinical results of current colonoscopic hemostasis are compared with medical management, angiography, and surgery for treatment of acute diverticular hemorrhage. These results will be described and discussed in detail in this article.

The specific aims of this report all relate to acute TIC hemorrhage and include(1) to present the rationale, methods, and results for early colonoscopic diagnosis and treatment, (2) to review the short-term natural history of definitive TIC hemorrhage based upon SRH and DEP monitoring, (3) to describe short-term and long-term rebleeding rates after colonoscopic hemostasis in comparison with medical treatment, angiographic embolization, and surgery, (4) to discuss a new approach for earlier diagnosis of definitive TIC hemorrhage in patients with severe LGI bleeding, (5) to describe new treatment techniques to improve colonoscopic hemostasis so that TIC rebleeding can be reduced when compared to older colonoscopic treatments, and (6) to provide recommendations about salvage treatments for severe or recurrent TIC bleeding, including angiographic embolization, surgery, and repeat colonoscopic hemostasis by an expert endoscopist.

Definitions of TIC Hemorrhage

The classification of colon diverticulosis as the cause of severe LGI hemorrhage is important to put into context with the different ways "diverticular hemorrhage" is defined and reported elsewhere. Elderly patients commonly have colon diverticulosis but most do not develop diverticular hemorrhage. Prior to presenting to the hospital with an acute LGI bleed, many elderly patients have colon diverticula diagnosed by previous colonoscopy, barium enema, computerized tomography (CT), or MRI. After discharge, International Classification of Diseases (ICD) coding of patients with LGI hemorrhage and diverticulosis is often not classified or reported accurately. For example, patients who stop bleeding and do not have a GI evaluation with colonoscopy or have one that is non-diagnostic are usually coded as *diverticular hemorrhage* for billing purposes. However, such ICD coding is neither sufficiently accurate for classification of true diverticular hemorrhage (eg, as definitive or presumptive diverticular hemorrhage or incidental diverticulosis, as detailed later) nor for reporting these ICD-based results in evidence-based research.

A more accurate classification for colon diverticulosis as the cause of an acute severe LGI hemorrhage is detailed in **Box 1**.[2] These diagnoses are based upon whether or not there are colonic diverticula with SRH or other lesions that are found as the cause of the GI hemorrhage. This classification is highly recommended for investigators and colonoscopists who report about diagnosis, management, and clinical outcomes of patients with an acute TIC hemorrhage. If utilized, this TIC classification as it relates to an acute LGI hemorrhage will facilitate communication, interpretation, and comparisons of diagnostic findings and clinical outcomes of different subgroups of patients with colon diverticulosis and acute LGI bleeding.[2]

Box 1
Classification of diverticulosis as cause[a] (or not) of severe hematochezia

[a]Definitive diverticular bleed—stigmata of hemorrhage on a colon TIC found on urgent colonoscopy &/or surgery; or active bleeding on RBC scan or angiogram confirmed to be diverticulosis on colonoscopy.

[a]Presumptive diverticular bleed—diverticulosis without stigmata & no other bleeding lesions found by colonoscopy, anoscopy, enteroscopy, & capsule endoscopy.

Incidental diverticulosis—diverticulosis present but another source of bleeding is identified in the colon, anorectum, foregut, or small intestine.

[a]These are true diverticular hemorrhage. See Ref.[2]

METHODS
Classification of TIC Hemorrhage Based upon Stigmata of Recent Hemorrhage

For a diagnosis of *definite diverticular hemorrhage*, our patients have an SRH in a colon diverticulum on urgent colonoscopy, such as active bleeding, non-bleeding visible vessel (NBVV), an adherent clot (eg, resistant to washing off), or a flat spot. TIC SRH are illustrated in **Fig. 1**. Some other patients classified as definitive diverticular hemorrhage have extravasation of contrast on angiography (eg, CT angiogram–CTA, standard interventional radiology -(IR)–angiogram, or MRI angiogram), or extravasation of technetium-labeled red blood cells (RBC) on an RBC scan while finding colon diverticula and no other lesions that could cause bleeding in that colon segment on colonoscopy performed during the same LGI hemorrhage.[2] A diagnosis of *presumptive diverticular hemorrhage* is made if non-bleeding colon diverticula without SRH are found on urgent colonoscopy and other GI procedures are negative for a definitive lesion diagnosis in the colon, anorectum, foregut, or small intestine by anoscopy, pan-endoscopy, push enteroscopy, and capsule endoscopy, performed during the same hospitalization for diagnosis of a bleeding site. *Incidental diverticulosis* is the diagnosis if colon diverticula without SRH are seen on colonoscopy and another definitive GI source is found in the colon, anorectum, foregut, and small bowel.[2]

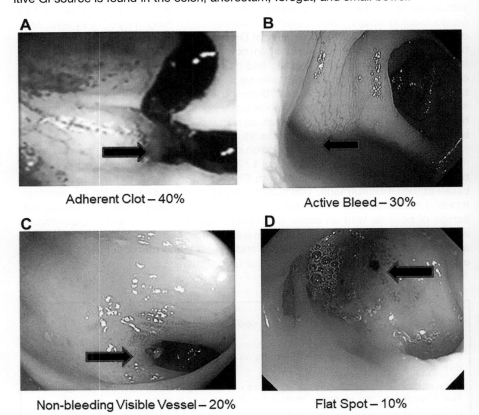

A Adherent Clot – 40%

B Active Bleed – 30%

C Non-bleeding Visible Vessel – 20%

D Flat Spot – 10%

Fig. 1. Stigmata of recent hemorrhage and their prevalence rates as found in 160 patients with severe diverticular hemorrhage. These identify the diverticular bleeding site and are all criteria for diagnosis of a definitive diverticular bleed. (*A-D*) are the TIC stigmata of hemorrhage placed in order of prevalance as diagnosed on urgent colonoscopy.

Patient Resuscitation, Colon Preparation, and Timing of Colonoscopy

Patients should be hemodynamically resuscitated and medically stable before urgent colonoscopy is performed.[1,2] After a rapid bowel preparation with a polyethylene glycol (PEG)-based balanced electrolyte solution,[1,23] urgent colonoscopy is feasible, safe, and often diagnostic for patients with an acute, severe LGI bleed, including those with suspected diverticular hemorrhage.[24] For severe hematochezia in hospitalized patients, 6 to 8 L of a PEG solution is recommended for the patient to drink or to be given via a nasogastric (NG) tube as a liter every 30 to 45 minutes to clear the colon of stool, blood, clots, and food fiber prior to urgent colonoscopy.[18,24] To facilitate gastric emptying and reduce nausea, metoclopramide (5–10 mg intravenously–IV) 1 to 2 hours before starting the colon purge and 4 to 6 hours later is also recommended.[2,24]

To optimize finding SRH in a diverticulum or on other colon lesions during hospitalization for an acute, severe, LGI bleed, urgent colonoscopy for diagnosis and treatment is recommended within 12 to 24 hours after the patient is hospitalized and evaluated by a GI bleeding team.[2,5,24] Depending upon the hemodynamic stability of the patient, treatment status of active co-morbidities, and availability of anesthesia support, the colonoscopy can be performed in an operating room (OR), an intensive care unit (ICU), in a monitored bed, or in the medical procedure unit (MPU). Best results of urgent colonoscopy in finding a lesion with SRH will be when the rectal effluent is clear of blood, clots, stool, and food fiber.[2,5,24]

Gastrointestinal Bleed Team, Equipment, and Accessories

Invaluable members of a GI bleeding team are an experienced and well-trained staff including a GI endoscopy nurse, an endoscopy technician, and an anesthesiologist or nurse anesthetist. The team should be led by a gastroenterologist who is a well-trained clinician with expertise in urgent colonoscopy, GI bleeding, and colonoscopic hemostasis. All of these will contribute to successful results of urgent colonoscopies and other emergency GI procedures.[25]

The choice of a standard size or smaller pediatric colonoscope depends upon the size of the patient, the completeness of colon purge, and whether colon stenosis is suspected. Current video colonoscopies have relatively large suction ports (eg, 3.2–3.8 mm), adequate fields of view, and good tip angulation. These instruments also have a separate channel for target irrigation. Placing a cap on the colonoscope tip facilitates visualization, suctioning, and eversion of diverticula which are all useful during urgent colonoscopy for identification of SRH and diagnosis of a definitive TIC hemorrhage.

Various accessories are helpful for bedside utilization during urgent colonoscopy. These include a needle to pre-inject active bleeding or an adherent clot with epinephrine and a rotatable snare to cold guillotine the clot off prior to thermal coagulation or hemoclipping of the pedicle or underlying SRH. A colon length DEP probe with control unit is recommended for interrogation of non-bleeding TIC SRH before endoscopic hemostasis.[5,18] The DEP is also useful after hemostasis of both active bleeding TICs and non-bleeding SRH to confirm obliteration of underlying arterial blood flow, which correlates with definitive TIC hemostasis and reduced TIC rebleeding rates.[5,18] Through-the-scope hemoclips, both small (8 mm, when open) or larger (11–12 mm), are useful for focal hemostasis especially for SRH in the base of the diverticulum.[5,18] Multipolar thermal coagulation (MPEC) probes in 7 and 10 French sizes are recommended with a bipolar generator for treatment of SRH at the neck of the TIC.

Over-the-scope-clips (OTSC) of various sizes, tip lengths, and different teeth configurations are also useful for hemostasis of definitive TIC bleeding and other focal colon lesions, as they are for non-variceal UGI hemorrhage.[26] OTSCs grasp more tissue than through-the-scope hemoclips and this results in high rates of definitive hemostasis of bleeding lesions by obliterating arterial blood flow underneath SRH of focal lesions.[26]

Injection needles and a tattoo solution to label 3 to 4 areas around the TIC with the SRH will facilitate identification of the bleeding site for rebleeding or surveillance colonoscopy. Multi-shot rubber band ligation (RBL) kits which fit on a colonoscope are also recommended by some colonoscopists.[10–12] Other accessories which are useful in removing large clots from diverticula are a foreign body grasper and a Roth net.

Hemostasis technique application for different TIC stigmata of recent hemorrhage

For active TIC hemorrhage, after target irrigation and suctioning of blood and clots from the bleeding site, pre-injection with dilute epinephrine (1:20,000 in saline) in 3 to 4 quadrants around the bleeding point in 1 to 2 cc aliquots is useful to temporarily stop the bleeding. If the bleeding point is on the neck of the diverticulum, MPEC for applying moderate, lateral pressure on the active bleeder to tamponade and to coagulate it is recommended, with a low-power setting (eg, 12–14 W) with either a 7 or 10 French size probe. Coagulation with short pulses (2–4 sec) is recommended for coaptive coagulation of the underlying artery.[27] Refer to **Figs. 2–4**.

If the bleeding site is in the base of the TIC, pre-injection of epinephrine followed by deployment of hemoclips, OTSC, or rubber band ligation (RBL) is recommended. Refer to **Figs. 5** and **6**. With a cap on the colonoscope or with the OTSC or RBL, TICs with the SRH in the base can be everted so that the hemoclips or band can be placed on the SRH and/or on either side of it to obliterate underlying arterial blood flow.[5,10–12,24] Because the OTSCs stay on the TIC longer than through-the-scope clips or rubber bands, these large clips usually result in long-term definitive hemostasis when deployed on the SRH.[5,15,16]

If either OTSC or RBL treatment of TIC SRH is used, initial colonoscopic diagnosis without these devices on the tip is required to first localize SRH and mark this TIC.[10–12,15,16] Then a colonoscope with the OTSC or bander on the tip is reinserted to treat the SRH. For active bleeding, pre-injection with epinephrine and placement of a clip adjacent to the TIC with the SRH will help the endoscopist locate it again. Pre-loading of the OTSC or bander on the tip of another colonoscope will hasten the process of diagnostic colonoscope removal and re-intubation of a colonoscope with the OTSC or RBL attached.

For an adherent clot either in the base or neck of the diverticulum, DEP interrogation and pre-injection with epinephrine are recommended prior to shaving the clot down with a rotatable snare to a small pedicle or to expose an underlying NBVV or spot.[5] If the clot is in the base of the TIC, standard hemoclipping, OTSC, or RBL are

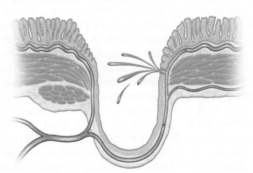

Fig. 2. Active bleeding from the neck of a colon diverticulum.

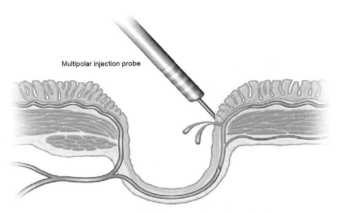

Fig. 3. Pre-injection of a dilute epinephrine around the bleeding site will stop active bleeding prior to use of the multipolar thermal coagulation (MPEC) probe for definitive hemostasis.

recommended but not MPEC. If the clot is at the neck, MPEC or hemoclipping are safe and effective.[5] RBL or OTSC may result in definitive hemostasis more often than through-the-scope- hemoclips because these usually fall off.[12,15,16]

NBVVs and flat spots at the neck or in the base of the TIC are treated to similar to adherent clots.[5,20] However, for these SRH, pre-injection with epinephrine is not necessary unless bleeding is induced. DEP interrogation of the SRH before treatment of non-bleeding SRH and after treatment of both non-bleeding and active bleeding is recommended.[5,18] If there is residual arterial blood flow detected by DEP after visually guided hemostasis, either additional MPEC treatment or hemoclipping to obliterate the arterial blood flow underneath SRH will result in definitive hemostasis and will reduce the risk of rebleeding.[5,18]

Tattooing the adjacent mucosa around the TIC with the SRH in 4 quadrants after colon hemostasis is recommended. This will facilitate identifying the TIC in case of early rebleeding or during surveillance colonoscopy.

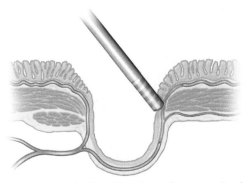

Fig. 4. Firm tamponade pressure on the bleeding site and compression laterally halts arterial blood flows in the artery at the neck of the diverticulum and facilitates thermal coaptive coagulation and definitive hemostasis.

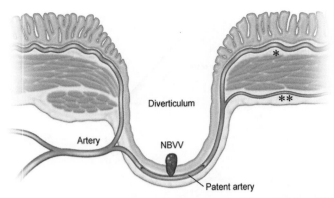

Fig. 5. Diagram of colon diverticulum with a non-bleeding visible vessel (NBVV) in the base. The arterial anatomy is shown including a submucosal artery (*asterisk*) and an interconnected subserosal artery (*double asterisk*).

Medical Treatment

Medical treatment to control constipation with daily supplemental fiber, a stool softener, and drinking an extra liter of fluid (without alcohol or caffeine) is recommended.[2,5,18] Anti-thrombotic drugs (eg, aspirin or clopidogrel), anti-coagulants, and non-steroidal anti-inflammatory drugs (NSAIDs) should be stopped in the short term and longer if the prescribing subspecialist (eg, cardiologist, neurologist, or vascular surgeon) agrees that this is safe.[5,18,28]

RESULTS
Non-colonoscopy Tests and Results

Although RBC scanning has been reported to detect active bleeding at a very low rate of 0.04 cc/min,[29] this test is not readily available as an emergency procedure in most smaller hospitals and there are other limitations for diagnosis of diverticular hemorrhage. First, an anatomic diagnosis is not possible without other imaging. Second, because

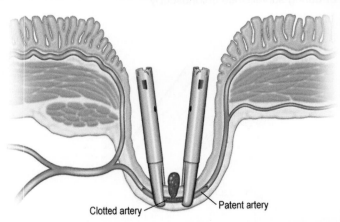

Fig. 6. Successful colonoscopic hemostasis with hemoclip placement on either side of the NBVV in the base of the diverticulum to obliterate blood flow between the clips and to prevent rebleeding.

only about 30% of patients with definitive diverticular hemorrhage have active bleeding on urgent colonoscopy and because RBC scanning and other radionuclide tests do not detect nonbleeding SRH, 70% or more of the RBC scans will be negative and not detect a bleeding site, including a definitive diverticular hemorrhage.[2,5,18] A positive RBC scan within 30 to 60 minutes after radionuclide injection is helpful as a screening test prior to angiography to potentially increase the yield of angiography.[1,2,24] However, scans that are positive later (eg, 4–24 hours) after injection of the radionuclide may be inaccurate for lesion localization because of movement of the label in the colon with peristalsis in between scheduled scans.[30] Although the diagnostic yield for patients with different types of GI hemorrhage is reported to be as high as 45%,[29,30] Center for Ulcer Research and Education (CURE) Hemostasis studies of TIC hemorrhage report that the RBC scan yield is less than 20%.[1,2,5,24,25]

CT angiograms (CTAs) are usually available in larger referral hospitals and are often ordered from the emergency room (ER) for patients presenting with acute severe LGI hemorrhage. Although there are reports of diagnostic yields of 50% or higher,[31,32] CTAs have many of the same limitations as RBC scans. First, only active bleeding can be detected by CTA and not non-bleeding SRH in TICs and on other LGI lesions.[1,2,5,18,33] Second, CTA is not recommended in patients with renal insufficiency because acute worsening of renal function may result. Third, CTAs which are not therapeutic expose the patient to radiation when other tests such as colonoscopy or angiography may be more useful clinically because they can be both diagnostic and therapeutic for TIC hemorrhage.

Angiography has theoretic advantages of detecting bleeding when active bleeding is 0.5 cc/min or more.[34] When extravasation of contrast is seen, embolization of the focal bleeding site is feasible.[34–36] Disadvantages and limitations are lack of availability of urgent angiography in smaller hospitals and a low pre-test probability of a positive test since only about 30% of definitive TIC hemorrhage has active bleeding on urgent colonoscopy (see **Fig. 1**). Also, angiography is expensive and major complications can occur. Complications include acute kidney injury, bowel ischemia, hematomas, artery thrombosis, and allergic reactions to contrast agents.[36] As an example, in 1 study where acute LGI bleeding was controlled by emergency angiographic embolization, severe gut ischemia and death were reported for several patients.[36] Also, angiography may not be clinically useful because it is only diagnostic for a bleeding site in less than 25% of patients with severe LGI bleeds[1] and less than 20% of patients with colonoscopically documented definitive diverticular hemorrhage.[2] However, angiography with embolization is particularly useful as salvage treatment after a definitive TIC hemorrhage is treated with hemoclips and early rebleeding (eg, within 30 days) occurs. Even if active bleeding is not seen on the angiogram, the hemoclips can serve as a target for super selective embolization of the TIC with the rebleeding.[18,37]

Surgery

With current colonoscopic, radionuclide scanning, and angiographic techniques, surgery is now rarely required as a first line for diagnosis and treatment of TIC hemorrhage.[1,2,5,18,37] It is indicated as a salvage treatment for TIC hemorrhage which is ongoing or recurrent and when colonoscopic hemostasis and angiography with embolization are unsuccessful.[18,37] Surgery is also indicated for severe colon ischemia after IR embolization or for a perforation after colonoscopic hemostasis. Permanent hemostasis can be expected after resection of the bleeding TIC segment, but the complication rate of urgent surgery is significantly higher than IR embolization or urgent colonoscopy in a recent report.[37]

Colonoscopy

Diagnostic yield

Colonoscopy has the advantages of being widely available, safe, and often diagnostic in patients hospitalized with acute LGI bleeding.[1,2,5,18,24,38,39] Colon hemostasis is also safe and effective when a definitive TIC bleed is diagnosed on urgent colonoscopy based upon SRH and supplemented by DEP monitoring of underlying arterial blood flow.[5,18] In an initial report of urgent colonoscopy for acute severe LGI hemorrhage, the diagnostic yield was 80% compared to a 20% yield by angiography when these tests were both performed in the same patient.[1] Refer to **Fig. 1** which documents the SRH findings on urgent colonoscopic for 160 patients with definitive TIC hemorrhage. An adherent clot was found in 40% of patients, active bleeding in 30%, an NBVV in 20%, and a flat spot in 10%.

When the DEP probe became available for monitoring arterial blood flow in the colon, TIC SRH were evaluated to potentially improve risk stratification and to increase the rate that definitive diverticular hemorrhage was diagnosed during urgent colonoscopy.[18,20] Recent results are shown in **Table 2** that include flat spots as a major SRH. Detection rates of arterial blood flow were very high underneath TIC SRH, varying from 80% for flat spots or adherent clots to 93% for NBVV and 100% for active bleeding. The overall detection rate of arterial blood flow for these SRH was 88%, which contrasted with a 0% detection rate in presumptive TIC bleeds when the base of the TICs with small visible arteries without SRH was interrogated.[18]

In a report from 2016 of 436 patients hospitalized with colon diverticulosis and severe hematochezia, the distribution by final TIC diagnosis is illustrated in **Fig. 7**. Incidental diverticulosis (eg, a non-diverticular source was the cause of the LGI bleed) was the final diagnosis in 45.6%. Presumptive diverticular bleeding was the diagnosis in 28%. Definitive diverticular TIC bleed was diagnosed in 26.4% of patients based upon finding an SRH in a colon diverticulum. Subsequently, the CURE Hemostasis Research group updated their results for the diagnosis of diverticular hemorrhage as shown in **Fig. 8**. For 100 patients recently hospitalized with severe LGI bleeding and a final diagnosis of diverticular hemorrhage after evaluation with urgent colonoscopy, SRH, and DEP, 75% had presumptive TIC hemorrhage and 25% had definitive TIC hemorrhage.

Table 2
Arterial blood flow by Doppler probe for definitive versus. presumptive diverticular hemorrhage

Stigmata of Hemorrhage	Number	+ DEP	Totals (Rate + DEP %)
Major SRH			
Active Bleeding	5	5	5/5 (100)
NBVV	14	13	13/14 (93)
Clot	5	4	4/5 (80)
Flat spot	10	8	8/10 (80)
Definitive TIC Bleed	34	30	30/34 (88)[a]
Clean Base			
Presumptive TIC Bleed	32	0	0/32 (0)

TIC is diverticular (bleed). (Adapted from Jensen DM, Machicado GA, Jutabha R, et al. Urgent colonoscopy for the diagnosis and treatment of severe diverticular hemorrhage. N Engl J Med 2000;342:78–82.

Abbreviations: NBVV, non-bleeding; SRH, stigmata of recent hemorrhage.

[a] $P < .05$. + DEP is positive Doppler endoscopic probe signal for arterial blood flow.

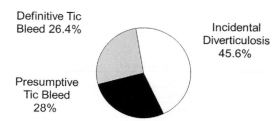

Fig. 7. Prevalence of definitive, presumptive, and incidental diverticular hemorrhage. A total of 436 patients hospitalized with diverticulosis and severe hematochezia.

Definitive TIC Hemorrhage: Natural History and Colonoscopic Hemostasis Results

In a 2016 report about the natural history of definitive diverticular hemorrhage in patients treated medically without colon hemostasis, results are summarized in **Table 3**. For patients with definitive diverticular bleeds, the rates of more, severe TIC bleeding within 30 days varied by SRH. That is from 43% for adherent clot patients to 84% for those with active TIC bleeding. Rates of intervention within 30 days to control TIC bleeding also varied by SRH from 29% for adherent clot patients to 58% for those with actively bleeding TICs.[18,20] Based upon these high rates of rebleeding on medical therapy and high rates of major intervention (eg, with angiography or surgery in most patients or more recently repeat urgent colonoscopy by an expert colonoscopist), colonoscopic hemostasis is highly recommended when any of these SRH are found during urgent (or later) colonoscopy.

In a 2018 report of 118 patients with definitive diverticular hemorrhage, early rebleeding rates were compared for patients treated with colonoscopic hemostasis or medical therapy alone.[5] The definitive TIC treatment groups included patients with active bleeding, NBVV, or adherent clots, but not flat spots.[5] For 81 patients with colonoscopic hemostasis, the 30-day rebleeding rate was 6.2%, whereas 37 patients treated medically had a rebleeding rate of 64.9%.[5] For the medical and colonoscopic hemostasis groups, the rates of surgery or embolization for control of severe rebleeding within 30 days were 43.2% and 2.5%, respectively. The median days to discharge after treatment were also significantly higher in the medical group than the colon hemostasis group (8.5 vs 2 days).

In a recent report, 162 patients with definitive TIC hemorrhage and 3 or more months of follow-up had clinical outcomes compared according to medical treatment alone, embolization angiographic, surgery, or colon hemostasis.[37] The rebleeding rates within 30 days of angiographic embolization, surgery, colonoscopic hemostasis, or medical treatment alone were 6.7%, 0%, 8.7%, and 41.7%, respectively. The respective complication rates were 13.3%, 36.9%, 2.9%, and 0%, respectively. The median hospital days were 6 days, 12 days, 2 days, and 4 days, respectively. During 1 year of

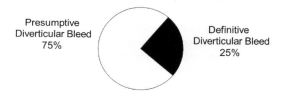

Fig. 8. Proven diverticular hemorrhage: recent prevalence of definitive and presumptive bleeding based on urgent colonoscopy. A total of 100 consecutive patients with severe hematochezia were evaluated by urgent colonoscopy by the Center for Ulcer Research and Education (CURE) hemostasis Research Group.

Table 3
Natural history and 30 day outcomes of definitive diverticular hemorrhage on medical therapy

	Major Rebleed	Intervention for Rebleed
Active bleed (N = 19)	84%	58%
NBVV (N = 5)	60%	40%
Clot (N = 14)	43%	29%
Flat spot (N = 6)	60%	33%
TOTALS (N = 44)	64%	43%

Interventions were either angiography with embolization, surgery, or repeat urgent colonoscopy and hemostasis by an expert colonoscopist.

Abbreviations: Clot, adherent clot; N, number of patients; NBVV, non-bleeding visible vessel.

follow-up, the rates of rebleeding were 0% for surgery, 13.3% for IR embolization, 17.3% for colonic hemostasis, and 50% for medical treatment. Based upon these studies, urgent colonoscopy was strongly recommended for early diagnosis and hemostasis of definitive TIC hemorrhage. These recommendations are similar to those of the Japan Gastroenterological Association.[38] In the CURE TIC study, either DEP monitored treatment or OTSC appeared to yield higher long-term rates of definitive TIC hemorrhage.[37] However, no RCTs have been reported which compare these newer treatments with other older TIC treatments.

Presumptive TIC Hemorrhage

The CURE Hemostasis Group recently reported on the natural history of 158 patients with a colonoscopic diagnosis of presumptive TIC hemorrhage.[39] During a median follow-up of 59 months, 71.5% of patients had no TIC rebleeds and 28.5% had 1 or more TIC rebleeds. For rebleeds, 40% were diagnosed as definitive and 60% were presumptive again. Definitive TIC hemorrhage diagnosis was made by urgent colonoscopy in 44.4%, RBC scanning in 27.6%, angiography in 16.2%, and surgery in 11.1%.[39]

DISCUSSION

Most patients with diverticular hemorrhage are elderly with the mean age of 74 years.[1,2,5,18,24] Not all patients who present to the hospital with severe hematochezia have colonoscopy within 6 to 24 hours when TIC SRH are the most prevalent.[1,2,5,18] However, when urgent colonoscopy is performed by experienced colonoscopists such as in the United States or Japan, the rate of diagnosing definitive TIC hemorrhage is approximately 25%.[18,23,38] Even though the rate of diagnosing definitive TIC hemorrhage is higher during long-term follow-up of patients with a prior presumptive TIC hemorrhage at 40%,[39] this is much lower than the definitive diagnosis rate of urgent pan endoscopy for severe UGI hemorrhage.[40]

Definitive diagnosis during colonoscopy of TIC hemorrhage depends upon the quality of the colon prep, the timing of the colonoscopy after the LGI bleed, and most of all the expertise of the colonoscopist in recognizing SRH.[5,18,25] When there is a dedicated GI bleeding team prepared to perform urgent colonoscopy, higher rates of diagnosis and colonoscopic hemostasis are more likely.[2,5,18,25,38] However, without other major advances to improve early diagnosis of definitive TIC hemorrhage, it is unlikely that the rate of definitive TIC hemorrhage diagnosis will exceed 40%.

There is a lack of consensus about the yield of urgent colonoscopy for diagnosis of acute LGI bleeding and whether the timing makes a difference in rates of finding SRH on diverticula.[25,38,41–43] In a retrospective report from the Mayo Clinic in 2003, there was no difference in the rate of finding TIC SRH (eg, active bleeding, NBVV, or adherent clot), for different colonoscopy times–either early, later, or elective.[41] In an RCT from 2010, Laine and colleagues reported that there was no difference in outcomes (eg, more bleeding, transfusions, hospital stay, or hospital changes) for patients with acute LGI bleeding who had urgent colonoscopy within 12 hours, or elective colonoscopy more than 36 hours after hospitalization.[42] Limitations of this RCT are that most patients did not have diverticular hemorrhage and those with severe LGI hemorrhage were excluded from enrollment.[42] In a recent guideline from the American College of Gastroenterology (ACG), urgent colonoscopy was not recommended for patients with acute LGI hemorrhage.[43] That contrasts with the recommendations of the CURE Hemostasis Research Group,[1,2,5,18] some reports by experts from Japan,[10–12] and the Japan GI Association.[38]

In another report of acute LGI bleeding, early colonoscopy resulted in shorter hospitalization.[44] In CURE prospective studies of acute LGI hemorrhage, the hospitalization time and cost of urgent colonoscopy cases were less than elective colonoscopy or other treatments.[6] Also, in a more recent report of patients with definitive diverticular hemorrhage, the length of hospitalization with colonoscopic hemostasis was significantly shorter than for those patients treated medically.[5]

As future directions, there are 3 recommendations which are complementary. The first is to amplify the didactic and procedural training in LGI bleeding.[25] Because of earlier reports[41,42] and a recent ACG guideline on LGI bleeding,[43] urgent colonoscopy is not currently recommended for diagnosis by some gastroenterologists or the ACG. This will contribute to limiting the training about acute LGI hemorrhage, deemphasizing discussion about this topic in GI meetings, and ultimately reducing the utilization rate of urgent colonoscopy for diagnosis of definitive diverticular hemorrhage in the United States. In addition, most hospitals do not support funding of a GI bleeding team which can improve patient care, clinical outcomes, promote teaching of GI trainees, and reduce patient care costs.[25] Such funding should be available, particularly for large referral centers.

Second, there is a need for innovations for earlier diagnosis of definitive TIC and other colon bleeding sites by detecting either active bleeding and other nonbleeding SRH before these disappear. One candidate is urgent colon capsule endoscopy which can be performed when a patient presents to the ER with a severe acute LGI bleeding. In initial results by the CURE hemostasis group, more than 80% of patients had a lesion diagnosis and/or bleeding site localization by urgent colon capsule compared to less than 25% for CTA or RBC scanning.[45] Colonoscopy or other tests confirmed the final diagnosis which included TIC hemorrhage and other colorectal lesions. The advantages of colon capsule for urgent diagnosis and localization of the bleeding site are multiple. First, colon capsule endoscopy is ingested without sedation and the procedure can be performed in either small or larger hospitals. After downloading images, telemedicine can be utilized for remote image review and diagnosis by experts. Second, this can be performed early while waiting for other procedures to be scheduled. Also, the colon capsule results can be utilized as a management guide for decisions about ordering other GI endoscopic procedures, IR embolization, or surgery. Last, urgent colon capsule endoscopy is relatively inexpensive compared to CTA, standard angiography, or colonoscopy and is less labor intensive. Future studies are warranted to determine what the role of urgent colon capsule endoscopy may be and whether it can increase the diagnostic yield of definitive diverticular hemorrhage and other colon sites.

Last, the role of elective colon surgery with laparoscopic resection of segmental diverticulosis for patients with recurrent diverticular hemorrhage should be evaluated. In the CURE Hemostasis Group's experience, there are several relevant results and reasons to recommend this. First, most patients with definitive diverticular hemorrhage have the TIC bleeding site located at or proximal to the splenic flexure. However, most colon diverticula are anatomically distributed distal to the splenic flexure in most US patients.[2,5,18] Second, most early or recurrent diverticular rebleeds are from the same colon TIC and not another region of the colon.[5,24] Third, elective laparoscopic segmental colectomy is much safer than emergency colon resection and should be as effective in preventing long-term TIC rebleeding.[1,2,24] Last, in patients having colon surgery for a definitive diverticular hemorrhage, the CURE Hemostasis Group reported no TIC rebleeding during long-term follow-up.[37] For long-term prevention of TIC rebleeding, surgery is more definitive treatment than colonoscopic hemostasis or IR embolization.[37] For patients with recurrent TIC hemorrhage who are surgical candidates, a new algorithm should be evaluated for elective laparoscopic resection of the colon segment where the bleeding site was localized preoperatively. That is particularly relevant in patients with risk factors for TIC rebleeding, including those on chronic NSAIDs, aspirin, other anti-platelet drugs, or anti-coagulants risk.[46,47]

SUMMARY

There are multiple conclusions of this analysis about the diagnosis and treatment of diverticular hemorrhage. First, when urgent colonoscopy after adequate colon purge is performed by an expert colonoscopist, the diagnostic rate of definitive diverticular hemorrhage will be about 25% and for patients with a prior presumptive diverticular hemorrhage who rebleed will be about 40%.[2,39] Second, when definitive diverticulosis is based upon SRH, the most common findings will be adherent clot (about 40%), active bleeding (30%), NBVV (20%), and a flat spot (10%). Third, DEP supplements SRH for risk stratification before hemostasis and for documenting definitive hemostasis with obliteration of arterial blood flow underneath TIC SRH.[5,18] Fourth, when colonoscopic hemostasis is successful, shorter hospitalization and lower complications are reported when compared to medical treatment, IR embolization, or surgery.[2,5,6,18,44] Fifth, for failures of colonoscopic diagnosis and hemostasis, angiographic embolization or colonic surgery is recommended.[37] Last, improvements in early diagnosis of definitive TIC hemorrhage are warranted and so is evaluation of an algorithm to incorporate elective surgery with segmental resection in patients with recurrent TIC hemorrhage when the bleeding TIC or colon segment has been localized pre-operatively.

CLINICS CARE POINTS

- With urgent colonoscopy in well prepped patients with colon diverticulosis and severe LGI bleeding, experienced colonoscopists can expect to find TIC stigmata in about 25% of cases, for a diagnosis of definitive TIC hemorrhage. If no TIC stigmata or other lesions are found, presumptive TIC hemorrhage will be the diagnosis in about 75% of patients with true diverticular hemorrhage.
- The expected prevalence of TIC stigmata in definitive TIC hemorrhage cases is adherent clots (40%), active bleeding (30%), visible vessels (20%), and flat spots (10%).

- Don't expect any type of angiography (CTA, MRI, or standard types) or RBC scan to be able to diagnose more than the 30% of definitive TIC hemorrhages because non-bleeding stigmata are not identified by these imaging techniques.
- Expect to find about 50% of TIC stigmata in the diverticulum base and the other 50% at the neck of the TIC. You may have to use a cap to evert the TIC to see and treat SRH in the base.
- For efficacy and safety, use hemoclips, OTSC, or rubber band ligation to treat stigmata in the TIC base and MPEC or OTSC at the neck. If you confirm absence of arterial blood flow under the SRH after hemostasis, the TIC rebleed rate will be very low unless the hemoclips or rubber bands fall off early.
- Embolization and surgery are effective as salvage therapies for severe rebleeding.

DISCLOSURE

The CURE Hemostasis research studies included in this article were funded by the following research grants: (1) NIH-NIDDK. P30 DK041301 CURE Digestive Diseases Research Core Center (DDRCC). CORE Grant. (2) VA Clinical Merit Review Grant – 5I01CX001403, (3) VA Merit Review Grant–CLIN-013-07F, (4) an American College of Gastroenterology Research Institute Clinical Research Award. Other disclosures are: Research support also from Vascular Technology Inc and Medtronic. Speakers bureau for AstraZeneca.

REFERENCES

1. Jensen DM, Machicado GA. Diagnosis and treatment of severe hematochezia - the role of urgent colonoscopy after purge. Gastroenterol 1988;95:1569–74.
2. Jensen DM, Machicado GA, Jutabha R, et al. Urgent colonoscopy for the diagnosis and treatment of severe diverticular hemorrhage. N Engl J Med 2000; 342:78–82.
3. Longstreth GF. Epidemiology and outcome of patients hospitalized with acute lower gastrointestinal hemorrhage: a population-based study. Am J Gastroenterol 1997;92:419–24.
4. Jensen D. Management of patients with severe hematochezia—with all current evidence available. Am J Gastroenterol 2005;100:2403–6.
5. Jensen DM. Diagnosis and treatment of definitive diverticular hemorrhage (DDH). Amer J Gastroenterol 2018;113:1570–3.
6. Jensen DM, Machicado GA. Colonoscopy for Diagnosis and Treatment of Severe Lower Gastrointestinal Bleeding: Routine Outcomes and Cost Analysis. Gastrointest Endosc Cl N Am 1997;7:477–98.
7. Ramirez FC, Johnson DA, Zierer ST, et al. Successful endoscopic hemostasis of bleeding colonic diverticula with epinephrine injection. Gastrointest Endosc 1996;43:167–70.
8. Savides TJ, Jensen DM. Colonoscopic hemostasis for recurrent diverticular hemorrhage associated with a visible vessel: a report of three cases. Gastrointest Endosc 1994;40:70–3.
9. Lara LF, Bloomfeld RS. Endoscopic therapy for acute diverticular hemorrhage. Gastrointest Endosc 2001;53:492.
10. Ishii N, Setoyama T, Deshpande GA, et al. Endoscopic band ligation for colonic diverticular hemorrhage. Gastrointest Endosc 2012;75:382–7.
11. Barker KB, Arnold HL, Fillman EP, et al. Safety of band ligator use in the small bowel and the colon. Gastrointest Endosc 2005;62:224–7.

12. Nagata N, Ishii N, Kaise M, et al. Long-term recurrent bleeding risk after endoscopic therapy for definitive colonic diverticular bleeding: band ligation versus clipping. Gastrointest Endsoc 2018;88:841–53.
13. Yoshikane H, Sakakibara A, Ayakawa T, et al. Hemostasis by capping bleeding diverticulum of the colon with clips. Endoscopy 1997;29:S33–4.
14. Yen E, Ladabaum U, Muthusamy V, et al. Colonoscopic treatment of acute diverticular hemorrhage using endoclips. Dig Dis Sci 2008;53:2480–5.
15. Kaltenbach T, Asokkumar R, Kolb JM, et al. Use of the endoscopic clipping over the scope technique to treat acute severe lower gastrointestinal bleeding in the colon and anal transition zone. Gastrointest Endosc Clin N Am 2020;30:13–23.
16. Yamazaki K, Maruta A, Taniguchi H, et al. Endoscopic treatment of colonic diverticular bleeding with an over-the-scope clip after failure of endoscopic band ligation. VideoGIE 2020;5:252–4.
17. Forrest JA, Finlayson ND, Shearman DJ. Endoscopy in gastrointestinal bleeding. Lancet 1974;2:394–7, 6736-1770.
18. Jensen DM, Ohning GV, Kovacs TO, et al. Natural history of definitive diverticular hemorrhage based upon stigmata of recent hemorrhage and colonoscopic Doppler blood flow monitoring for risk stratification on definitive hemostasis. Gastrointest Endosc 2016;83:416–23.
19. Foutch PG, Zimmerman K. Diverticular bleeding and the pigmented protuberance (sentinel clot): clinical implications, histopathological correlation, and results of endoscopic intervention. Am J Gastroenterol 1996;91:2589–93.
20. Jensen DM, Jensen ME, Kovacs TOG, et al. Flat spots are unrecognized as stigmata for diagnosis of definitive diverticular hemorrhage in the colon. Gastrointest Endosc 2017;85:AB247.
21. McGuire HH Jr. Bleeding colonic diverticula. a reappraisal of natural history and management. Ann Surg 1994;220:653–6.
22. Jensen DM, Kovacs TOG, Ohning GV, et al. Doppler endoscopic probe monitoring for blood flow improves risk stratification and outcomes of patients with severe non-variceal UGI hemorrhage. Gastroenterology 2017;152:1310–8.
23. Davis GR, Santa Ana CA, Morawski SG, et al. Development of a large solution associated with minimal water and electrolyte absorption or secretion. Gastroenterology 1980;78:991–5.
24. Jensen DM. Diverticular Bleeding: An appraisal based upon stigmata of recent hemorrhage. Tech Gastrointest Endosc 2001;3:192–8.
25. Jensen DM. Training in GI Hemostasis. In: Cohen J, editor. Successful training in gastrointestinal endoscopy. 2nd Edition. Hoboken, NJ: Wiley Blackwell; 2022. p. 195–214.
26. Jensen DM, Kovacs TOG, Ghassemi KA, et al. Randomized controlled trial of over-the-scope clip as initial treatment of severe non-variceal upper gastrointestinal bleeding. Clin Gastroenterol Hepatol 2021;19:2315–23.
27. Johnston JH, Jensen DM, Auth D. Experimental comparison of endoscopic Yttrium aluminum-Garnet laser, electrosurgery, and heater probe for canine gut arterial coagulation: The importance of vessel compression and avoidance of tissue erosion. Gastroenterology 1987;92:1101–8.
28. Khrucharoen U, Wangrattanapranee P, Jensen DM, et al. Definitive diverticular hemorrhage: 90 day outcome comparisons of colonoscopic hemostasis and medical treatment. Gastrointest Endosc 2022;95:AB192–3.
29. Thorne DA, Datz FL, Remley K, et al. Bleeding rates necessary for detecting acute gastrointestinal bleeding with technetium-99m-labeled red blood cells in an experimental model. J Nucl Med 1987;28:514–20.

30. Zuckerman GR, Prakash C. Acute lower intestinal bleeding: part I: clinical presentation and diagnosis. Gastrointest Endosc 1998;48:606–17.
31. Zink S, Ohki S, Stein B, et al. Noninvasive evaluation of active lower gastrointestinal bleeding: comparison between contrast-enhanced MDCT and 99mTc-labeled RBC scintigraphy. Am J Roentgerol 2008;191:1107–14.
32. Copland A, Munroe CA, Friedland S, et al. Integrating urgent multidetector CT scanning in the diagnostic algorithm of active lower GI bleeding. Gastrointest Endosc 2010;72:402–5.
33. Camus-Duboc M, Khungar V, Jensen DM, et al. Origin, clinical characteristics and 30-day outcomes of severe hematochezia in cirrhotics and non-cirrhotics. Dig Dis Sc 2016;61:2732–40.
34. Baum S. Angiography and the gastrointestinal bleeder. Radiology 1982;143:569–72.
35. Egglin TK, O'Moore PV, Feinstein AR, et al. Complications of peripheral arteriography: a new system to identify patients at increased risk. J Vasc Surg 1995;22:787–94.
36. Cohn SM, Moller BA, Zieg PM, et al. Angiography for preoperative evaluation in patients with lower gastrointestinal bleeding: are the benefits worth the risks? Arch Surg 1998;133:50–5.
37. Khrucharoen U, Jensen DM, Wangrattanapranee P, et al. Definitive diverticular hemorrhage: outcomes up to one year after medical treatment, colonoscopic hemostasis, embolization, or colon surgery. Gastrointest Endosc 2023;97:AB548–9.
38. Nagata N, Ishii N, Manabe N, et al. Guideline for colonic diverticular bleeding and colon diverticulitis: japan gastroenterological association. Digestion 2019;99(Supplement 1):1–16.
39. Wangrattanapranee P, Khrucharoen U, Jensen DM, et al. Natural history of presumptive diverticular (TIC) hemorrhage during long-term prospective follow-up. Gastrointest Endosc 2022;95:AB202–3.
40. Kovacs TOG, Jensen DM. Gastrointestinal hemorrhage. In: Goldman L, Shafer AI-, editors. Goldman cecil medicine. 27th Edition. Philadelphia: Elsevier Saunders; 2023. p. 840–5. Chapter 126.
41. Smoot R, Gostout C, Rajan E, et al. Is early colonoscopy after admission for acute diverticular bleeding needed? Am J Gastroenterol 2003;98:1996.
42. Laine L, Shah A. Randomized trial of urgent vs. elective colonoscopy in patients hospitalized with lower GI bleeding. Am J Gastroenterol 2010;105:2636–41, quiz 2642.
43. Sengupta N, Feuerstein JD, Jairath V, et al. Management of patients with Acute Lower Gastrointestinal Bleeding: An Updated ACG Guideline. Am J Gastroenterol 2023;118:208–31.
44. Strate LL, Syngal S. Timing of colonoscopy: impact on length of hospital stay in patients with acute lower intestinal bleeding. Am J Gastroenterol 2003;98:317–22.
45. Camus M, Jensen DM, Ohning GV, et al. Urgent capsule endoscopy for bleeding site localization & lesion diagnosis of patients with severe hematochezia. Gastrointest Endosc 2013;77:AB274.
46. Foutch P. Diverticular bleeding: Are nonsteroidal anti-inflammatory drugs risk factors and can colonoscopy predict outcome for patients? Am J Gastroenterol 1995;90:1779–84.
47. Strate LL, Liu YL, Huang ES, et al. Use of aspirin or nonsteroidal anti-inflammatory drugs increases risk for diverticulitis and diverticular bleeding. Gastroenterol 2011;140:1427–33.

Updates on the Prevention and Management of Post-Polypectomy Bleeding in the Colon

Hisham Wehbe, MD[a], Aditya Gutta, MD[b], Mark A. Gromski, MD[b,*]

KEYWORDS

- Polypectomy • GI bleed • Snare resection • Bleeding prevention

KEY POINTS

- Patient demographics and polyp characteristics along with the use of antithrombotic agents peri-endoscopically play an important role in determining the risk of post-polypectomy bleeding.
- Reducing the risk of post-polypectomy bleeding depends on the type of polypectomy and involves inspection, use of clips, endoloops, and hemostatic powders and/or gels.
- Treatment of immediate and delayed post-polypectomy bleeding can be achieved with various modalities, primarily mechanical therapy with hemostatic clips and thermal therapy. Topical hemostatic powders and gels are also increasingly being used and studied with significant interest.
- Delayed post-polypectomy bleeding carries high morbidity and mortality if not recognized promptly.

INTRODUCTION

Colorectal cancer (CRC) remains the third most common cancer in the United States.[1] Colonoscopy is the gold standard for prevention of diagnosing CRC. It allows for resection of precancerous polyps and earlier detection of malignancies; however, polypectomy carries a risk of complications primarily post-polypectomy bleeding (PPB), post-polypectomy syndrome, and perforation. PPB is classified as immediate which occurs at the time of procedure and is often managed intra-procedurally and delayed which occurs hours to days after colonoscopy and usually presents with signs or

[a] Department of Internal Medicine, Indiana University School of Medicine, 550 University Boulevard, UH 3533, Indianapolis, IN 46202, USA; [b] Department of Medicine, Division of Gastroenterology and Hepatology, Indiana University School of Medicine, 550 North University Boulevard, Suite 4100 Indianapolis, IN 46202, USA
* Corresponding author. Department of Medicine, Division of Gastroenterology and Hepatology, Indiana University School of Medicine, 550 North University Boulevard, Suite 4100, Indianapolis, IN 46202.
E-mail address: mgromski@iu.edu

Gastrointest Endoscopy Clin N Am 34 (2024) 363–381
https://doi.org/10.1016/j.giec.2023.09.008
1052-5157/24/© 2023 Elsevier Inc. All rights reserved.

symptoms of hematochezia and acute blood loss anemia.[2] This review aims at understanding the risk factors, prevention, and management of PPB in the colon.

RISK FACTORS

Multiple factors have been associated with an increased risk of immediate and/or delayed PPB including polyp-related factors and patient-related factors.

POLYP-RELATED FACTORS

One major polyp-related factor includes polyp size. A systematic review and meta-analysis demonstrated that the rate of bleeding with polypectomy of large polyps ($\geq$20 mm) was 6.5%, significantly higher than small polyps.[3] Another meta-analysis showed that polyp size is a strong risk factor for delayed PPB and a size of $\geq$10 mm was associated with a 3.4-fold risk of PPB.[4] Multiple other studies also revealed an association between polyp size and risk for PPB with an increase in risk with each additional 1 mm increase in polyp size.[5-7]

Polyp location has also been identified as an important risk factor for PPB. Studies have shown that right-sided polyps, particularly cecal polyps, carry a higher risk for PPB. A meta-analysis showed a significant association between right-sided polypectomy and PPB (OR = 1.6, 95% CI 1.12–2.3).[4] A study by Rutter and colleagues demonstrated a 13.5-fold increase of bleeding requiring transfusion after cecal polypectomy compared with distal colon polypectomy,[8] in line with other studies.[7,9] Interestingly, one study showed that right-sided polyps were associated with a reduced risk of immediate PPB by 61% (OR = 0.39; 95% CI 0.21–0.74; P = .0057).[10] It is not entirely clear why right-sided polypectomy carries a higher risk for PPB. A study by Sorbi and colleagues hypothesized that the wall of the cecum is thinner, which increases the risk of damage to the larger vessels in the deep submucosal layer.[11] Another study suggested that fresh ileal fluids may contain digestive enzymes and bile acids, which may dissolve the clot that maintains hemostasis post-polypectomy.[7]

In addition, multiple studies demonstrated that polyp morphology and/or pathology may play a role in increasing the risk of PPB. A study by Kim and colleagues (in which more than 9000 polyps in 5152 patients were removed) showed that laterally spreading polyps and pedunculated polyps with thick stalks are risk factors for PPB.[12] A retrospective case-control study revealed that pedunculated polyps carry a higher risk for delayed PPB (OR 3.47, 95% CI 1.58–7.66).[13] Another large study by Zhang and colleagues that included 15,553 polypectomies showed multiple risk factors for delayed PPB, most notable was polyp pathology where both juvenile (OR 4.3, 95% CI 1.8–11.0) and Peutz–Jeghers (P-J) polyps (OR 3.3, 95% CI 1.0–10.7) were associated with higher risk for delayed PPB when compared with inflammatory/hyperplastic polyps.[14] The association between pedunculated polyps and increased risk for PPB may be explained by the fact that pedunculated polyps tend to have large caliber vessels in their stalks, which increases the risk for PPB. Moreover, juvenile and P-J polyps being hamartomatous polyps[15] may also play a role in increasing the risk of PPB.

PATIENT-RELATED FACTORS

Demographic data have not been consistently associated with increased risk for PPB. The meta-analysis by Jaruvongvanich revealed that age was not associated with increased risk of PPB.[4] Another study by Park and colleagues demonstrated an increased odds of delayed PPB with younger age less than 50 years (OR 2.6; 95% CI 1.35–5.12),[16] which conflicts with other studies where increased age was associated with higher risk for PPB.[13] Multiple studies have commented on the increased risk of PPB associated with comorbidities such as hypertension, cardiovascular disease, and chronic kidney disease.[4,13,17]

The use of antiplatelets and antithrombotic agents is also an important aspect to consider due to the increased use among patients. The risk of PPB is affected by multiple factors, including the type of antithrombotic used, the duration withheld prior and after the polypectomy, the use of bridging therapy, and the technique of polypectomy (thermal/hot vs nonthermal/cold).

Studies have shown no increased risk of immediate PPB in patients who underwent polypectomy on aspirin; however, the chance of delayed PPB was increased.[18] Current guidelines do not recommend the discontinuation of aspirin at low doses (81 mg) before endoscopic procedures.[19–21] A recent randomized trial (RCT) by Won and colleagues found no significant difference in the rates of intraprocedural bleeding between those receiving dual antiplatelet therapy (P2Y12 inhibitor + aspirin) and those receiving aspirin alone (4.8% vs 2.2%, $P = .608$).[22] Another RCT by Chang and colleagues compared clopidogrel with placebo and found no significance difference between the two groups in terms of delayed (3.8% vs 3.6%, $P = .945$) and immediate (8.5% vs 5.5%, $P = .38$) PPB.[23] A recent meta-analysis, however, found an increased risk of immediate PPB in patients with uninterrupted P2Y 12 inhibitor use (OR 4.43, 95% CI 1.40–14.00) with highest risk in clopidogrel users compared with other P2Y 12 inhibitors (OR 13.28 vs OR 2.59). The risk of delayed PPB was also increased in those with uninterrupted P2Y12 inhibitors (OR 10.80, 95% CI 4.63–25.16).[24]

The incidence of PPB in patients on unfractionated heparin bridge has been reported to be as high as 22% in one study by Ishigami and colleagues compared with 1.9% in those who were not on a heparin bridge, independent of polyp size,[25] consistent with multiple other studies.[26–28] Warfarin has been associated with an increased risk of PPB. A study by Hui and colleagues revealed an increased risk of both immediate and delayed PPB with warfarin use (OR 13.37, 95% CI 4.10–43.65).[29] Another study noted that the presence of low-molecular weight heparin bridge is an independent risk factor for PPB even in the presence of warfarin (OR 12.27, $P = .0001$).[30]

Direct oral anticoagulants (DOACs) have also been extensively studied with respect to PPB. A recent study by Lau and colleagues showed that apixaban was associated with a lower risk of PPB compared with warfarin (adjusted HR [aHR] 0.39, 95% CI 0.24 to 0.63), whereas both dabigatran (aHR 2.23, 95% CI 1.04–4.77) and rivaroxaban (aHR 2.72, 95% CI 1.35–5.48) were associated with a higher PPB risk than apixaban.[31] This is in contrast to another study which demonstrated a higher risk for PPB in patients taking DOACs compared with those on warfarin (HR 1.97, 95% CI 1.16–3.33); however, the risk of overall gastrointestinal bleed was lower in those on DOACs compared with warfarin (HR 0.86, 95% CI 0.78–0.94).[32] Another study by Kim and colleagues compared DOACs to clopidogrel and found no significant difference in delayed PPB (OR 0.929, 95% CI 0.436–1.975), which occurred in 3% in both groups.[33]

PREVENTION

The periendoscopic management of antiplatelet and anticoagulant use can be challenging. Several guidelines have been published on this topic, including those by the American and Canadian Societies of Gastroenterology in 2022 and the British Society of Gastroenterology/European Society of Gastrointestinal Endoscopy (ESGE) in 2021. Both guidelines classified polypectomy (thermal and nonthermal) and endoscopic mucosal resection (EMR) as high-risk procedures for PPB.[19,20] Relevant guidelines are summarized in **Table 1**. To manage the risk, both guidelines recommend

Table 1
Summary of guidelines regarding antiplatelets and anticoagulant use before endoscopic procedures

Drug	American College of Gastroenterology[18]	Canadian Gastroenterology Association[18]	British Society of Gastroenterology[19]	European Society of Gastrointestinal Endoscopy[19]
Aspirin	Continue use	Continue use	Continue use	Continue use
P2Y12 inhibitors: clopidogrel, prasugrel, ticagrelor	Temporarily interrupt if used in combination with aspirin No consensus regarding P2Y12 monotherapy	Temporarily interrupt if used in combination with aspirin No consensus regarding P2Y12 monotherapy	Low-risk procedure: Continue therapy High-risk procedure without cardiac stents: stop 7 d before endoscopy High-risk procedure with cardiac stents: discuss with interventional cardiologist	Low-risk procedure: Continue therapy High-risk procedure without cardiac stents: stop 7 d before endoscopy High-risk procedure with cardiac stents: discuss with interventional cardiologist
Warfarin	Elective and planned outpatient endoscopic procedures: Continue use High-risk procedure: temporarily discontinue for 5 d without bridging	Elective and planned outpatient endoscopic procedures: Continue use High-risk procedure: temporarily discontinue for 5 d without bridging	Low-risk procedure: Continue warfarin if International Normalized Ratio (INR) within therapeutic range High-risk procedure: Stop warfarin 5 d before endoscopy	Low-risk procedure: Continue warfarin if INR within therapeutic range High-risk procedure: Stop warfarin 5 d before endoscopy
DOAC	Temporarily interrupt 1–2 d before procedure	Temporarily interrupt 1–2 d before procedure	Low-risk procedure: Omit DOAC on morning of procedure High-risk procedure: Take last dose of drug 3 d before endoscopy	Low-risk procedure: Omit DOAC on morning of procedure High-risk procedure: Take last dose of drug 3 d before endoscopy

| Heparin | Recommend against bridging unless mechanical valves, atrial fibrillation with CHADs (Congestive heart failure, Hypertension, Age ≥ 75, Diabetes mellitus, Stroke or TIA symptoms) score >5, previous thromboembolism, or certain types of surgery (cardiac valve replacement, vascular surgery, or carotid endarterectomy) | Recommend against bridging unless mechanical valves, atrial fibrillation with CHADs score>5, previous thromboembolism, or certain types of surgery (cardiac valve replacement, vascular surgery, or carotid endarterectomy) | High-risk procedure at high thrombosis risk: substitute warfarin with low molecular weight heparin (LMWH) | High-risk procedure at high thrombosis risk: substitute warfarin with LMWH |

High-risk procedures: endoscopic polypectomy, endoscopic retrograde cholangiopancreatography (ERCP) with sphincterotomy, ampullectomy, endoscopic mucosal resection, endoscopic submucosal dissection, endoscopic dilation of strictures, endoscopic therapy of varices, percutaneous endoscopic gastrostomy, and endoscopic ultrasound-guided sampling.

Low-risk procedures: diagnostic procedures ± biopsy sampling, biliary or pancreatic stenting, device-assisted enteroscopy without polypectomy, esophageal, enteral, or colonic tenting, endoscopic ultrasound.

creating individual plans for patients based on their comorbidities and individual characteristics. The guidelines also consider the individual risk of the antithrombotic agents used, the risks associated with their discontinuation, the need for heparin bridging, and the timing of their resumption after the procedure.

Cold Snare Versus Hot Snare Polypectomy

Over the last few years, there have been multiple studies to assess the difference in risk of PPB between cold snare polypectomy (CSP) and hot snare polypectomy (HSP). Cold forceps polypectomy (CFP) has previously been used for diminutive polyps (<5 mm); CSP has been found to be superior to cold biopsy forceps for histologic eradication and shorter polypectomy time.[34] However, a recent RCT showed CFP to be non-inferior and faster compared with CSP for polyps ≤3 mm in size.[35] Current ESGE guidelines recommend CSP for the removal of diminutive polyps (<5 mm) or noncancerous polyps up to 10 mm as it has shown a high rate of complete resection, low complication rates, and the ability to obtain adequate tissue for histology.[20] The risk of immediate bleeding with CSP is higher, owing to capillary and venule injury; however, this can be recognized at the time of polypectomy and can be managed during the procedure. The risk of immediate PPB with HSP lower, but due to the thermal injury to deeper layers of the colon wall and involvement of larger blood vessels, there is a higher risk of delayed PPB.[36] A recent meta-analysis revealed that CSP had a higher rate of immediate bleeding than HSP (54% vs 14%), though there was no significant difference in bleeding needing intervention (OR 1.99, 95% CI 0.59–6.75).[37] Another meta-analysis revealed comparable or higher rates of intraprocedural bleeding in CSP, with higher rates of delayed bleeding in HSP.[38] A recent RCT showed a decreased risk of delayed PPB (risk difference −1.1%, 95% CI −1.7% to −0.5%) with CSP for polyps 4 to 10 mm compared with HSP along with a shorter polypectomy time, with no difference in complete histologic resection.[39] This is similar to another meta-analysis, which also showed longer procedure times in HSP.[40] The use of anticoagulation before procedures plays an independent factor as well and an RCT found that patients on anticoagulation undergoing HSP had higher rates of delayed PPB compared with CSP.[41] Other studies supported that the use of antiplatelet and antithrombotic agents did not increase the risk of delayed PPB in CSP compared with HSP.[41,42] A recent multicenter RCT compared the outcomes between continuous administration of anticoagulants with CSP and periprocedural heparin bridging with HSP and found that patients who were receiving oral anticoagulants did not have an increased incidence of PPB, and procedure time and hospitalization were shorter than those on heparin bridge.[43]

CSP has been considered for larger nonpedunculated polyps (>10 mm). An RCT demonstrated higher rates of clinically significant bleeding, post-polypectomy syndrome, and abdominal pain in HSP compared with CSP.[44] A recent RCT demonstrated superiority of CSP over other techniques for non-pedunculated polyps 6 to 15 mm with less procedure time and lower risk of PPB.[45] A systematic review/meta-analysis also demonstrated the safety and efficacy of CSP compared with HSP for non-pedunculated polyps greater than 10 mm as well as serrated polyps greater than 10 mm in regard to PPB, complete resection, and residual/recurrent polyp rate.[46] One major caveat for CSP is the recurrence rate, which is being addressed in two large ongoing trials.[47,48]

The use of CSP for small pedunculated polyps (<10 mm) with thin stalks has also been evaluated and a recent study revealed that CSP carried a higher risk for intraprocedural bleeding (38.2% [39/102] versus 3.5% [3/86]; P < .001), whereas HSP demonstrated higher rates of delayed PPB (4.7% [4/86] versus 0% [0/102]; P < .001)[49] despite the use of prophylactic clipping both before and after the procedure. CSP for pedunculated polyps less than 10 mm with a technique of squeezing the stalk for at least 10 seconds before transection was shown to reduce the likelihood of immediate bleeding by 97%.[10] A combination of techniques may therefore be used to reduce the risk of PPB for these types of polyps. The current guidelines continue to recommend HSP for pedunculated polyps given the risk of bleeding, especially the larger polyps with anticipated larger vessels in the stalk.[2]

There is a debate among endoscopists over which type of electrosurgical setting should be used for HSP. There are two types of commonly used settings, either a blended and cutting current (Endocut Q) or a pure coagulation current (forced coagulation).[50] An RCT by Pohl and colleagues showed no significant difference in the rate of serious adverse events, complete resection, or risk of recurrence between the two groups; however, more patients in the Endocut group had immediate bleeding requiring an intervention as compared with the forced coagulation group (17% vs 11%, $P = .006$).[51] An older study also showed no difference in the complication rates between the two groups; however, there was a significant difference in the timing of PPB between the groups. All immediate hemorrhages occurred when blended current was used, whereas all delayed PPB occurred with the use of coagulation current.[52] Guidelines do not weigh in on this detail, and electrosurgical settings could be selected based on endoscopist preference and expertise.

Prophylactic Clipping

Mechanically closing the mucosal defect of polyp resection sites has been hypothesized to decrease the risk of delayed PPB. The data on PPB after prophylactic endoscopic clipping using through-the-scope (TTS) clips have been conflicting. A study by Feagins and colleagues found no significant difference in the rates of delayed PPB between the hemoclip group (12 out of 530 [2.3%]) compared with no hemoclip one (15 out of 520 [2.9%]) (RR 0.79, 95% CI 0.37–1.66),[53] consistent with the results of another study which showed no significant difference in PPB between prophylactic clipping versus no clipping in all polyps (OR 1.49, 95% CI 0.56–4.00).[54] On the other hand, a meta-analysis concluded that there is a lower risk of delayed PPB with the use of hemoclips for polyps ≥2 cm (RR 0.55, 95% CI 0.36–0.86) with even a lower risk if located in the proximal colon (RR 0.41, 95% CI 0.24–0.70).[55] A meta-analysis with a total of 71,897 colorectal lesions found that the benefit of clipping in reducing PPB was significant for polyps ≥20 mm (RR 0.51, 95% CI 0.33–0.78), and for proximal lesions greater than 20 cm (OR 0.37, 95% CI 0.22–0.61).[56] **Figs. 1–5** demonstrate examples of prophylactic clipping after EMR.

The risk of PPB differs between pedunculated and non-pedunculated polyps. As for non-pedunculated polyps alone, a study by Pohl and colleagues found an absolute risk difference of 3.6% (95% CI 0.7% to 6.5%) for PPB between the clip and the control groups, with the protective effect being restricted to large polyps localized to the proximal colon.[57] A meta-analysis demonstrated a benefit of prophylactic clipping large (≥20 mm) non-pedunculated polyps especially if on anti-thrombotic, with no clear benefit in the distal colon.[58] A very recent RCT showed no clear benefit with prophylactic clip closure for large (≥20 mm) non-pedunculated polyps in general, although there was some suggestion of benefit specifically for adenomatous polyps greater than 20 mm in the proximal colon.[59] Another meta-analysis showed some benefit with prophylactic clip closure in preventing delayed PPB, modest benefit in polyps greater than 10 mm with a more pronounced benefit in polyps greater than 20 mm and those in the proximal colon.[60]

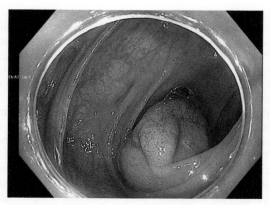

Fig. 1. Endoscopic images of sessile colonic polyp lifted in preparation for endoscopic mucosal resection (EMR).

When it comes to pedunculated polyps, an RCT of 105 polypectomies found that the total rate of complications was 10.6% in the clipping group which included early and delayed PPB, perforation, and mucosal burns (compared with 7.7% in the non-clipping group).[61] The American Society for Gastrointestinal Endoscopy (ASGE) guidelines recommend the use of prophylactic endoclips for polyps with a pedicle greater than 5 mm,[62] whereas ESGE recommends the additional use of diluted adrenaline and/or mechanical hemostasis for large pedunculated polyps with thick stalks ≥10 mm.[2] As for the cost, a study by Shah and colleagues showed that prophylactic clip closure after resection of large colon polyps, particularly in the right colon, was cost saving but only if the clip costs less than $100.[63] Studies are lacking to demonstrate superiority of one type of TTS clips over others.

In summary, the benefit of prophylactic clip closure in preventing delayed PPB remains unclear and likely depends most of the polyp characteristics. Based on current data, the use of prophylactic clipping may be beneficial and selectively used in polyps ≥ 2 cm and in the proximal colon; however, other considerations including patient's characteristics, use of anticoagulation ± antiplatelet agents,[21] and polyp morphology should be taken into account.

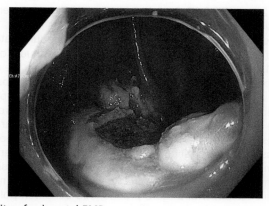

Fig. 2. Resection site of colorectal EMR.

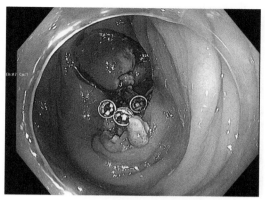

Fig. 3. Prophylactic endoscopic clipping of EMR resection site.

Epinephrine

Other preventative measures have been studied including the use of adrenaline injection into the stalk of pedunculated polyps before polypectomy. Individual studies have shown that the injection of the stalk with 0.01% epinephrine before conventional snare polypectomy is associated with lower risk of PPB.[64,65] A meta-analysis of six RCTs demonstrated that prophylactic use of epinephrine is associated with significant reduction in the immediate PPB (OR 0.38, 95% CI, 0.20–0.69) but not with delayed PPB (OR 0.45, 95% CI 0.11–1.81).[66]

Endoloops

The use of detachable snare loops such as endoloops has also been studied. A previous RCT demonstrated that the use of detachable snare significantly reduced the rate of PPB when compared with conventional polypectomy (0% vs 12%, $P<.05$).[67] The previously mentioned meta-analysis also compared epinephrine to the use of mechanical hemostasis (endoloops or clips) and found that the risk for overall and early bleeding is reduced with use of mechanical methods for larger polyps ($\geq$20 mm) when compared with injection of epinephrine alone but this was not seen for delayed bleeding,[66] which was consistent with other studies.[68,69] In addition, the

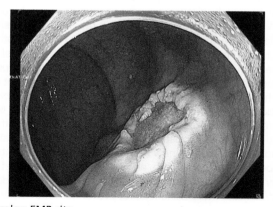

Fig. 4. Right side colon EMR site.

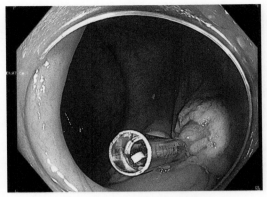

Fig. 5. Prophylactic endoscopic clipping of post-EMR resection site.

overall bleeding rates were similar for those receiving clip ligation when compared with endoloop placement (5.1% vs 5.7%, P = .847) in another RCT with 203 pedunculated colorectal polyps with heads ≥10 mm and stalks ≥5 mm.[70]

Inspection

Inspection of the post-polypectomy site has also important implications on the prevention of PPB. Visible defects such as visible muscle fibers and the presence of a "cherry red spot" have been shown to correlate with increased risk for PPB.[71] In addition, inspecting for a bleeding vessel after the polyp removal has been shown to reduce the rates of delayed PPB compared with controls (0.4% vs 1.1%), though the effect is less pronounced in the presence of antithrombotics or the use of HSP.[72] The time of inspection was 30 seconds, though other studies advocated for a longer observation time especially after use of prophylactic argon plasma coagulation (APC).[73]

Topical Gels

The use of gels and topical applicants is a newer category with many recent commercially available products. A recent RCT assessed the application of PuraStat (3-D Matrix, Boston, USA), which is a topical self-assembling peptide for hemostasis during endoscopic submucosal dissection (ESD), and found a significant reduction in the need for use of heat therapy for intraprocedural hemostasis when compared with the control group in which diathermy was used to control bleeding (49.3% vs 99.6%, P<.001).[74] Another recent RCT showed a rate of hemostasis of 62.2% with the use of PuraStat with a mean dosage of 1.75 ± 2.14 mL.[75] Other agents have been studied including modified cyanoacrylate glue,[76] which showed potential benefit, and platelet-rich plasma[77] which failed to show benefit in preventing bleeding after ESD, likely due to lack of adherence to larger wounds. EndoClot (Olympus America, Boston, USA) has also shown promising results in prevention of bleeding following various endoscopic interventions.[78,79] Hemostatic powder, which is an absorbable and modified polymer particle powder, was evaluated as well, and although the results of the RCT showed lower rates of post-ESD bleeding in the hemostasis powder group, the results were not significant.[80] A new mucoadhesive gel that contains epinephrine nanoparticles is being developed with ability to maintain hemostasis as long as 72 hours.[81] Further studies including head-to-head analysis to elucidate which hemostatic powder and/or gel is more beneficial for prevention of PPB, and the exact role for them in bleeding prevention is needed.

TREATMENT
Early Post-Polypectomy Bleeding

Immediate PPB can be detected and addressed at the time of the procedure. As previously mentioned, inspection of the site after polypectomy allows for detection of bleeding vessels, perforation, and residual polyps. In most cases, observation with water lavage results in self-limited cessation of oozing. Occasionally, a direct pressure using the scope tip for suctioning may be applied on the mucosal defect to treat slow oozing. However, for more brisk bleeds, targeted deployment of endoscopic therapy becomes essential.

One of the most used options in the management of immediate PPB is the use of clips. TTS clips have been widely used for the initial management of PPB.[82,83] The method of deployment depends on the type of polyp removed. In general, if PPB results after a pedunculated polyp removal, then the clip is deployed perpendicular to the stalk to ligate the feeding vessels.[84] As for sessile polyps, the clip should be maneuvered to tamponade the bleeding vessels, usually followed by closure of the mucosal defect.[84,85] Following closure of the clip, the area is washed, and if no active bleeding is noted, then the clip can be safely deployed. Immediate bleeding can also be managed using snare tip soft coagulation (STSC) or coagulation grasping forceps[86,87]; however, there are no comparative studies of clipping versus thermal therapies for PPB. STSC has been shown to be safe and effective during wide-field EMR, which also reduces the incidence of adenoma recurrence when used.[86,88] The ultimate decision to use a certain method depends on the endoscopist's expertise and the available equipment.

Over-the-scope clip (OTSC; Ovesco Endoscopy, Tubingen, Germany) may play a selective role in the management of PPB. This has been extensively studied in the management of upper gastrointestinal (GI) bleeding but has also been found effective in the management of lower GI bleed.[89–92] A major limitation of OTSC in management of PPB is the ability to pass the endoscope with the OTSC device to the right colon which is the more common location of PPB.

Hemostatic powders have gained interest for their excellent efficacy in the initial hemostasis if PPB occurs. Among the first studies on Hemospray or TC-325 (Cook Medical, Winston-Salem, NC) was the one by Soulellis and colleagues which was the first to report the use of Hemospray as salvage therapy in two patients who failed to respond to clips and thermal therapy, without evidence of recurrence at day 14 and 104 of follow-up.[93] Hemospray has also been shown to be a safe and effective option either as a monotherapy, part of a combination approach, or as a rescue therapeutic option, with 5 out of 50 patients demonstrating recurrence of bleeding.[94] Other agents such as EndoClot (Olympus America, Boston, USA)[95] and Ankaferd Blood Stopper[96] have also been studied. A meta-analysis by Facciorusso and colleagues noted that initial hemostasis was achieved in 95.3% of patients regardless of which agent was used.[97] Newer agents, including UI-EWD (NexPowder, Medtronic, Minneapolis, USA)[98] and a self-propelling thrombin powder (American Elements, Los Angeles, USA),[99] are also being studied, mostly in upper GI bleed, and have shown promising results in initial trials. Despite the growing interest, the use of hemostatic powders is limited by their rapid sloughing off resulting in higher rates of rebleeding[100,101] and the need for repeat colonoscopy for a more definitive therapy. Some experts recommend the use of Hemospray as a temporary bridge to achieve initial hemostasis before a repeat colonoscopy with a more definitive treatment in 24 to 48 hours.[102]

Delayed Post-Polypectomy Bleeding

As mentioned previously, HSP is associated with a higher risk of delayed PPB. PPB occurs if the tissue necrosis that follows HSP extends beyond the mucosa into the submucosal blood vessels resulting in bleeding that is not visualized at the time of polypectomy. There are currently no guidelines for the management of delayed PPB; however, the decision to proceed with colonoscopy and the timing of colonoscopy should be individualized. Hemodynamic stability should precede any intervention, and this would include assessing for blood loss duration, quantity, and resultant intravascular depletion. Sonnenberg modeled delayed PPB as a decision tree which suggested that repeat colonoscopy to treat bleeding is beneficial in 22% of patients, with a number needed to treat of 4.5.[103] Another study also showed that colonoscopy may be overused in patients with delayed PPB.[104] A recent study assessed the safety and efficacy of prompt colonoscopy for delayed PPB for colon polyps ≤10 mm and found an 89.9% success rate of initial colonoscopic hemostasis with at least two clips placement as an independent prognostic factor for this success.[105] Hemoclip placement is the most commonly used modality for the management of delayed PPB. Several studies have demonstrated the efficacy of using hemoclips as an initial approach for hemostasis[105,106]; though one study by Lee and colleagues found that a large number of clips correlate with a higher rate of rebleeding.[107] Other therapeutic measures including OTSC, and hemostatic spray powders have been used.[94,108] Thermal therapy is generally avoided in the post-polypectomy site due to the risk of perforation, though the risk of perforation has also been reported with clipping.[109] The failure of initial hemostasis resulting in persistent hemodynamic instability should prompt urgent interventional radiology and/or surgical evaluation.

SUMMARY

PPB is one of the most common complications after polypectomy. Multiple risk factors relating to the polyp characteristics, patient demographics, and comorbid medical conditions along with endoscopist's expertise have been identified and should be accounted for during the evaluation. PPB can occur immediately, and this is generally managed promptly. Delayed PPB can occur and can result in hemodynamic instability. In delayed PPB, hemodynamic stabilization should take precedence before any intervention. CSP is associated with a higher immediate PPB rate and a lower delayed PPB rate. The role for prophylactic clipping of polypectomy sites is likely best reserved for polyps greater than 20 mm located in the right colon.

CLINICS CARE POINTS

- Polyp-related factors associated with an increased risk of PPB include polyp size ≥20 mm, right-sided polyps, and pedunculated polyps with thick stalks.
- Pre-procedural use of aspirin has not been associated with an increased risk of immediate PPB, but risk of delayed PPB may be increased. P2Y12 inhibitor and warfarin use has been associated with an increased risk of immediate and delayed PPB. Studies on risk with direct oral anticoagulant use yielded conflicting results.
- Cold snare polypectomy (CSP) is currently recommended for polyps ≤10 mm but is associated with higher risk of immediate PPB and has been studied for large non-pedunculated polyps (≥10 mm) with lower rates of PPB compared with hot snare polypectomy (HSP).
- Some studies noted increased risk of immediate PPB with CSP for pedunculated polyps while increased risk of delayed PPB with HSP. Current guidelines continue to recommend HSP for pedunculated polyps.
- The data on PPB after prophylactic clipping have been conflicting with some studies showing the benefit of clipping reducing PPB was significant for polyps ≥20 mm.

- Epinephrine injection into the stalk of pedunculated polyps before polypectomy is associated with decreased risk for immediate PPB.
- Novel topical gels and hemostatic powders are currently being evaluated for this purpose.
- Through-the-scope clips are widely used for the initial management of PPB.
- The use of over-the-scope clip may play a role in the management of certain PPB scenarios, but navigating to bleeding in right colon can be difficult.
- There are currently no guidelines on the management of delayed PPB; however, hemodynamic stability should precede any intervention.

CONFLICT OF INTEREST

M.A. Gromski: Consultant (Boston Scientific). None of the other contributing authors have any conflict of interest, including specific financial interests or relationships and affiliations relevant to the subject matter or materials discussed in this article.

REFERENCES

1. Siegel RL, Miller KD, Fuchs HE, et al. Cancer statistics, 2022. CA Cancer J Clin 2022;72(1):7–33 (In eng).
2. Ferlitsch M, Moss A, Hassan C, et al. Colorectal polypectomy and endoscopic mucosal resection (EMR): European Society of Gastrointestinal Endoscopy (ESGE) Clinical Guideline. Endoscopy 2017;49(3):270–97 (In eng).
3. Hassan C, Repici A, Sharma P, et al. Efficacy and safety of endoscopic resection of large colorectal polyps: a systematic review and meta-analysis. Gut 2016;65(5):806–20 (In eng).
4. Jaruvongvanich V, Prasitlumkum N, Assavapongpaiboon B, et al. Risk factors for delayed colonic post-polypectomy bleeding: a systematic review and meta-analysis. Int J Colorectal Dis 2017;32(10):1399–406 (In eng).
5. Tsuruta S, Tominaga N, Ogata S, et al. Risk Factors for Delayed Hemorrhage after Colonic Endoscopic Mucosal Resection in Patients Not on Antithrombotic Therapy: Retrospective Analysis of 3,844 Polyps of 1,660 Patients. Digestion 2019;100(2):86–92 (In eng).
6. Sawhney MS, Salfiti N, Nelson DB, et al. Risk factors for severe delayed postpolypectomy bleeding. Endoscopy 2008;40(2):115–9 (In eng).
7. Buddingh KT, Herngreen T, Haringsma J, et al. Location in the right hemi-colon is an independent risk factor for delayed post-polypectomy hemorrhage: a multi-center case-control study. Am J Gastroenterol 2011;106(6):1119–24 (In eng).
8. Rutter MD, Nickerson C, Rees CJ, et al. Risk factors for adverse events related to polypectomy in the English Bowel Cancer Screening Programme. Endoscopy 2014;46(2):90–7 (In eng).
9. Choung BS, Kim SH, Ahn DS, et al. Incidence and risk factors of delayed postpolypectomy bleeding: a retrospective cohort study. J Clin Gastroenterol 2014; 48(9):784–9 (In eng).
10. Fatima H, Tariq T, Gilmore A, et al. Bleeding Risk With Cold Snare Polypectomy of ≤10 mm Pedunculated Colon Polyps. J Clin Gastroenterol 2023;57(3):294–9. https://doi.org/10.1097/mcg.0000000000001699 (In eng).
11. Sorbi D, Norton I, Conio M, et al. Postpolypectomy lower GI bleeding: descriptive analysis. Gastrointest Endosc 2000;51(6):690–6 (In eng).

12. Kim HS, Kim TI, Kim WH, et al. Risk factors for immediate postpolypectomy bleeding of the colon: a multicenter study. Am J Gastroenterol 2006;101(6): 1333–41 (In eng).

13. Kim JH, Lee HJ, Ahn JW, et al. Risk factors for delayed post-polypectomy hemorrhage: a case-control study. J Gastroenterol Hepatol 2013;28(4):645–9 (In eng).

14. Zhang Q, An S, Chen Z, et al. Assessment of risk factors for delayed colonic post-polypectomy hemorrhage: a study of 15553 polypectomies from 2005 to 2013. PLoS One 2014;9(10):e108290 (In eng).

15. Jelsig AM, Qvist N, Brusgaard K, et al. Hamartomatous polyposis syndromes: A review. Orphanet J Rare Dis 2014;9(1):101.

16. Park SK, Seo JY, Lee MG, et al. Prospective analysis of delayed colorectal post-polypectomy bleeding. Surg Endosc 2018;32(7):3282–9 (In eng).

17. Paszat LF, Sutradhar R, Luo J, et al. Perforation and post-polypectomy bleeding complicating colonoscopy in a population-based screening program. Endosc Int Open 2021;9(4):E637–45 (In eng).

18. Pigò F, Bertani H, Grande G, et al. Post-polypectomy bleeding after colonoscopy on uninterrupted aspirin/non steroideal antiflammatory drugs: Systematic review and meta-analysis. Dig Liver Dis 2018;50(1):20–6 (In eng).

19. Acosta RD, Abraham NS, Chandrasekhara V, et al. The management of antithrombotic agents for patients undergoing GI endoscopy. Gastrointest Endosc 2016;83(1):3–16 (In eng).

20. Veitch AM, Radaelli F, Alikhan R, et al. Endoscopy in patients on antiplatelet or anticoagulant therapy: British Society of Gastroenterology (BSG) and European Society of Gastrointestinal Endoscopy (ESGE) guideline update. Gut 2021; 70(9):1611–28 (In eng).

21. Lau LHS, Jiang W, Guo CLT, et al. Effectiveness of prophylactic clipping in preventing postpolypectomy bleeding in aspirin users: a propensity-score analysis. Gastrointest Endosc 2023;97(3):517–27.e1 (In eng).

22. Won D, Kim JS, Ji JS, et al. Cold Snare Polypectomy in Patients Taking Dual Antiplatelet Therapy: A Randomized Trial of Discontinuation of Thienopyridines. Clin Transl Gastroenterol 2019;10(10):e00091 (In eng).

23. Chan FKL, Kyaw MH, Hsiang JC, et al. Risk of Postpolypectomy Bleeding With Uninterrupted Clopidogrel Therapy in an Industry-Independent, Double-Blind, Randomized Trial. Gastroenterology 2019;156(4):918–25.e1 (In eng).

24. Valvano M, Fabiani S, Magistroni M, et al. Risk of colonoscopic post-polypectomy bleeding in patients on single antiplatelet therapy: systematic review with meta-analysis. Surg Endosc 2022;36(4):2258–70 (In eng).

25. Ishigami H, Arai M, Matsumura T, et al. Heparin-bridging therapy is associated with a high risk of post-polypectomy bleeding regardless of polyp size. Dig Endosc 2017;29(1):65–72 (In eng).

26. Inoue T, Nishida T, Maekawa A, et al. Clinical features of post-polypectomy bleeding associated with heparin bridge therapy. Dig Endosc 2014;26(2): 243–9 (In eng).

27. Kubo T, Yamashita K, Onodera K, et al. Heparin bridge therapy and post-polypectomy bleeding. World J Gastroenterol 2016;22(45):10009–14 (In eng).

28. Sakai T, Nagami Y, Shiba M, et al. Heparin-bridging therapy is associated with post-colorectal polypectomy bleeding in patients whose oral anticoagulation therapy is interrupted. Scand J Gastroenterol 2018;53(10–11):1304–10 (In eng).

29. Hui AJ, Wong RM, Ching JY, et al. Risk of colonoscopic polypectomy bleeding with anticoagulants and antiplatelet agents: analysis of 1657 cases. Gastrointest Endosc 2004;59(1):44–8 (In eng).

30. Lin D, Soetikno RM, McQuaid K, et al. Risk factors for postpolypectomy bleeding in patients receiving anticoagulation or antiplatelet medications. Gastrointest Endosc 2018;87(4):1106–13 (In eng).

31. Lau LH, Guo CL, Yip TC, et al. Risks of post-colonoscopic polypectomy bleeding and thromboembolism with warfarin and direct oral anticoagulants: a population-based analysis. Gut 2022;71(1):100–10 (In eng).

32. Pae JY, Kim ES, Kim SK, et al. Gastrointestinal bleeding risk of non-vitamin K antagonist oral anticoagulants versus warfarin in general and after polypectomy: a population-based study with propensity score matching analysis. Intest Res 2022;20(4):482–94 (In eng).

33. Kim GU, Lee S, Choe J, et al. Risk of postpolypectomy bleeding in patients taking direct oral anticoagulants or clopidogrel. Sci Rep 2021;11(1):2634 (In eng).

34. Lee CK, Shim JJ, Jang JY. Cold snare polypectomy vs. Cold forceps polypectomy using double-biopsy technique for removal of diminutive colorectal polyps: a prospective randomized study. Am J Gastroenterol 2013;108(10):1593–600 (In eng).

35. Wei MT, Louie CY, Chen Y, et al. Randomized Controlled Trial Investigating Cold Snare and Forceps Polypectomy Among Small POLYPs in Rates of Complete Resection: The TINYPOLYP Trial. Am J Gastroenterol 2022;117(8):1305–10 (In eng).

36. Takayanagi D, Nemoto D, Isohata N, et al. Histological Comparison of Cold versus Hot Snare Resections of the Colorectal Mucosa. Dis Colon Rectum 2018;61(8):964–70 (In eng).

37. Qu J, Jian H, Li L, et al. Effectiveness and safety of cold versus hot snare polypectomy: A meta-analysis. J Gastroenterol Hepatol 2019;34(1):49–58 (In eng).

38. Takeuchi Y, Shichijo S, Uedo N, et al. Safety and efficacy of cold versus hot snare polypectomy including colorectal polyps ≥1 cm in size. Dig Endosc 2022;34(2):274–83 (In eng).

39. Chang LC, Chang CY, Chen CY, et al. Cold Versus Hot Snare Polypectomy for Small Colorectal Polyps : A Pragmatic Randomized Controlled Trial. Ann Intern Med 2023;176(3):311–9 (In eng).

40. Shinozaki S, Kobayashi Y, Hayashi Y, et al. Efficacy and safety of cold versus hot snare polypectomy for resecting small colorectal polyps: Systematic review and meta-analysis. Dig Endosc 2018;30(5):592–9 (In eng).

41. Horiuchi A, Nakayama Y, Kajiyama M, et al. Removal of small colorectal polyps in anticoagulated patients: a prospective randomized comparison of cold snare and conventional polypectomy. Gastrointest Endosc 2014;79(3):417–23 (In eng).

42. Arimoto J, Chiba H, Ashikari K, et al. Safety of Cold Snare Polypectomy in Patients Receiving Treatment with Antithrombotic Agents. Dig Dis Sci 2019; 64(11):3247–55 (In eng).

43. Takeuchi Y, Mabe K, Shimodate Y, et al. Continuous Anticoagulation and Cold Snare Polypectomy Versus Heparin Bridging and Hot Snare Polypectomy in Patients on Anticoagulants With Subcentimeter Polyps: A Randomized Controlled Trial. Ann Intern Med 2019;171(4):229–37 (In eng).

44. Ket SN, Mangira D, Ng A, et al. Complications of cold versus hot snare polypectomy of 10-20 mm polyps: A retrospective cohort study. JGH Open 2020;4(2): 172–7 (In eng).

45. Rex DK, Anderson JC, Pohl H, et al. Cold versus hot snare resection with or without submucosal injection of 6- to 15-mm colorectal polyps: a randomized controlled trial. Gastrointest Endosc 2022;96(2):330–8 (In eng).

46. Thoguluva Chandrasekar V, Spadaccini M, Aziz M, et al. Cold snare endoscopic resection of nonpedunculated colorectal polyps larger than 10 mm: a systematic review and pooled-analysis. Gastrointest Endosc 2019;89(5):929–36.e3 (In eng).

47. Rotermund C, Djinbachian R, Taghiakbari M, et al. Recurrence rates after endoscopic resection of large colorectal polyps: A systematic review and meta-analysis. World J Gastroenterol 2022;28(29):4007–18 (In eng).

48. Tziatzios G, Papaefthymiou A, Facciorusso A, et al. Comparative efficacy and safety of resection techniques for treating 6 to 20mm, nonpedunculated colorectal polyps: A systematic review and network meta-analysis. Dig Liver Dis 2023;55(7):856–64 (In eng).

49. Arimoto J, Chiba H, Ashikari K, et al. Management of Less Than 10-mm-Sized Pedunculated (Ip) Polyps with Thin Stalk: Hot Snare Polypectomy Versus Cold Snare Polypectomy. Dig Dis Sci 2021;66(7):2353–61 (In eng).

50. Morris ML, Tucker RD, Baron TH, et al. Electrosurgery in gastrointestinal endoscopy: principles to practice. Am J Gastroenterol 2009;104(6):1563–74 (In eng).

51. Pohl H, Grimm IS, Moyer MT, et al. Effects of Blended (Yellow) vs Forced Coagulation (Blue) Currents on Adverse Events, Complete Resection, or Polyp Recurrence After Polypectomy in a Large Randomized Trial. Gastroenterology 2020; 159(1):119–28.e2 (In eng).

52. Van Gossum A, Cozzoli A, Adler M, et al. Colonoscopic snare polypectomy: analysis of 1485 resections comparing two types of current. Gastrointest Endosc 1992;38(4):472–5 (In eng).

53. Feagins LA, Smith AD, Kim D, et al. Efficacy of Prophylactic Hemoclips in Prevention of Delayed Post-Polypectomy Bleeding in Patients With Large Colonic Polyps. Gastroenterology 2019;157(4):967–76.e1 (In eng).

54. Boumitri C, Mir FA, Ashraf I, et al. Prophylactic clipping and post-polypectomy bleeding: a meta-analysis and systematic review. Ann Gastroenterol 2016;29(4): 502–8 (In eng).

55. Kamal F, Khan MA, Khan S, et al. Prophylactic hemoclips in prevention of delayed post-polypectomy bleeding for $\geq$ 1 cm colorectal polyps: meta-analysis of randomized controlled trials. Endosc Int Open 2020;8(9):E1102–10 (In eng).

56. Spadaccini M, Albéniz E, Pohl H, et al. Prophylactic Clipping After Colorectal Endoscopic Resection Prevents Bleeding of Large, Proximal Polyps: Meta-analysis of Randomized Trials. Gastroenterology 2020;159(1):148–58.e11 (In eng).

57. Pohl H, Grimm IS, Moyer MT, et al. Clip Closure Prevents Bleeding After Endoscopic Resection of Large Colon Polyps in a Randomized Trial. Gastroenterology 2019;157(4):977–84.e3 (In eng).

58. Turan AS, Pohl H, Matsumoto M, et al. The Role of Clips in Preventing Delayed Bleeding After Colorectal Polyp Resection: An Individual Patient Data Meta-Analysis. Clin Gastroenterol Hepatol 2022;20(2):362–71.e23 (In eng).

59. Crockett SD, Khashab M, Rex DK, et al. Clip Closure Does Not Reduce Risk of Bleeding After Resection of Large Serrated Polyps: Results From a Randomized Trial. Clin Gastroenterol Hepatol 2022;20(8):1757–65.e4 (In eng).

60. Chen B, Du L, Luo L, et al. Prophylactic clips to reduce delayed polypectomy bleeding after resection of large colorectal polyps: a systematic review and

meta-analysis of randomized trials. Gastrointest Endosc 2021;93(4):807–15 (In eng).

61. Quintanilla E, Castro JL, Rábago LR, et al. Is the use of prophylactic hemoclips in the endoscopic resection of large pedunculated polyps useful? A prospective and randomized study. J Interv Gastroenterol 2012;2(4):183–8 (In eng).

62. Kaltenbach T, Anderson JC, Burke CA, et al. Endoscopic Removal of Colorectal Lesions: Recommendations by the US Multi-Society Task Force on Colorectal Cancer. Am J Gastroenterol 2020;115(3):435–64 (In eng).

63. Shah ED, Pohl H, Rex DK, et al. Valuing innovative endoscopic techniques: prophylactic clip closure after endoscopic resection of large colon polyps. Gastrointest Endosc 2020;91(6):1353–60 (In eng).

64. Di Giorgio P, De Luca L, Calcagno G, et al. Detachable snare versus epinephrine injection in the prevention of postpolypectomy bleeding: a randomized and controlled study. Endoscopy 2004;36(10):860–3 (In eng).

65. Dobrowolski S, Dobosz M, Babicki A, et al. Prophylactic submucosal saline-adrenaline injection in colonoscopic polypectomy: prospective randomized study. Surg Endosc 2004;18(6):990–3 (In eng).

66. Tullavardhana T, Akranurakkul P, Ungkitphaiboon W, et al. Efficacy of submucosal epinephrine injection for the prevention of postpolypectomy bleeding: A meta-analysis of randomized controlled studies. Ann Med Surg (Lond) 2017; 19:65–73 (In eng).

67. Iishi H, Tatsuta M, Narahara H, et al. Endoscopic resection of large pedunculated colorectal polyps using a detachable snare. Gastrointest Endosc 1996; 44(5):594–7 (In eng).

68. Paspatis GA, Paraskeva K, Theodoropoulou A, et al. A prospective, randomized comparison of adrenaline injection in combination with detachable snare versus adrenaline injection alone in the prevention of postpolypectomy bleeding in large colonic polyps. Am J Gastroenterol 2006;101(12):2805 [quiz: 2913]. (In eng).

69. Kouklakis G, Mpoumponaris A, Gatopoulou A, et al. Endoscopic resection of large pedunculated colonic polyps and risk of postpolypectomy bleeding with adrenaline injection versus endoloop and hemoclip: a prospective, randomized study. Surg Endosc 2009;23(12):2732–7 (In eng).

70. Ji JS, Lee SW, Kim TH, et al. Comparison of prophylactic clip and endoloop application for the prevention of postpolypectomy bleeding in pedunculated colonic polyps: a prospective, randomized, multicenter study. Endoscopy 2014;46(7):598–604 (In eng).

71. Elliott TR, Tsiamoulos ZP, Thomas-Gibson S, et al. Factors associated with delayed bleeding after resection of large nonpedunculated colorectal polyps. Endoscopy 2018;50(8):790–9 (In eng).

72. Okugawa T, Oshima T, Nakai K, et al. Effect of Instruction on Preventing Delayed Bleeding after Colorectal Polypectomy and Endoscopic Mucosal Resection. J Clin Med 2021;10(5) (In eng).

73. Jung Y, Chung IK, Cho YS, et al. Do We Perform a Perfect Endoscopic Hemostasis Prophylactically with Argon Plasma Coagulation in Colonic Endoscopic Mucosal Resection? Dig Dis Sci 2015;60(10):3100–7 (In eng).

74. Subramaniam S, Kandiah K, Chedgy F, et al. A novel self-assembling peptide for hemostasis during endoscopic submucosal dissection: a randomized controlled trial. Endoscopy 2021;53(1):27–35 (In eng).

75. Uraoka T, Uedo N, Oyama T, et al. Efficacy and Safety of a Novel Hemostatic Peptide Solution During Endoscopic Submucosal Dissection: A Multicenter Randomized Controlled Trial. Am J Gastroenterol 2023;118(2):276–83 (In eng).

76. Martines G, Picciariello A, Dibra R, et al. Efficacy of cyanoacrylate in the prevention of delayed bleeding after endoscopic mucosal resection of large colorectal polyps: a pilot study. Int J Colorectal Dis 2020;35(11):2141–4 (In eng).

77. Lorenzo-Zúñiga V, Moreno de Vega V, Bartolí R. Endoscopic Shielding With Platelet-rich Plasma After Resection Of Large Colorectal Lesions. Surg Laparosc Endosc Percutan Tech 2021;31(3):376–7 (In eng).

78. Hagel AF, Raithel M, Hempen P, et al. Multicenter analysis of endoclot as hemostatic powder in different endoscopic settings of the upper gastrointestinal tract. J Physiol Pharmacol 2020;71(5). https://doi.org/10.26402/jpp.2020.5.06 (In eng).

79. Mourad FH, Leong RW. Role of hemostatic powders in the management of lower gastrointestinal bleeding: A review. J Gastroenterol Hepatol 2018;33(8):1445–53 (In eng).

80. Jung DH, Moon HS, Park CH, et al. Polysaccharide hemostatic powder to prevent bleeding after endoscopic submucosal dissection in high risk patients: a randomized controlled trial. Endoscopy 2021;53(10):994–1002 (In eng).

81. Medicine J.H., Gastroenterologist Develops Gel to Stop Bleeding After Precancerous Polyp Removal. Available at: https://clinicalconnection.hopkinsmedicine.org/news/gastroenterologist-develops-gel-to-stop-bleeding-after-precancerous-polyp-removal. Accessed July 10, 2023.

82. Parra-Blanco A, Kaminaga N, Kojima T, et al. Hemoclipping for postpolypectomy and postbiopsy colonic bleeding. Gastrointest Endosc 2000;51(1):37–41 (In eng).

83. Sobrino-Faya M, Martínez S, Gómez Balado M, et al. Clips for the prevention and treatment of postpolypectomy bleeding (hemoclips in polypectomy). Rev Esp Enferm Dig 2002;94(8):457–62 (In eng spa).

84. Hokama A, Kishimoto K, Kinjo F, et al. Endoscopic clipping in the lower gastrointestinal tract. World J Gastrointest Endosc 2009;1(1):7–11 (In eng).

85. Ma MX, Bourke MJ. Complications of endoscopic polypectomy, endoscopic mucosal resection and endoscopic submucosal dissection in the colon. Best Pract Res Clin Gastroenterol 2016;30(5):749–67 (In eng).

86. Fahrtash-Bahin F, Holt BA, Jayasekeran V, et al. Snare tip soft coagulation achieves effective and safe endoscopic hemostasis during wide-field endoscopic resection of large colonic lesions (with videos). Gastrointest Endosc 2013;78(1):158–63.e1 (In eng).

87. Burgess NG, Bahin FF, Bourke MJ. Colonic polypectomy (with videos). Gastrointest Endosc 2015;81(4):813–35 (In eng).

88. Chandan S, Facciorusso A, Ramai D, et al. Snare tip soft coagulation (STSC) after endoscopic mucosal resection (EMR) of large (> 20 mm) non pedunculated colorectal polyps: a systematic review and meta-analysis. Endosc Int Open 2022;10(1):E74–81 (In eng).

89. Dinelli M, Omazzi B, Andreozzi P, et al. First clinical experiences with a novel endoscopic over-the-scope clip system. Endosc Int Open 2017;5(3):E151–6 (In eng).

90. Goenka MK, Rodge GA, Tiwary IK. Endoscopic Management with a Novel Over-The-Scope Padlock Clip System. Clin Endosc 2019;52(6):574–80 (In eng).

91. Nishiyama N, Mori H, Kobara H, et al. Efficacy and safety of over-the-scope clip: including complications after endoscopic submucosal dissection. World J Gastroenterol 2013;19(18):2752–60 (In eng).

92. Prosst RL, Kratt T. A randomized comparative trial of OTSC and Padlock for upper GI hemostasis in a standardized experimental setting. Minim Invasive Ther Allied Technol 2017;26(2):65–70 (In eng).
93. Soulellis CA, Carpentier S, Chen YI, et al. Lower GI hemorrhage controlled with endoscopically applied TC-325 (with videos). Gastrointest Endosc 2013;77(3):504–7 (In eng).
94. Hookey L, Barkun A, Sultanian R, et al. Successful hemostasis of active lower GI bleeding using a hemostatic powder as monotherapy, combination therapy, or rescue therapy. Gastrointest Endosc 2019;89(4):865–71 (In eng).
95. Huang R, Pan Y, Hui N, et al. Polysaccharide hemostatic system for hemostasis management in colorectal endoscopic mucosal resection. Dig Endosc 2014;26(1):63–8 (In eng).
96. Karaman A, Torun E, Gürsoy S, et al. Efficacy of Ankaferd Blood Stopper in post-polypectomy bleeding. J Altern Complement Med 2010;16(10):1027–8 (In eng).
97. Facciorusso A, Straus Takahashi M, Eyileten Postula C, et al. Efficacy of hemostatic powders in upper gastrointestinal bleeding: A systematic review and meta-analysis. Dig Liver Dis 2019;51(12):1633–40 (In eng).
98. Park JS, Bang BW, Hong SJ, et al. Efficacy of a novel hemostatic adhesive powder in patients with refractory upper gastrointestinal bleeding: a pilot study. Endoscopy 2019;51(5):458–62 (In eng).
99. Ali-Mohamad N, Cau M, Baylis J, et al. Severe upper gastrointestinal bleeding is halted by endoscopically delivered self-propelling thrombin powder: A porcine pilot study. Endosc Int Open 2021;9(5):E693–8 (In eng).
100. Chahal D, Lee JGH, Ali-Mohamad N, et al. High rate of re-bleeding after application of Hemospray for upper and lower gastrointestinal bleeds. Dig Liver Dis 2020;52(7):768–72 (In eng).
101. Rodríguez de Santiago E, Burgos-Santamaría D, Pérez-Carazo L, et al. Hemostatic spray powder TC-325 for GI bleeding in a nationwide study: survival and predictors of failure via competing risks analysis. Gastrointest Endosc 2019;90(4):581–90.e6 (In eng).
102. Gutta A, Gromski MA. Endoscopic Management of Post-Polypectomy Bleeding. Clin Endosc 2020;53(3):302–10 (In eng).
103. Sonnenberg A. Management of delayed postpolypectomy bleeding: a decision analysis. Am J Gastroenterol 2012;107(3):339–42 (In eng).
104. Rodríguez de Santiago E, Hernández-Tejero M, Rivero-Sánchez L, et al. Management and Outcomes of Bleeding Within 30 Days of Colonic Polypectomy in a Large, Real-Life, Multicenter Cohort Study. Clin Gastroenterol Hepatol 2021;19(4):732–42.e6 (In eng).
105. Guo XF, Yu XA, Hu JC, et al. Endoscopic management of delayed bleeding after polypectomy of small colorectal polyps: two or more clips may be safe. Gastroenterol Rep (Oxf) 2022;10:goab051 (In eng).
106. Binmoeller KF, Thonke F, Soehendra N. Endoscopic hemoclip treatment for gastrointestinal bleeding. Endoscopy 1993;25(2):167–70 (In eng).
107. Lee JM, Kim WS, Kwak MS, et al. Clinical outcome of endoscopic management in delayed postpolypectomy bleeding. Intest Res 2017;15(2):221–7 (In eng).
108. Alcaide N, Peñas-Herrero I, Sancho-del-Val L, et al. Ovesco system for treatment of postpolypectomy bleeding after failure of conventional treatment. Rev Esp Enferm Dig 2014;106(1):55–8 (In eng).
109. Metz AJ, Bourke MJ, Moss A, et al. Factors that predict bleeding following endoscopic mucosal resection of large colonic lesions. Endoscopy 2011;43(6):506–11 (In eng).

Moving?

Make sure your subscription moves with you!

To notify us of your new address, find your **Clinics Account Number** (located on your mailing label above your name), and contact customer service at:

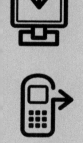

Email: journalscustomerservice-usa@elsevier.com

800-654-2452 (subscribers in the U.S. & Canada)
314-447-8871 (subscribers outside of the U.S. & Canada)

Fax number: 314-447-8029

Elsevier Health Sciences Division
Subscription Customer Service
3251 Riverport Lane
Maryland Heights, MO 63043

*To ensure uninterrupted delivery of your subscription, please notify us at least 4 weeks in advance of move.

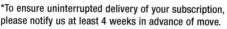
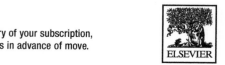

Printed and bound by CPI Group (UK) Ltd, Croydon, CR0 4YY

08/05/2025

01864748-0001